CW01270412

303 Yummy Pasta Recipes

(303 Yummy Pasta Recipes - Volume 1)

Rosalie Walston

Content

303 Awesome Pasta Recipes

***

1. $4 Spaghetti That's Almost As Good As $24 Spaghetti

Serving: 4 to 6 servings plus 4 cups of sauce | Prep: | Cook: | Ready in: 180mins

Ingredients

- 4 ounces white button mushrooms, thinly sliced
- 3/4 cup (4 ounces, from about 4 heads) peeled garlic cloves
- 2/3 cup extra-virgin olive oil
- 56 ounces (2 cans) peeled Italian tomatoes with their juices
- Salt
- Freshly ground pepper
- 1 pound spaghetti
- 1/4 cup basil leaves, torn
- Parmigiano-Reggiano cheese, freshly grated; for serving

Direction

- In a saucepan, bring the mushrooms and 3 cups of water to a boil. Simmer over moderate heat until the broth is reduced to 1 cup, 1 hour. Strain and discard the mushrooms.
- Meanwhile, in a small saucepan, bring the garlic and olive oil to a boil. Simmer over moderately low heat, stirring, until the garlic is very tender and golden, about 30 minutes.
- In a large enameled cast-iron casserole or Dutch oven, bring the tomatoes and the garlic and oil to a boil. Add the mushroom broth and, using an immersion blender, puree the sauce until smooth. Bring the sauce back to a boil, then simmer over moderately low heat until thickened, about 1 hour. Season the sauce with salt and pepper.
- Cook the spaghetti in a large pot of salted boiling water until al dente. Drain the spaghetti and return to the pot. Add 2 cups of the sauce and cook, tossing, for 1 minute. Transfer the spaghetti to bowls, top with the basil and serve with grated cheese.

2. Angel Hair Pasta Delight

Serving: 4 servings (serving size: 1 cup spinach mixture, 1 cup pasta, and 1 tablespoon cheese) | Prep: | Cook: | Ready in:

Ingredients

- 2 teaspoons olive oil
- 1 1/2 cups chopped Vidalia or other sweet onion
- 3 garlic cloves, minced
- 1/4 cup water
- 1 (10-ounce) package fresh spinach, chopped
- 2 cups chopped plum tomato
- 2 cups chopped cooked chicken breast (about 1/2 pound)
- 1/4 cup chopped cooked bacon (about 2 slices)
- 3 tablespoons balsamic vinegar
- 4 cups hot cooked angel hair (about 8 ounces uncooked pasta)
- 1/4 cup (1 ounce) shredded Asiago cheese

Direction

- Heat oil in a large nonstick skillet over medium-high heat. Add onion; sauté 2 minutes. Add garlic; sauté 1 minute. Add water and spinach; cover and cook 2 minutes or until spinach wilts.

- Stir in tomato, chicken, bacon, and vinegar; cook 1 minute or until thoroughly heated. Serve over pasta; sprinkle with cheese.

Nutrition Information

- Calories: 350
- Fiber: 4.7 g
- Saturated Fat: 2.4 g
- Total Fat: 8.1 g
- Sodium: 433 mg
- Total Carbohydrate: 44.7 g
- Protein: 26.4 g
- Cholesterol: 42 mg

3. Angel Hair Pasta With Mussels And Red Pepper Sauce

Serving: 4 servings (serving size: 9 mussels, about 1 cup pasta, and about 2 teaspoons parsley) | Prep: 37mins | Cook: | Ready in:

Ingredients

- 8 ounces uncooked angel hair pasta
- 2 teaspoons olive oil
- 1/3 cup diced onion
- 1 garlic clove, minced
- 2 cups diced red bell pepper (about 2 medium)
- 1/2 teaspoon salt
- Dash of ground red pepper
- 1 (14.5-ounce) can whole tomatoes, undrained and chopped
- 1/2 cup white wine
- 36 mussels (about 3 pounds), scrubbed and debearded
- 3 tablespoons chopped fresh parsley

Direction

- Cook pasta according to package directions, omitting salt and fat. Drain; keep warm.
- Heat oil in a large saucepan over medium-high heat. Add the onion and garlic; sauté 5 minutes or until tender. Add bell pepper, salt, and ground red pepper; sauté 2 minutes. Add tomatoes and wine; bring to a boil. Reduce heat to low, and simmer 10 minutes. Add mussels, and increase heat to medium. Cover and simmer for 7 minutes or until shells open. Discard any unopened shells. Serve mussel mixture over pasta; sprinkle with parsley.

Nutrition Information

- Calories: 372
- Protein: 24.9 g
- Saturated Fat: 1 g
- Sodium: 809 mg
- Cholesterol: 40 mg
- Total Carbohydrate: 46.9 g
- Fiber: 4.5 g
- Total Fat: 7.4 g

4. Angel Hair Pasta With Shrimp And Green Garlic

Serving: Serves 4 | Prep: | Cook: | Ready in: 35mins

Ingredients

- 1 1/2 tablespoons butter
- 5 or 6 green garlic* stalks, trimmed (see "Tips for Cooks," below) and cut into 3-in.-long slivers to make 1 cup
- 1/4 cup dry white wine
- 1 cup heavy whipping cream
- 1/2 cup reduced-sodium chicken broth
- 1/4 cup grated parmesan cheese
- 1/4 teaspoon nutmeg, preferably freshly grated
- About 1 tsp. kosher salt
- About 1 tsp. pepper
- 10 ounce angel hair pasta
- 1 pound raw peeled, deveined medium shrimp (40 to 50 per lb.)
- 2 tablespoons sliced fresh chives

Direction

- Melt butter in a 12-in. frying pan over medium heat. Add green garlic and cook, stirring often, until softened and fragrant, 4 to 5 minutes. Add wine, increase heat to medium-high, and cook until it has nearly evaporated, about 1 minute. Stir in cream, broth, parmesan, nutmeg, and 1 tsp. each salt and pepper. Bring to a simmer, reduce heat to medium-low, and cook until cream is slightly thickened, about 3 minutes.
- Cook pasta according to package instructions until just tender, 3 to 4 minutes. Reserve 1 cup cooking water, then drain pasta.
- Meanwhile, add shrimp to cream sauce, increase heat to medium, and cook, stirring occasionally, just until pink, 3 to 4 minutes. Add pasta to frying pan and stir to coat. Stir in reserved pasta water (mixture will be soupy, then thicken as it stands) and toss in chives. Add more salt and pepper if you like.
- Tips for cooks
- Green garlic is simply immature regular garlic and tastes fresher and more delicate. It has juicy, edible stalks with no bulbs at the base (if picked quite young), or bulbs with tiny cloves that don't need peeling.
- FIND Look for slender pale green stalks in springtime at farmers' markets and some supermarkets. Or substitute green onions plus regular garlic (see the recipe).
- PREP Trim green garlic as you would green onions, removing tough tops (save to flavor soup) and roots, plus any tough outer layers. Ten stalks yield 2 cups chopped.
- *If you can't find green garlic, use 1 cup slivered green onions plus 3 minced garlic cloves.

Nutrition Information

- Calories: 671
- Saturated Fat: 18 g
- Protein: 32 g
- Sodium: 966 mg
- Cholesterol: 274 mg
- Fiber: 1.3 g
- Total Carbohydrate: 64 g
- Total Fat: 32 g

5. Angel Hair With Green And Yellow Tomato Sauce

Serving: 4 first-course servings | Prep: | Cook: | Ready in: 20mins

Ingredients

- 2 tablespoons pure olive oil
- 4 cloves garlic, minced
- 2 (large) shallots, minced
- 1 pound yellow tomatoes, diced
- 1 pound ripe green heirloom tomatoes such as Green Zebra, diced
- 1/4 cup chopped basil
- 2 sage leaves, finely chopped
- Salt
- 1/2 pound angel hair pasta
- 2 tablespoons unsalted butter, at room temperature, or 2 tablespoons extra-virgin olive oil

Direction

- In a skillet, heat the oil. Add the garlic and cook over low heat until fragrant, 2 minutes. Add the shallots and cook over moderate heat, stirring, until softened, 4 minutes.
- In a bowl, toss the tomatoes with the garlic, shallots, basil and sage. Season with salt.
- In a pot of boiling salted water, cook the pasta until al dente; drain and transfer to the large bowl. Toss well with the butter; serve.

6. Artichoke, Spinach, And Feta Stuffed Shells

Serving: 5 servings (serving size: 4 stuffed shells) | Prep: | Cook: | Ready in:

Ingredients

- 1 teaspoon dried oregano
- 1/4 cup chopped pepperoncini peppers
- 1 (28-ounce) can fire-roasted crushed tomatoes with added puree (such as Progresso)
- 1 (8-ounce) can no-salt-added tomato sauce
- 1 cup (4 ounces) shredded provolone cheese, divided
- 1 cup (4 ounces) crumbled feta cheese
- 1/2 cup (4 ounces) fat-free cream cheese, softened
- 1/4 teaspoon freshly ground black pepper
- 1 (9-ounce) package frozen artichoke hearts, thawed and chopped
- 1/2 (10-ounce) package frozen chopped spinach, thawed, drained, and squeezed dry
- 2 garlic cloves, minced
- 20 cooked jumbo shell pasta (about 8 ounces uncooked pasta)
- Cooking spray

Direction

- Preheat oven to 375°.
- Combine first 4 ingredients in a medium saucepan. Place over medium heat; cook 12 minutes or until slightly thick, stirring occasionally. Remove from heat; set aside.
- Combine 1/2 cup provolone and the next 6 ingredients (through garlic) in a medium bowl. Spoon or pipe about 1 1/2 tablespoons cheese mixture into each pasta shell; place stuffed shells in a 13 x 9-inch baking dish coated with cooking spray. Spoon tomato mixture over shells; sprinkle with remaining 1/2 cup provolone. Bake at 375° for 25 minutes or until thoroughly heated and cheese melts.

Nutrition Information

- Calories: 394
- Cholesterol: 38 mg
- Protein: 21.3 g
- Saturated Fat: 7.7 g
- Fiber: 8.7 g
- Sodium: 954 mg
- Total Fat: 12.4 g
- Total Carbohydrate: 48.9 g

7. Asian Chicken And Rice Noodle Salad

Serving: 4 Servings | Prep: 20mins | Cook: 5mins | Ready in:

Ingredients

- 3 tablespoons fish sauce
- 2 tablespoons fresh lime juice
- 11/2 tablespoons sugar
- 1/8 teaspoon crushed red pepper flakes
- 1 garlic clove, minced
- 8 ounces rice noodles
- 3 cups diced cooked chicken (about 10 oz.)
- 1 cup mung bean sprouts
- 4 scallions, thinly sliced
- 1 carrot, peeled and grated
- 1/4 cup chopped fresh coriander
- 1/3 cup chopped unsalted, dry-roasted peanuts (optional)

Direction

- Whisk together fish sauce, lime juice, sugar, red pepper flakes, and garlic. Set aside.
- Place noodles in a large bowl in sink; cover them with hot water and let stand for 10 minutes. Meanwhile, bring a large pot of water to a boil. Drain noodles and add to pot; cook, stirring, until tender, 3 to 4 minutes. Drain and rinse with cold water until cool.
- Transfer noodles to a large salad bowl. Add chicken and remaining ingredients; toss well.

Pour half of dressing on salad and toss again. Add more dressing as desired.

Nutrition Information

- Calories: 486
- Fiber: 2 g
- Sodium: 1 mg
- Total Fat: 8 g
- Protein: 35 g
- Saturated Fat: 2 g
- Total Carbohydrate: 66 g
- Cholesterol: 93 mg

8. Asian Meatballs With Mushrooms And Rice Noodles

Serving: 2 servings (serving size: 8 meatballs, 1 1/2 cups noodles, and 1 teaspoon cilantro) | Prep: | Cook: | Ready in:

Ingredients

- 1 regular-size foil oven bag
- Cooking spray
- 1/2 pound ground turkey breast
- 1/4 cup finely diced mushrooms
- 2 tablespoons thinly sliced green onions
- 1 tablespoon cornstarch, divided
- 1 tablespoon low-sodium soy sauce, divided
- 1 teaspoon dark sesame oil
- 4 cups hot water
- 4 ounces uncooked rice sticks (rice-flour noodles) or cooked vermicelli
- 1/4 cup fat-free, less-sodium chicken broth
- 2 tablespoons dry sherry
- 1 tablespoon fresh lime juice
- 1 1/2 cups sliced mushrooms
- 2 teaspoons minced peeled fresh ginger
- 1 1/4 teaspoons curry powder
- 1 garlic clove, minced
- 2 teaspoons minced fresh cilantro

Direction

- Preheat oven to 450°.
- Coat the inside of the oven bag with cooking spray. Place bag on a large shallow baking pan.
- Combine ground turkey, diced mushrooms, green onions, 2 teaspoons cornstarch, 1 teaspoon soy sauce, and sesame oil in a bowl, and shape into 16 (1-inch) meatballs. Place meatballs on a single layer of wax paper.
- Combine hot water and rice sticks in a bowl, and let stand 15 minutes. Drain well, and snip with scissors twice. Combine 1 teaspoon cornstarch and broth in a large bowl. Add 2 teaspoons soy sauce, sherry, and lime juice. Add rice sticks, sliced mushrooms, ginger, curry, and garlic, and toss well.
- Place the noodle mixture in the prepared oven bag. Place the meatballs on noodle mixture, and fold edges of bag over to seal. Bake at 450° for 20 minutes or until the meatballs are done. Place the oven bag on platter, cut open with a sharp knife, and peel back foil. Sprinkle with minced cilantro.

Nutrition Information

- Calories: 383
- Fiber: 1.8 g
- Saturated Fat: 0.9 g
- Sodium: 630 mg
- Cholesterol: 60 mg
- Total Fat: 4.2 g
- Total Carbohydrate: 59.5 g
- Protein: 28 g

9. Asian Noodles With Roast Pork

Serving: 6 servings | Prep: | Cook: | Ready in: 60mins

Ingredients

- 2 tablespoons canola oil
- 2 large shallots, finely chopped
- 2 garlic cloves, minced

- 1 pound ground pork
- 1 tablespoon light brown sugar
- 1 1/2 tablespoons Chinese black bean sauce
- 4 dried hot chiles
- 2 teaspoons Maggi sauce (a vegetable-based liquid seasoning) or soy sauce
- 2 teaspoons Asian fish sauce
- 1 1/4 cups low-sodium chicken broth
- 1 1/2 tablespoons unseasoned rice vinegar
- 2 tablespoons oyster sauce
- 1 teaspoon toasted sesame oil
- 1 tablespoon sambal oelek (hot chile sauce)
- 1 pound Chinese broccoli
- 1 pound fresh Chinese egg noodles, linguine or spaghetti
- 1/2 pound Chinese roast pork, thinly sliced
- 1 scallion, thinly sliced

Direction

- In a very large nonstick skillet, heat 1 tablespoon of the canola oil. Add the shallots and garlic and stir-fry over moderately high heat until lightly browned, about 2 minutes. Add the ground pork, brown sugar, black bean sauce, dried chiles, Maggi sauce and fish sauce and cook, breaking up the meat with a spoon, until it is browned in spots, about 10 minutes. Add 3/4 cup of the chicken broth and cook over moderately low heat until the broth has evaporated, about 8 minutes. Stir in 1 tablespoon of the vinegar. Transfer the ground pork mixture to a bowl and wipe out the skillet.
- In a jar, combine the remaining 1/2 cup of chicken broth and 1/2 tablespoon of vinegar with the oyster sauce, sesame oil and sambal oelek. Seal the jar and shake the sauce to blend.
- Bring a large pot of water to a boil. Add the Chinese broccoli and cook until it is crisp-tender, about 2 minutes. Using tongs, transfer the broccoli to a work surface and cut it into 1-inch pieces. Return the water to a boil and add the noodles. Cook just until al dente. Drain the noodles, shaking off the excess water.
- Heat the remaining 1 tablespoon of oil in the skillet. Add the roast pork, ground pork, broccoli and noodles and toss to combine. Add the sauce and cook, tossing, until the noodles are evenly coated, 5 minutes. Add the scallion, transfer to a large platter and serve.

10. Bacon And Shrimp Pasta Toss

Serving: Serves 4 (serving size: about 1 3/4 cups) | Prep: | Cook: | Ready in: 22mins

Ingredients

- 8 ounces uncooked penne
- 2 applewood-smoked bacon slices
- 5 garlic cloves, minced
- 1 pound large shrimp, peeled and deveined
- 2 tablespoons extra-virgin olive oil
- 5 cups baby spinach leaves
- 1/2 teaspoon kosher salt

Direction

- Cook pasta according to package directions until almost al dente, omitting salt and fat; drain, reserving 3/4 cup cooking liquid.
- Cook bacon in a large skillet over medium-high heat 10 minutes or until crisp, turning once. Remove from pan; reserve drippings. Crumble bacon. Add garlic to drippings in pan; cook 30 seconds, stirring constantly. Add shrimp; cook 1 1/2 minutes on each side or until done. Remove shrimp from pan; set aside.
- Add reserved 3/4 cup cooking liquid and oil to pan; bring to a boil. Boil 30 seconds, stirring with a whisk. Add pasta to pan; cook 1 minute, tossing to combine. Stir in spinach, shrimp, and salt. Top with bacon. Serve immediately.

Nutrition Information

- Calories: 396

- Sodium: 570 mg
- Total Fat: 11 g
- Total Carbohydrate: 48 g
- Fiber: 3 g
- Protein: 26 g
- Cholesterol: 148 mg
- Saturated Fat: 2.1 g

11. Bacon, Ranch, And Chicken Mac And Cheese

Serving: 4 servings (serving size: about 2 cups) | Prep: | Cook: | Ready in: 45mins

Ingredients

- 8 ounces uncooked elbow macaroni
- 1 slice applewood-smoked bacon
- 8 ounces skinless, boneless chicken breast, cut into 1/2-inch pieces
- 1 tablespoon canola oil
- 1 tablespoon all-purpose flour
- 1 1/2 cups fat-free milk
- 1/3 cup condensed 45% reduced-sodium 98% fat-free cream of mushroom soup, undiluted
- 3/4 cup (3 ounces) shredded six-cheese Italian blend (such as Sargento)
- 1/2 teaspoon onion powder
- 1/2 teaspoon garlic powder
- 1/2 teaspoon chopped fresh dill
- 1/8 teaspoon salt
- Cooking spray
- 1/2 cup (2 ounces) shredded colby-Jack cheese

Direction

- Cook pasta according to package directions, omitting salt and fat; drain.
- Cook bacon in a large nonstick skillet over medium heat until crisp. Remove bacon from pan, reserving drippings in pan. Finely chop bacon; set aside. Increase heat to medium-high. Add chicken to drippings in pan; sauté 6 minutes or until done.
- Heat oil in a large saucepan over medium heat; sprinkle flour evenly into pan. Cook 2 minutes, stirring constantly with a whisk. Combine milk and soup, stirring with a whisk; gradually add milk mixture to saucepan, stirring with a whisk. Bring to a boil; cook 2 minutes or until thick. Remove from heat; let stand 4 minutes or until sauce cools to 155°. Add Italian cheese blend, onion powder, garlic powder, dill, and salt, stirring until cheese melts. Stir in pasta and chicken.
- Preheat broiler.
- Spoon mixture into an 8-inch square baking dish coated with cooking spray. Sprinkle evenly with reserved bacon and colby-Jack cheese. Broil 3 minutes or until cheese melts.

Nutrition Information

- Calories: 497
- Cholesterol: 74 mg
- Saturated Fat: 7.4 g
- Total Carbohydrate: 51.7 g
- Protein: 33.3 g
- Fiber: 2 g
- Total Fat: 17 g
- Sodium: 545 mg

12. Baked Linguine With Meat Sauce

Serving: 8 servings | Prep: 40mins | Cook: 30mins | Ready in:

Ingredients

- 2 pounds lean ground beef
- 2 garlic cloves, minced
- 1 (28-ounce) can crushed tomatoes
- 1 (8-ounce) can tomato sauce
- 1 (6-ounce) can tomato paste
- 1 teaspoon salt
- 2 teaspoons sugar
- 8 ounces uncooked linguine

- 1 (16-ounce) container sour cream
- 1 (8-ounce) package cream cheese, softened
- 1 bunch green onions, chopped
- 2 cups (8 ounces) shredded sharp Cheddar cheese

Direction

- Cook beef and garlic in a Dutch oven, stirring until beef crumbles and is no longer pink. Stir in tomatoes and next 4 ingredients; simmer 30 minutes. Set mixture aside.
- Cook pasta according to package directions; drain. Place pasta in a lightly greased 13- x 9-inch baking dish.
- Stir together sour cream, cream cheese, and green onions. Spread over pasta. Top with meat sauce.
- Bake at 350° for 20 to 25 minutes or until thoroughly heated. Sprinkle with Cheddar cheese, and bake 5 more minutes or until cheese melts. Let stand 5 minutes. Serve with a salad and bread, if desired.
- Note: To lighten dish, use no-salt-added tomato products, light sour cream, light cream cheese, and reduced-fat Cheddr cheese.

13. Baked Mac And Cheese

Serving: Serves 12 (serving size: about 2/3 cup) | Prep: | Cook: | Ready in: 50mins

Ingredients

- 10 ounce uncooked large elbow macaroni
- 1/2 cup canola mayonnaise
- 1 tablespoon all-purpose flour
- 1 teaspoon dry mustard
- 1 teaspoon garlic powder
- 3/4 teaspoon kosher salt
- 3/4 teaspoon black pepper
- 1/2 teaspoon paprika
- 1 large egg
- 1 (12-ounce) can 2% evaporated milk
- 6 ounces colby-Jack cheese, shredded (about 1 1/2 cups)
- Cooking spray
- 1 1/2 tablespoons canola oil
- 1 tablespoon melted butter
- 2/3 cup panko breadcrumbs
- 1 tablespoon minced fresh parsley

Direction

- Preheat oven to 350°.
- Cook pasta according to package directions. Drain.
- Combine mayo and next 7 ingredients (through egg) in a large bowl; stir with a whisk. Gradually whisk in milk. Stir in cheese and pasta. Spoon into an 11 x 7-inch baking dish coated with cooking spray.
- Combine oil and butter in a medium bowl. Add panko and parsley; toss. Sprinkle over pasta mixture. Bake at 350° for 30 minutes or until lightly browned.

Nutrition Information

- Calories: 241
- Protein: 10 g
- Saturated Fat: 3.5 g
- Fiber: 1 g
- Sodium: 332 mg
- Total Carbohydrate: 24 g
- Cholesterol: 37 mg
- Total Fat: 11.3 g

14. Baked Rigatoni With Beef

Serving: 8 servings (serving size: 1 cup) | Prep: | Cook: | Ready in:

Ingredients

- 4 cups Tomato Sauce
- 1 pound ground round

- 4 cups cooked rigatoni (about 2 1/2 cups uncooked pasta)
- 1 1/2 cups (6 ounces) shredded part-skim mozzarella cheese, divided
- Cooking spray
- 1/4 cup (1 ounce) grated fresh Parmesan cheese

Direction

- Prepare Tomato Sauce.
- Preheat oven to 350°.
- Cook beef in a large nonstick skillet over medium-high heat until browned; stir to crumble. Drain well. Combine beef, rigatoni, Tomato Sauce, and 1 cup mozzarella in an 11 x 7-inch baking dish coated with cooking spray. Top with 1/2 cup mozzarella and Parmesan. Bake at 350° for 20 minutes or until thoroughly heated.

Nutrition Information

- Calories: 305
- Total Fat: 9.6 g
- Protein: 24 g
- Sodium: 438 mg
- Cholesterol: 50 mg
- Total Carbohydrate: 30.5 g
- Saturated Fat: 4.3 g
- Fiber: 2.3 g

15. Baked Stuffed Shells

Serving: 6 servings (serving size: 3 stuffed shells and about 1 cup sauce) | Prep: | Cook: | Ready in:

Ingredients

- Stuffing:
- 1/4 cup boiling water
- 6 sun-dried tomatoes
- 1 cup (4 ounces) shredded part-skim mozzarella cheese
- 1/4 cup (1 ounce) grated fresh Parmesan cheese
- 1 tablespoon chopped fresh parsley
- 1/4 teaspoon freshly ground black pepper
- 1/8 teaspoon salt
- 1 (14-ounce) package reduced-fat firm tofu
- 1 egg, lightly beaten
- 18 cooked jumbo pasta shells
- Sauce:
- 1 tablespoon olive oil
- 1 3/4 cups chopped onion (about 1 large)
- 1 cup chopped green bell pepper (about 1 medium)
- 1 cup chopped red bell pepper (about 1 medium)
- 3 garlic cloves, minced
- Cooking spray
- 3/4 pound low-fat turkey breakfast sausage, casings removed
- 1/4 cup red wine
- 2 tablespoons no-salt-added tomato paste
- 1 teaspoon dried oregano
- 1 teaspoon dried basil
- 1/2 teaspoon freshly ground black pepper
- 1/8 teaspoon salt
- 1 (28-ounce) can organic crushed tomatoes
- 2 tablespoons grated fresh Parmesan cheese

Direction

- Preheat oven to 350°.
- To prepare stuffing, combine 1/4 cup boiling water and sun-dried tomatoes in a small bowl; let stand 20 minutes or until tomatoes soften. Drain and finely chop. Combine tomatoes, mozzarella, and next 6 ingredients (through egg) in a food processor; process until smooth. Spoon 2 tablespoons stuffing into each shell. Set stuffed shells aside.
- To prepare sauce, heat oil in a large skillet over medium-high heat. Add onion, bell peppers, and garlic; sauté 6 minutes or until tender. Place onion mixture in a bowl.
- Coat pan with cooking spray; return pan to heat. Add sausage, and cook 6 minutes or until browned, stirring to crumble. Add wine; cook until wine is reduced to 2 tablespoons (about 3

minutes). Stir in onion mixture, tomato paste, and next 5 ingredients (through tomatoes); bring to a simmer. Cook 25 minutes or until slightly thick.

- Spread 2 cups sauce over bottom of an 11 x 7-inch baking dish coated with cooking spray. Arrange stuffed shells in a single layer in pan; top with remaining sauce. Sprinkle 2 tablespoons Parmesan over sauce. Bake at 350° for 40 minutes or until bubbly.

Nutrition Information

- Calories: 391
- Cholesterol: 84 mg
- Total Fat: 13.8 g
- Protein: 27 g
- Saturated Fat: 4.8 g
- Total Carbohydrate: 37.1 g
- Sodium: 892 mg
- Fiber: 4.7 g

16. Baked Ziti With Sausage

Serving: Makes 8 servings | Prep: | Cook: | Ready in: 55mins

Ingredients

- 12 ounces uncooked ziti pasta
- 4 ounces pancetta or bacon, diced
- 1 large onion, chopped
- 3 garlic cloves, chopped
- 1 (1-lb.) package ground Italian sausage
- 1 cup dry red wine
- 1 (28-oz.) can crushed tomatoes
- 1/2 cup firmly packed torn fresh basil
- 1/2 teaspoon kosher salt
- 1/2 teaspoon dried crushed red pepper
- 1 cup ricotta cheese
- 1 (8-oz.) package shredded mozzarella cheese, divided
- Vegetable cooking spray
- 1/2 cup grated Parmesan cheese

Direction

- Preheat oven to 350°. Prepare ziti according to package directions for al dente.
- Meanwhile, cook pancetta in a large skillet over medium-high heat 3 minutes. Add onion and garlic, and sauté 3 minutes or until onion is tender. Add sausage, and sauté 5 minutes or until meat is no longer pink. Add wine, and cook 3 minutes. Stir in tomatoes and next 3 ingredients. Reduce heat to low, and cook, stirring occasionally, 3 minutes.
- Stir ricotta and 1 cup mozzarella cheese into hot cooked pasta. Lightly grease a 13- x 9-inch baking dish with cooking spray. Transfer pasta mixture to prepared dish, and top with sausage mixture. Sprinkle with Parmesan cheese and remaining 1 cup mozzarella cheese.
- Bake at 350° for 25 to 30 minutes or until bubbly.

17. Baked Ziti With Shrimp And Scallops

Serving: 4 servings | Prep: | Cook: | Ready in:

Ingredients

- 8 ounces uncooked ziti (short tube-shaped pasta)
- 1/2 cup hot water
- 1 (12-ounce) bottle roasted red bell peppers, drained
- 1 (8-ounce) block fat-free cream cheese, softened
- 1 tablespoon olive oil
- 1/8 teaspoon salt
- 8 ounces large shrimp, peeled, deveined, and chopped
- 8 ounces bay scallops
- 4 garlic cloves, minced
- 1 tablespoon chopped fresh parsley
- Cooking spray

- 3/4 cup (3 ounces) shredded sharp provolone cheese

Direction

- Preheat oven to 400°.
- Cook pasta according to the package directions, omitting salt and fat. Drain well.
- Combine hot water, roasted red bell peppers, and cream cheese in a food processor; process until smooth, scraping sides.
- Heat the oil in a Dutch oven over medium-high heat. Add salt, shrimp, scallops, and garlic; sauté 2 minutes or until shrimp and scallops are almost done. Add pepper mixture to pan; bring to a simmer. Reduce heat; cook 2 minutes, stirring frequently. Add pasta and parsley to shrimp mixture, tossing well to combine. Spoon pasta mixture into an 8-inch square baking dish lightly coated with cooking spray, and sprinkle evenly with cheese. Bake at 400° for 20 minutes or until cheese melts; remove from oven.
- Preheat broiler.
- Return dish to oven; broil 2 minutes or until cheese begins to brown. Remove from heat; let stand 10 minutes.

Nutrition Information

- Calories: 508
- Cholesterol: 130 mg
- Saturated Fat: 4.7 g
- Total Carbohydrate: 53.4 g
- Total Fat: 11.7 g
- Protein: 43.3 g
- Sodium: 977 mg
- Fiber: 2.4 g

18. Banh Mi Rice Noodle Bowl

Serving: Serves 4 to 6 | Prep: | Cook: | Ready in: 25mins

Ingredients

- Noodles
- 14 ounces medium-wide (linguine-style) rice noodles
- 1/2 cup lime juice
- 1/4 cup toasted sesame oil
- 2 tablespoons Thai or Vietnamese fish sauce
- 2 tablespoons sugar
- 1 teaspoon salt
- 1 teaspoon Sriracha
- Toppings
- Pâté, roast chicken, or seasoned, cooked tofu
- Shredded carrots
- Slivered green onions
- Chopped cilantro
- Diced cucumber
- Sliced jalapeño
- Toasted sesame seeds
- 1 to 2 limes, cut in wedges

Direction

- Cook rice noodles according to package directions. In a large bowl, whisk together lime juice, sesame oil, fish sauce, sugar, salt, and Sriracha. Add cooked noodles and toss to coat.
- Arrange noodles in individual bowls, topped with choice of protein, then garnish with carrots, green onions, cilantro, cucumber, and jalapeños. Serve with additional sauce on side and lime wedges.

19. Barbecue Mac And Cheese

Serving: Makes 6 to 8 servings | Prep: | Cook: | Ready in: 20mins

Ingredients

- 1/4 cup plus 1 1/2 tsp. kosher salt, divided
- 1 qt. milk
- 6 tablespoons butter, cut into pieces
- 6 tablespoons all-purpose flour
- 1 pound pasta (such as penne, cavatappi, or rotini)

- 1 (8-oz.) package shredded extra-sharp Cheddar cheese
- 1 (8-oz.) package shredded Gouda cheese
- 1 teaspoon hot sauce (such as Tabasco)
- 1/2 teaspoon freshly ground black pepper
- 1 pound pulled pork barbecue (without sauce)
- 1 1/2 cups crumbled cornbread
- 2 teaspoons olive oil
- 1/2 cup chopped green onions
- 1/2 cup bottled barbecue sauce

Direction

- Preheat broiler with oven rack 8 to 9 inches from heat.
- Bring 1/4 cup salt and 4 qt. water to a boil in a large covered Dutch oven over high heat.
- Meanwhile, microwave milk in a microwave-safe 1-qt. glass measuring cup covered with plastic wrap at HIGH 3 minutes. While milk is heating, melt butter in a 12-inch cast-iron skillet over medium heat. Reduce heat to medium-low; add flour, and cook, whisking constantly, 2 minutes. Gradually whisk in hot milk. Increase heat to medium-high, and bring to a low boil, whisking often.
- Add pasta to boiling water, and cook 8 minutes.
- Meanwhile, continue to cook sauce, whisking often, 6 minutes. Remove from heat; whisk in cheeses, hot sauce, 1 1/2 tsp. salt, and 1/2 tsp. pepper. Cover.
- Stir together cornbread and olive oil.
- Drain pasta, and fold into cheese sauce. Stir in pulled pork barbecue. Sprinkle with cornbread mixture; sprinkle green onions over cornbread mixture.
- Broil 1 to 2 minutes or until breadcrumbs are golden brown. Drizzle with barbecue sauce. Serve immediately.

20. Basil Shrimp With Feta And Orzo

Serving: 2 servings (serving size: 1 cup orzo and about 5 ounces shrimp) | Prep: | Cook: | Ready in:

Ingredients

- 1 regular-size foil oven bag
- Cooking spray
- 1/2 cup uncooked orzo (rice-shaped pasta)
- 2 teaspoons olive oil, divided
- 1 cup diced tomato
- 3/4 cup sliced green onions
- 1/2 cup (2 ounces) crumbled feta cheese
- 1/2 teaspoon grated lemon rind
- 1 tablespoon fresh lemon juice
- 1/4 teaspoon salt
- 1/4 teaspoon black pepper
- 3/4 pound large shrimp, peeled and deveined
- 1/4 cup chopped fresh basil

Direction

- Preheat oven to 450°.
- Coat inside of oven bag with cooking spray. Place the bag on a large shallow baking pan.
- Cook the pasta in boiling water 5 minutes, omitting salt and fat; drain. Place the pasta in a large bowl. Stir in 1 teaspoon oil and next 7 ingredients (1 teaspoon oil through pepper). Place the orzo mixture in prepared oven bag. Combine shrimp and basil. Arrange shrimp mixture on orzo mixture. Fold edge of bag over to seal. Bake at 450° for 25 minutes or until the shrimp are done. Cut open bag with a sharp knife, and peel back the foil. Drizzle with 1 teaspoon oil.

Nutrition Information

- Calories: 498
- Saturated Fat: 5.5 g
- Cholesterol: 219 mg
- Total Fat: 14.4 g
- Sodium: 817 mg
- Total Carbohydrate: 52.7 g

- Protein: 38.8 g
- Fiber: 3.4 g

21. Black Pepper Bow Tie Pasta

Serving: Yields 3/4 lb. pasta | Prep: | Cook: | Ready in: 1500mins

Ingredients

- 1 2/3 cups all-purpose flour
- 2 large eggs
- 1 tablespoon olive oil
- 2 teaspoons pepper
- 1/2 teaspoon salt

Direction

- In a large bowl, using an electric hand mixer on medium speed with dough-hook attachments, combine flour, eggs, olive oil, pepper, salt and 2 Tbsp. lukewarm water. Mix until just combined.
- On a floured surface, knead dough until smooth and elastic, 8 to 10 minutes, adding more flour as necessary. Wrap dough in plastic and allow to rest for 15 minutes.
- Working with 1/2 of dough at a time, roll out on a floured surface until very thin. Transfer dough to a cutting board and use a sharp knife or pizza cutter to make 1-inch-wide strips. Slice strips at 1 1/2-inch intervals, creating small rectangles. Pinch centers of rectangles together to make bow-tie pasta. Let pasta dry for 24 hours on a floured towel or wire rack.
- Cook pasta in salted boiling water until al dente; about 5 minutes, then serve with your favorite sauce.

22. Bow Tie Pasta

Serving: Yields 3/4 lb. pasta | Prep: | Cook: | Ready in: 1500mins

Ingredients

- 1 2/3 cups all-purpose flour
- 2 large eggs
- 1 tablespoon olive oil
- 1/2 teaspoon salt

Direction

- In a large bowl, using an electric hand mixer on medium speed with dough-hook attachments, combine flour, eggs, olive oil, salt and 2 Tbsp. lukewarm water. Mix until just combined.
- On a floured surface, knead dough until smooth and elastic, 8 to 10 minutes, adding more flour as necessary. Wrap dough in plastic and allow to rest for 15 minutes.
- Working with 1/2 of dough at a time, roll out on a floured surface until very thin. Transfer dough to a cutting board and use a sharp knife or pizza cutter to make 1-inch-wide strips. Slice strips at 1 1/2-inch intervals, creating small rectangles. Pinch centers of rectangles together to make bow-tie pasta. Let pasta dry for 24 hours on a floured towel or wire rack.
- FLAVOR IT! Black Pepper Pasta: Add 2 tsp. pepper to ingredients before mixing. Spinach Pasta: Squeeze excess liquid from 1 10-oz. package frozen, thawed spinach. Pulse in a food processor and add to ingredients (after salt) before mixing. Omit 2 Tbsp. water.
- GIVE IT
- Spoon 1 1/2-cup portion of pasta into each of 2 cellophane bags. On a piece of card stock, write "Cook pasta in salted boiling water until al dente, about 5 minutes, then serve with your favorite sauce." Place card in bag. Using adhesive labels, create a label for each bag. Fold top edge of bag over and seal with label. We dressed up bags with mini clothespins and rick-rack bows.

23. Browned Butter Gnocchi With Broccoli And Nuts

Serving: Serves 6 | Prep: | Cook: | Ready in:

Ingredients

- 2 (16-ounce) packages prepared gnocchi (such as Gia Russa)
- 5 cups chopped broccoli florets
- 2 tablespoons unsalted butter
- 2 tablespoons extra-virgin olive oil
- 1/4 teaspoon freshly ground black pepper
- 3 tablespoons pine nuts, toasted
- 1.5 ounces shaved fresh pecorino Romano cheese (about 1/3 cup)

Direction

- Cook gnocchi in a large Dutch oven according to package directions. Add broccoli during last minute of cooking; cook 1 minute. Drain.
- Heat a large skillet over medium heat. Add butter and oil; cook 7 minutes or until butter browns. Add gnocchi mixture and pepper to pan; toss to coat. Spoon about 1 1/2 cups gnocchi mixture into each of 6 shallow bowls. Sprinkle each serving with 1 1/2 teaspoons pine nuts and about 2 teaspoons cheese.

Nutrition Information

- Calories: 368
- Fiber: 5.7 g
- Sodium: 614 mg
- Protein: 7.9 g
- Saturated Fat: 3.8 g
- Total Carbohydrate: 56.6 g
- Cholesterol: 13 mg
- Total Fat: 12.8 g

24. Bucatini Puttanesca

Serving: Serves 6 (serving size: about 1 1/2 cups) | Prep: | Cook: | Ready in: 24mins

Ingredients

- 1/4 cup extra-virgin olive oil
- 6 garlic cloves, minced
- 4 anchovy fillets
- 1 1/2 teaspoons dried oregano
- 3/4 teaspoon crushed red pepper
- 4 cups unsalted chicken stock
- 12 ounces bucatini or thick spaghetti
- 3 pints multicolored cherry or grape tomatoes, halved
- 2 tablespoons unsalted tomato paste
- 1/4 cup chopped fresh basil
- 1/4 cup chopped fresh parsley
- 24 pitted kalamata olives, chopped
- 3 tablespoons capers
- 1/8 teaspoon salt

Direction

- Heat a large high-sided sauté pan over medium heat. Add oil to pan; swirl to coat. Add garlic, anchovies, oregano, and red pepper; cook 2 minutes, stirring constantly to break up anchovies. Add stock and pasta to pan; bring to a boil. Cook 10 minutes, stirring occasionally. Add tomatoes and tomato paste. Cook 2 to 3 minutes or until pasta is done. Remove pan from heat; add remaining ingredients, tossing to combine.

Nutrition Information

- Calories: 368
- Cholesterol: 2 mg
- Fiber: 4 g
- Protein: 14 g
- Sodium: 569 mg
- Saturated Fat: 1.5 g
- Total Carbohydrate: 52 g
- Sugar: 7 g
- Total Fat: 12.2 g

25. Butternut Squash Ravioli With Pancetta And Sage

Serving: 4 servings (serving size: 5 ravioli) | Prep: | Cook: | Ready in:

Ingredients

- 1/4 cup dried porcini mushrooms (about 1/4 ounce)
- 1 1/2 tablespoons olive oil
- 2/3 cup chopped pancetta (about 2 1/2 ounces)
- 1 cup mashed cooked butternut squash (about 1 pound uncooked)
- 5 tablespoons dry breadcrumbs
- 1/4 cup (1 ounce) grated fresh Parmesan cheese
- 2 teaspoons grated lemon rind
- 1/4 teaspoon salt
- 1/8 teaspoon ground nutmeg
- 1 large egg, lightly beaten
- 40 won ton wrappers
- 2 teaspoons chopped fresh sage
- 1/4 teaspoon freshly ground black pepper

Direction

- Pour boiling water over mushrooms in a bowl. Cover and let stand 30 minutes or until tender, and drain. Squeeze mushrooms to remove excess moisture. Chop mushrooms.
- Heat oil in a medium saucepan over medium-high heat. Add pancetta; cook until crisp. Remove half of pancetta from pan with a slotted spoon, and place in a medium bowl, reserving remaining pancetta and drippings. Add the mushrooms, squash, breadcrumbs, cheese, rind, salt, nutmeg, and egg to bowl, stirring to combine.
- Working with 1 won ton wrapper at a time (cover remaining wrappers with a damp towel to keep them from drying), spoon about 1 tablespoon squash mixture into center of each wrapper. Brush edges of wrapper with water, and top with another wrapper, stretching top wrapper slightly to meet edges of bottom wrapper. Press the edges together firmly with fingers, and cut edges with a 2 1/2-inch round cutter. Repeat the procedure with remaining won ton wrappers and squash mixture.
- Fill a large Dutch oven with water; bring to a simmer. Add half of ravioli; cook 3 minutes or until done (do not boil). Remove the ravioli with a slotted spoon. Keep warm. Repeat procedure with remaining ravioli.
- Reheat remaining pancetta and drippings over medium-low heat; drizzle over ravioli. Sprinkle with sage and pepper.

Nutrition Information

- Calories: 389
- Cholesterol: 74 mg
- Sodium: 961 mg
- Total Fat: 11.6 g
- Fiber: 4.6 g
- Protein: 18.4 g
- Total Carbohydrate: 52.5 g
- Saturated Fat: 3.1 g

26. Butternut Squash Ravioli With Sage Butter Sauce

Serving: 8 servings | Prep: | Cook: | Ready in:

Ingredients

- 1/2 cup crushed gingersnaps (about 8 cookies)
- 2 tablespoons milk
- 1 (2-pound) butternut squash
- 1 cup (4 ounces) freshly grated Parmigiano-Reggiano cheese, divided
- 2 tablespoons butter, softened
- 1/2 teaspoon salt
- 1 (12-ounce) package won ton wrappers
- Sage Butter Sauce
- Freshly ground pepper

Direction

- Stir together gingersnaps and milk in a medium bowl. Let stand until cookies are softened (about 10 minutes).
- Cut squash in half lengthwise; remove seeds. Line a baking sheet with aluminum foil. Coat foil with cooking spray. Place squash, cut side down, on foil. Bake, uncovered, at 400° for 30 to 40 minutes or until tender. Scoop out pulp; mash. Discard shell. Measure 1 3/4 cups pulp; reserve any remaining pulp for another use.
- Stir 1 3/4 cups squash pulp, 1/2 cup cheese, butter, and salt into softened gingersnaps. Working with 6 won ton wrappers at a time (keeping remaining wrappers covered), spoon about 1 tablespoon squash filling into center of each wrapper. Moisten edges of each wrapper with water; bring 2 opposite corners together. Press edges together with a fork to seal, forming a triangle. Cover ravioli with a damp towel to keep them from drying.
- Bring 2 quarts water to a boil in a large saucepan. Cook ravioli, 6 at a time, uncovered, 1 to 2 minutes. Quickly remove from water with a slotted spoon. Keep warm. Place 6 ravioli in each serving bowl. Top each with 1 tablespoon Sage Butter Sauce. Sprinkle evenly with remaining 1/2 cup cheese and pepper.

27. Butternut Squash Ravioli With Spinach Pesto

Serving: Serves 6 | Prep: | Cook: | Ready in: 75mins

Ingredients

- 1 butternut squash, halved lengthwise and seeded (about 1 1/2 pounds)
- Cooking spray
- 1 tablespoon chopped fresh oregano
- 2 tablespoons unsalted butter, melted
- 2.5 ounces Parmesan cheese, grated and divided
- 3/8 teaspoon salt, divided
- 1/2 teaspoon freshly ground black pepper, divided
- 36 wonton wrappers
- 1 large egg, lightly beaten
- 2 garlic cloves
- 1 1/2 cups fresh baby spinach
- 1/2 cup fresh basil
- 1/4 cup walnuts, toasted, chopped, and divided
- 2 tablespoons extra-virgin olive oil
- 2 tablespoons organic vegetable broth
- 1 teaspoon fresh lemon juice
- 6 quarts water

Direction

- Preheat oven to 400°.
- Place squash halves, cut sides down, on a foil-lined baking sheet coated with cooking spray. Bake at 400° for 30 minutes or until tender. Cool. Scoop out pulp; discard peel. Mash pulp. Combine oregano, squash pulp, and butter in a large bowl. Stir in 2 ounces (about 1/2 cup) cheese, 1/4 teaspoon salt, and 1/4 teaspoon pepper. Working with 1 wonton wrapper at a time (cover remaining wrappers with a damp towel to keep them from drying), spoon about 1 1/2 teaspoons squash mixture into center of each wrapper. Moisten edges of wrapper with beaten egg; bring 2 opposite corners together. Pinch edges together to seal, forming a triangle. Repeat procedure with remaining wrappers, squash mixture, and egg. Cover ravioli loosely with a towel to prevent drying.
- Place garlic in a food processor, and pulse until finely chopped. Add remaining 1/2 ounce (about 2 tablespoons) cheese, remaining 1/8 teaspoon salt, remaining 1/4 teaspoon pepper, spinach, basil, and 2 tablespoons walnuts. With processor on, slowly pour oil, broth, and juice through food chute. Process until well blended. Place pesto in a large bowl.
- Bring 6 quarts water to a boil in a large Dutch oven. Add half of ravioli; cook 3 minutes or until thoroughly cooked. Remove ravioli with a slotted spoon. Repeat procedure with remaining ravioli. Add ravioli to pesto; toss

gently to coat. Arrange 6 ravioli on each of 6 plates; sprinkle each serving with 1 teaspoon walnuts.

Nutrition Information

- Calories: 344
- Protein: 11.1 g
- Saturated Fat: 5.2 g
- Total Fat: 15.7 g
- Fiber: 3.6 g
- Sodium: 586 mg
- Total Carbohydrate: 41.8 g
- Cholesterol: 57 mg

28. Butternut Squash, Caramelized Onion, And Spinach Lasagna

Serving: Serves 8 (serving size: 1 piece) | Prep: | Cook: | Ready in: 120mins

Ingredients

- 6 cups (1/2-inch) cubed peeled butternut squash
- 2 tablespoons extra-virgin olive oil, divided
- 2 tablespoons chopped fresh sage
- 12 garlic cloves, unpeeled (about 1 head)
- 1 teaspoon kosher salt, divided
- 1/2 teaspoon black pepper
- Cooking spray
- 1 large onion, vertically sliced
- 2 tablespoons water
- 2 (9-ounce) packages fresh spinach
- 5 cups 1% low-fat milk, divided
- 1 bay leaf
- 1 thyme sprig
- 5 tablespoons all-purpose flour
- 1 1/2 cups (6 ounces) shredded fontina cheese, divided
- 3/8 teaspoon ground red pepper
- 1/4 teaspoon grated whole nutmeg
- 9 no-boil lasagna noodles

Direction

- Preheat oven to 425°.
- Combine squash, 1 tablespoon oil, sage, garlic, 1/2 teaspoon salt, and black pepper in a large bowl; toss to coat. Arrange squash mixture on a baking sheet coated with cooking spray. Bake at 425° for 30 minutes or until squash is tender. Cool slightly; peel garlic. Place squash and garlic in a bowl; partially mash with a fork.
- Heat remaining 1 tablespoon oil in a large Dutch oven over medium-high heat. Add onion, and sauté for 4 minutes. Reduce heat to medium-low; continue cooking for 20 minutes or until golden brown, stirring frequently. Place onion in a bowl.
- Add 2 tablespoons water and spinach to Dutch oven; increase heat to high. Cover and cook 2 minutes or until spinach wilts. Drain in a colander; cool. Squeeze excess liquid from spinach. Add spinach to onions.
- Heat 4 1/2 cups milk, bay leaf, and thyme in a medium saucepan over medium-high heat. Bring to a boil; remove from heat. Let stand for 10 minutes. Discard bay leaf and thyme. Return pan to medium heat. Combine remaining 1/2 cup milk and flour in a small bowl. Add to pan, stirring with a whisk until blended. Bring to a boil; reduce heat, and simmer for 5 minutes or until thickened, stirring constantly. Remove from heat; stir in remaining 1/2 teaspoon salt, 1 1/4 cups cheese, red pepper, and nutmeg.
- Spread 1/2 cup milk mixture in bottom of a 13 x 9-inch glass or ceramic baking dish coated with cooking spray. Arrange 3 noodles over milk mixture; top with half of squash mixture, half of spinach mixture, and 3/4 cup milk mixture. Repeat layers, ending with noodles. Spread remaining milk mixture over noodles. Bake at 425° for 30 minutes, and remove from oven. Sprinkle with remaining 1/4 cup cheese.
- Preheat broiler.
- Broil 2 minutes or until cheese is melted and lightly browned. Let stand 10 minutes before serving.

Nutrition Information

- Calories: 360
- Cholesterol: 31 mg
- Fiber: 6.5 g
- Total Carbohydrate: 50 g
- Total Fat: 11.9 g
- Protein: 16.6 g
- Saturated Fat: 5.4 g
- Sodium: 576 mg

29. Cabbage And Radish Couscous

Serving: Serves 4 (serving size: 1 cup) | Prep: | Cook: | Ready in:

Ingredients

- 3/4 cup unsalted chicken stock
- 3/4 cup uncooked couscous
- 1/4 teaspoon kosher salt
- 1 cup very thinly sliced green cabbage
- 3/4 cup very thinly sliced radishes
- 1/2 cup prepared refrigerated salsa fresca
- 2 tablespoons extra-virgin olive oil
- 1 tablespoon fresh lime juice
- 1/4 teaspoon freshly ground black pepper
- 1.5 ounces queso fresco

Direction

- Bring stock to a boil in a small saucepan over high heat. Place couscous and salt in a small baking dish. Pour stock over couscous; stir to combine. Cover tightly with plastic wrap; let stand 8 minutes. Fluff with a fork.
- Combine cabbage, radishes, salsa fresca, olive oil, lime juice, and black pepper in a large bowl. Stir in couscous. Sprinkle with queso fresco.

Nutrition Information

- Calories: 242
- Saturated Fat: 2.4 g
- Total Carbohydrate: 29 g
- Total Fat: 9.8 g
- Sodium: 315 mg
- Protein: 7 g
- Cholesterol: 7 mg
- Fiber: 3 g

30. Campanile's Spaghetti And Meatballs In Red Sauce

Serving: Serves 8 generously | Prep: | Cook: | Ready in: 120mins

Ingredients

- Sauce
- 6 tablespoons extra-virgin olive oil
- 6 large garlic cloves, halved and thinly sliced
- 3 cans (28 oz. each) diced tomatoes, preferably fire-roasted, such as Muir Glen
- About 1 1/2 tsp. kosher salt
- About 3/4 tsp. freshly ground black pepper
- 3 large fresh basil sprigs, plus 1/2 cup leaves
- Meatballs
- About 1/4 cup olive oil, divided
- 1 medium onion, finely chopped
- 2 garlic cloves, minced
- 4 ounces white or cremini mushrooms, chopped
- 2 teaspoons cracked fennel seeds*
- 1 1/2 teaspoons kosher salt
- 1/2 teaspoon freshly ground black pepper
- About 2/3 cup cold dry white wine, divided
- 4 ounces country bread such as pain au levain, crusts removed, cut into 1-in. cubes
- 3 tablespoons minced flat-leaf parsley
- 3/4 pound cold ground pork
- 3/4 pound cold ground turkey (dark meat)
- 3/4 pound cold ground beef chuck
- 2 tablespoons flour
- Spaghetti
- 1 1/2 pounds spaghetti

- About 1 cup freshly grated parmesan cheese

Direction

- Make sauce: In a 5- to 6-qt. pan, cook oil and garlic over medium-low heat until garlic softens, 5 to 6 minutes. Add tomatoes, salt, and pepper. Cover, bring to a boil over high heat, then reduce heat and simmer, stirring often, until thick, 45 minutes to 1 hour. If needed, crush tomatoes with a spoon to break up. Stir in basil sprigs. Turn off heat; keep warm.
- Meanwhile, make meatballs: Heat 1 tbsp. oil in a large frying pan over medium heat. Add onion and cook until tender, 5 to 8 minutes. Stir in garlic and cook until fragrant, about 1 minute more. Add mushrooms, fennel, salt, and pepper. Cook until mushrooms are tender, 5 minutes. Remove from heat and stir in 1/4 cup wine and the bread until liquid is absorbed.
- Transfer mixture to a food processor and pulse to finely chop. Scrape into bowl of a stand mixer and let cool. Add parsley, meats, and 1/3 cup wine and beat on low speed until well blended, 1 to 2 minutes.
- Using wet hands, shape meat into 1 1/2-in. balls. Heat 2 large frying pans over medium heat with 1 tbsp. oil each. Brown about a third of meatballs in each pan, turning once and adding oil if needed, 6 to 8 minutes per batch. With a slotted spatula, transfer meatballs to a platter. Repeat with remaining meatballs and oil.
- Scrape all the drippings into 1 pan. Whisk in flour, then cook over medium heat until bubbling, 1 to 2 minutes. Whisk in 2 cups sauce to loosen browned bits. Scrape into pan with rest of sauce and stir.
- Return sauce to a simmer. Gently stir in meatballs; simmer, covered, until flavors are blended, about 20 minutes. Discard basil sprigs. Cut remaining basil leaves into fine slivers and stir into sauce. Meanwhile, cook spaghetti as package directs.
- Drain pasta and transfer to a large shallow bowl. Ladle all the meatballs and about half the sauce on top, and toss to coat. Serve with cheese and extra sauce.
- *Crack fennel seeds with a mortar and pestle, or buzz in a clean coffee grinder.
- Make ahead: Chill sauce and meatballs up to 1 day, or freeze up to 1 month.
- Note: Nutritional analysis is per serving.

Nutrition Information

- Calories: 872
- Saturated Fat: 9.5 g
- Sodium: 2116 mg
- Total Fat: 36 g
- Protein: 47 g
- Fiber: 7.2 g
- Total Carbohydrate: 88 g
- Cholesterol: 92 mg

31. Caramelized Cabbage With Whole Wheat Penne And Provolone

Serving: Serves 4 (serving size: about 2 cups) | Prep: | Cook: | Ready in:

Ingredients

- 6 ounces uncooked whole-wheat penne
- 3 tablespoons olive oil
- 2 garlic cloves, thinly sliced
- 6 cups coarsely chopped green cabbage
- 1/2 teaspoon kosher salt
- 1/4 teaspoon freshly ground black pepper
- 1 Fresno chile, thinly sliced
- 2 teaspoons grated lemon rind
- 3 ounces aged provolone cheese, shredded and divided (about 3/4 cup)
- 1 tablespoon fresh thyme leaves

Direction

- Bring a large saucepan filled with water to a boil. Add pasta; cook 7 to 9 minutes or until al dente. Drain in a colander over a bowl, reserving 1/4 cup cooking liquid.
- Heat a large skillet over medium heat. Add oil; swirl to coat. Add garlic to pan; sauté 30 seconds or until beginning to brown. Remove garlic from pan with a slotted spoon; set aside. Increase heat to medium-high. Add cabbage to pan; cook 6 minutes or until browned and tender, stirring occasionally. Stir in salt, black pepper, and chile; cook 2 minutes. Stir in pasta, reserved 1/4 cup pasta cooking liquid, and reserved garlic. Stir in rind and 5 ounces cheese. Divide pasta mixture among 4 bowls. Sprinkle evenly with remaining 5 ounces cheese and thyme.

Nutrition Information

- Calories: 359
- Total Fat: 18.1 g
- Saturated Fat: 5.1 g
- Sodium: 471 mg
- Sugar: 2 g
- Cholesterol: 15 mg
- Fiber: 7 g
- Protein: 14 g
- Total Carbohydrate: 44 g

32. Cauliflower Alfredo

Serving: Serves 4 (serving size: 1 1/2 cups) | Prep: | Cook: | Ready in: 30mins

Ingredients

- 8 ounces uncooked whole-wheat fettuccine
- 3 cups chopped broccoli
- 3 cups chopped cauliflower, divided
- 1 tablespoon white whole-wheat flour
- 1 cup unsalted chicken stock
- 3 garlic cloves
- 2/3 cup 1% low-fat milk
- 1 1/2 tablespoons unsalted butter
- 1 teaspoon freshly ground black pepper
- 1 teaspoon fresh lemon juice
- 1/2 teaspoon kosher salt
- 2 ounces grated Parmigiano-Reggiano cheese, divided (about 1/2 cup)
- 1 teaspoon grated lemon rind

Direction

- Cook pasta according to package directions, omitting salt and fat. Add broccoli and 1 cup cauliflower during last 2 minutes of cooking; drain.
- Place flour in a large saucepan. Gradually add stock, stirring constantly with a whisk until blended. Bring to a boil over medium heat; cook 2 minutes or until thick, stirring constantly. Add remaining 2 cups cauliflower and garlic. Bring to a boil; cook 15 minutes or until very tender. Place cauliflower mixture in a blender. Add milk, butter, pepper, juice, salt, and 1 ounce cheese. Remove center piece of blender lid (to allow steam to escape); secure blender lid on blender. Place a clean towel over opening in blender lid (to avoid splatters); process until smooth. Return cauliflower mixture to pan over low heat. Add pasta mixture and lemon rind; toss well to coat noodles. Sprinkle with remaining 1 ounce cheese. Serve immediately.

Nutrition Information

- Calories: 380
- Sugar: 5 g
- Fiber: 10 g
- Protein: 21 g
- Saturated Fat: 5.5 g
- Total Fat: 10.2 g
- Sodium: 547 mg
- Cholesterol: 26 mg
- Total Carbohydrate: 53 g

33. Cauliflower Rotini

Serving: Makes 4 servings | Prep: | Cook: | Ready in:

Ingredients

- 2 tablespoons olive oil
- 4 cloves garlic, minced
- 1 head cauliflower (1 3/4 lb.), rinsed, trimmed from core, and separated into 1-inch pieces
- 12 ounces dried rotini pasta or another shape about 1 inch long
- 1 cup grated parmesan cheese (see notes)
- Salt and pepper

Direction

- Pour oil into a 12-inch frying pan with 2-inch-high sides over medium heat. When hot, add garlic and stir until fragrant but not brown, about 1 minute. Add cauliflower and stir to coat, about 1 minute.
- Stir in pasta and 3 1/2 cups water. Bring to a simmer over high heat, then cover, reduce heat, and cook, stirring often, until pasta is just tender to bite and liquid has reduced to a creamy sauce, 15 to 20 minutes; if mixture begins to stick before pasta is done, add more water 1/2 cup at a time. Stir in cheese and add salt and pepper to taste.

Nutrition Information

- Calories: 489
- Sodium: 390 mg
- Total Carbohydrate: 69 g
- Saturated Fat: 4.9 g
- Cholesterol: 16 mg
- Total Fat: 14 g
- Protein: 21 g
- Fiber: 4 g

34. Cauliflower Turkey Tetrazzini

Serving: Serves 6 (serving size: 1 1/2 cups) | Prep: | Cook: | Ready in: 65mins

Ingredients

- 6 ounces uncooked whole-wheat spaghetti
- 5 teaspoons olive oil, divided
- 1 cup chopped yellow onion
- 1 (8-ounce) package white mushrooms, sliced
- 2 tablespoons all-purpose flour
- 1/4 cup white wine
- 1 3/4 cups unsalted chicken stock, divided
- 1 cup whole milk
- 1 tablespoon chopped fresh thyme, divided
- 1/2 teaspoon kosher salt
- 1/2 teaspoon freshly ground black pepper
- 3 ounces Parmesan cheese, grated and divided (about 3/4 cup)
- 2 cups leftover Cauliflower Salad
- 12 ounces skinless, boneless roast turkey breast, cut into 1/2-inch cubes
- Cooking spray
- 1/4 cup whole-wheat panko (Japanese breadcrumbs)

Direction

- Cook pasta according to package directions, omitting salt and fat. Drain.
- Preheat oven to 375°.
- Heat 1 tablespoon olive oil in a large saucepan over medium heat. Add onion; cook 5 minutes or until softened, stirring occasionally. Add mushrooms; cook 5 minutes or until golden and most of liquid evaporates. Sprinkle flour over vegetables; cook 1 minute, stirring constantly. Stir in wine. Add 1 cup chicken stock. Increase heat to medium-high; cook 2 minutes, stirring until smooth. Add milk; bring to a boil. Cook 4 minutes or until sauce is thickened, stirring almost constantly. Stir in 2 teaspoons thyme, salt, pepper, and 2 ounces Parmesan cheese. Remove from heat.
- Place remaining 3/4 cup stock and Cauliflower Salad in a blender; process until

smooth. Stir into sauce. Add turkey and pasta; toss to combine. Spoon into a 2-quart glass or ceramic baking dish coated with cooking spray.

- Combine remaining 2 teaspoons oil, panko, and remaining 1 teaspoon thyme in a small skillet; cook over medium heat 2 minutes or until lightly toasted. Stir in remaining 1 ounce cheese; sprinkle over pasta mixture. Bake at 375° for 20 minutes or until browned and bubbly.

Nutrition Information

- Calories: 395
- Total Carbohydrate: 35 g
- Total Fat: 13.8 g
- Saturated Fat: 4.9 g
- Sodium: 621 mg
- Fiber: 5 g
- Cholesterol: 67 mg
- Protein: 33 g

35. Celery And Cashew Couscous

Serving: Serves 4 (serving size: 3/4 cup) | Prep: | Cook: | Ready in:

Ingredients

- 3/4 cup unsalted chicken stock
- 3/4 cup uncooked couscous
- 1/4 teaspoon kosher salt
- 2 tablespoons extra-virgin olive oil
- 1 tablespoon fresh lemon juice
- 1 tablespoon lower-sodium soy sauce
- 1/2 teaspoon brown sugar
- 1 cup sliced celery
- 1 cup mung bean sprouts
- 3 1/2 tablespoons chopped unsalted cashews
- 2 tablespoons fresh cilantro

Direction

- Bring stock to a boil in a small saucepan over high heat. Place couscous and salt in a small baking dish. Pour stock over couscous; stir to combine. Cover tightly with plastic wrap; let stand 8 minutes. Fluff with a fork.
- Combine olive oil, lemon juice, soy sauce, and brown sugar in a bowl, stirring. Add celery and sprouts; toss. Stir in couscous. Sprinkle with cashews and cilantro.

Nutrition Information

- Calories: 248
- Fiber: 3 g
- Sodium: 296 mg
- Cholesterol: 0.0 mg
- Total Fat: 10.8 g
- Protein: 7 g
- Total Carbohydrate: 31 g
- Saturated Fat: 1.7 g

36. Cheese Ravioli With Pesto

Serving: Serves 4 | Prep: | Cook: | Ready in: 12mins

Ingredients

- 1 (9-ounce) package fresh 3-cheese ravioli
- 1 1/3 cups fresh baby spinach
- 2/3 cup fresh basil leaves
- 1/2 teaspoon salt
- 1/4 teaspoon crushed red pepper
- 2 garlic cloves
- 2 tablespoons fat-free, lower-sodium chicken broth
- 2 tablespoons olive oil
- 1 tablespoon fresh lemon juice
- 1 plum tomato, diced
- 1/2 cup (2 ounces) shaved fresh Parmesan cheese
- 1/3 cup pine nuts, toasted
- Fresh basil leaves (optional)

Direction

- Cook ravioli according to package directions; omit salt and fat. Drain.
- Combine spinach, basil, salt, red pepper, and garlic in a food processor. With processor running, add broth, olive oil, and lemon juice through chute until mixture is smooth.
- Combine ravioli, pesto, and tomato in medium saucepan over medium-high heat; cook 1 minute or until warm. Spoon 3/4 cup into each of 4 bowls; sprinkle each serving with 2 tablespoons cheese and about 4 teaspoons nuts. Garnish with basil leaves, if desired.
- Wine Match: This rich dish needs a crisp white to refresh the palate. Costamolino Vermentino di Sardegna 2010 ($10) is zesty and refreshing with tropical fruit and an herbal edge to match the basil. --Jeffery Lindenmuth

Nutrition Information

- Calories: 389
- Total Carbohydrate: 31.7 g
- Cholesterol: 45 mg
- Total Fat: 23.4 g
- Fiber: 3 g
- Protein: 14.5 g
- Saturated Fat: 6.9 g
- Sodium: 811 mg

37. Cheese Ravioli With Toasted Walnuts

Serving: Makes 4 servings | Prep: 20mins | Cook: | Ready in:

Ingredients

- 1 14- to 16-ounce package cheese ravioli (frozen or fresh)
- 1/3 cup olive oil
- 1 clove garlic, sliced
- 1 cup (2 ounces) walnuts, roughly chopped
- 2 teaspoons lemon juice
- Kosher salt and pepper
- 1/2 cup fresh flat-leaf parsley, chopped
- 1/4 cup grated Parmesan

Direction

- Cook the ravioli according to the package directions. Drain, reserving 3 tablespoons of the cooking water.Heat the oil in a medium skillet over medium heat. Add the garlic and walnuts. Cook, stirring, until the nuts are lightly toasted and fragrant, about 5 minutes. Stir in the lemon juice, 1/2 teaspoon salt, 1/4 teaspoon pepper, the parsley, and the reserved cooking water. Add the ravioli and toss to coat. Divide among individual plates and sprinkle with the Parmesan.Substitution: For a hit of vegetables and a change of pace, use pumpkin or butternut-squash ravioli instead of cheese-filled. You can also replace the walnuts with pecans or almonds.

Nutrition Information

- Calories: 491
- Sodium: 595 mg
- Saturated Fat: 8 g
- Cholesterol: 55 mg
- Total Fat: 36 g
- Fiber: 2 g
- Protein: 15 g
- Total Carbohydrate: 29 g
- Sugar: 2 g

38. Cheesy Stuffed Shells With My Secret Tomato Sauce

Serving: Serves 10 (serving size: 3 stuffed shells) | Prep: | Cook: | Ready in: 64mins

Ingredients

- 30 uncooked jumbo shell pasta (about 8 ounces)

- 4 ounces shredded 6-cheese Italian-blend cheese, divided (about 1 cup)
- 8 ounces shredded part-skim mozzarella cheese (about 2 cups)
- 1/4 cup chopped fresh flat-leaf parsley
- 1/4 cup chopped fresh basil
- 1/2 teaspoon kosher salt
- 1/2 teaspoon freshly ground black pepper
- 1 (15-ounce) container part-skim ricotta cheese
- Cooking spray
- 3 cups My Secret Tomato Sauce or bottled pasta sauce

Direction

- Preheat oven to 350°.
- Cook pasta in boiling water 8 minutes or until almost al dente. Drain. Rinse with cold water; drain.
- Combine 1/2 cup Italian-blend cheese and next 6 ingredients (through ricotta) in a bowl. Spoon about 1 1/2 tablespoons cheese mixture into each pasta shell. Place shells, stuffed sides up, in a 13 x 9- inch glass or ceramic baking dish coated with cooking spray. Pour sauce over shells. Cover and bake at 350° for 30 minutes or until bubbly. Uncover; sprinkle with remaining 1/2 cup Italian-blend cheese. Bake 5 minutes or until cheese melts.
- Tip: If you don't have any My Secret Tomato Sauce prepared, the Organic Tomato Basil Sauce from Whole Foods Market is a great go-to option.

Nutrition Information

- Calories: 285
- Total Carbohydrate: 24.5 g
- Protein: 17.5 g
- Fiber: 1.5 g
- Sodium: 536 mg
- Cholesterol: 37 mg
- Saturated Fat: 6.5 g
- Total Fat: 13.1 g

39. Chicken Dan Dan Noodles

Serving: Serves 4 | Prep: | Cook: | Ready in: 35mins

Ingredients

- 1/2 pound fresh, thin Chinese-style egg noodles (chow mein)* or dried chow mein
- 1 tablespoon minced fresh ginger
- 2 teaspoons minced garlic
- 2 tablespoons cornstarch
- 3 tablespoons reduced-sodium soy sauce
- 3/4 pound ground chicken
- 2/3 cup low-sodium chicken broth
- 2 tablespoons creamy old-fashioned peanut butter
- 1 tablespoon unseasoned rice vinegar
- 2 teaspoons Asian chili garlic sauce, plus more to taste
- 2 teaspoons hot chili oil, plus more to taste
- 2 teaspoons toasted sesame oil
- 2 tablespoons canola or safflower oil
- 1/4 cup sliced green onions, plus more for garnish
- 1 1/2 red bell peppers, seeded and cut into slivers
- 1/2 pound snow peas, trimmed
- 1/2 cup chopped roasted salted peanuts

Direction

- Bring a large pot of water to a boil. Add noodles, stir to separate, and cook until very tender, 5 to 8 minutes or according to package instructions. Drain and rinse with cold water.
- Meanwhile, thoroughly mix ginger, garlic, cornstarch, soy sauce, and chicken in a bowl. In another bowl, whisk together broth, peanut butter, vinegar, chili garlic sauce, chili oil, and sesame oil.
- Heat a large (not nonstick) frying pan over high heat and swirl in canola oil. Add green onions and chicken mixture, stirring to break up the meat, until chicken is lightly browned and no longer pink, 4 to 5 minutes. Add bell peppers and stir for 1 minute. Add chicken

broth mixture; stir until slightly thickened, 2 minutes.

- Add snow peas and noodles to pan. With tongs, toss just until snow peas are brighter green and noodles are well combined and heated through, 1 to 2 minutes. Add 1/4 cup peanuts and toss. Top with more green onions and remaining peanuts, and serve with more chili garlic sauce and chili oil.
- *Look for fresh or dried Chinese-style egg noodles at well-stocked supermarkets or Asian markets.
- Wine pairing: A slightly off-dry white such as Zocker 2013 Paragon Vineyard Riesling (Edna Valley; $20), with vibrant florals that tame the heat. --Sara Schneider

Nutrition Information

- Calories: 604
- Saturated Fat: 5.4 g
- Total Carbohydrate: 48 g
- Sodium: 876 mg
- Total Fat: 33 g
- Protein: 31 g
- Cholesterol: 73 mg
- Fiber: 6 g

40. Chicken Noodle Bowl With Peanut Ginger Sauce

Serving: Serves 6 | Prep: | Cook: | Ready in: 20mins

Ingredients

- PEANUT-GINGER SAUCE
- 1/2 cup creamy peanut butter
- 4 1/2 tablespoons fresh lime juice
- 3 tablespoons soy sauce
- 3 tablespoons honey
- 2 tablespoons peeled and chopped fresh ginger
- 1 1/2 teaspoons sesame oil
- 1/4 teaspoon crushed red pepper
- 3 tablespoons rice vinegar
- 1/4 teaspoon kosher salt
- CHICKEN NOODLE BOWL
- 8 cups water
- 2 tablespoons rice vinegar
- 1 tablespoon kosher salt
- 6 ounces rice noodles or bean threads
- 3 cups shredded cooked chicken
- 3 cups shredded napa cabbage
- 1 1/2 cups halved and thinly sliced seedless cucumber
- 1 1/2 cups matchstick carrots
- 1 1/2 cups thinly sliced red bell pepper
- 6 tablespoons chopped lightly salted dry-roasted peanuts

Direction

- Prepare the Sauce: Process all 9 ingredients in a blender or food processor until smooth.
- Prepare the Chicken Noodle Bowl: Microwave water in a large bowl on HIGH 10 minutes. Stir vinegar and salt into boiling water. Add noodles and let stand until softened, about 5 minutes. Drain noodles.
- Divide noodles, chicken, cabbage, cucumber, carrots, and bell pepper among 6 bowls. Top each bowl with 1 tablespoon peanuts and 2 tablespoons Peanut-Ginger Sauce. Serve remaining sauce on the side.

41. Chicken Paillard With Citrus Salad And Couscous

Serving: Makes 4 servings | Prep: | Cook: | Ready in: 85mins

Ingredients

- VINAIGRETTE
- 1/4 cup fresh orange juice
- 2 tablespoons fresh lime juice
- 2 tablespoons fresh lemon juice
- 2 tablespoons rice wine vinegar
- 2 tablespoons honey

- 1/2 teaspoon kosher salt
- 1/3 cup olive oil
- 1 tablespoon chopped fresh flat-leaf parsley
- 1 teaspoon fresh thyme leaves
- CHICKEN
- 4 (6- to 8-oz.) skinned and boned chicken breasts
- COUSCOUS
- 1/2 tablespoon butter
- 1 1/2 teaspoons olive oil
- 1 cup uncooked Israeli couscous
- 1 1/2 cups chicken broth
- 1 teaspoon kosher salt, divided
- 1 teaspoon black pepper, divided
- SALAD
- 8 ounces haricots verts (French green beans), trimmed
- 1 cup arugula
- 1/2 cup thinly sliced celery
- 1/2 cup celery leaves
- 1 navel orange, peeled and sectioned
- 1 grapefruit, peeled and sectioned

Direction

- Prepare Vinaigrette: Whisk together first 6 ingredients in a medium bowl. Add olive oil in a slow, steady stream, whisking constantly until smooth and well blended. Stir in parsley and thyme leaves. Reserve 1/3 cup plus 2 Tbsp. vinaigrette for use in couscous and salad.
- Prepare Chicken: Place chicken between 2 sheets of plastic wrap, and flatten to about 1/2-inch thickness, using a rolling pin or flat side of a meat mallet. Place chicken in a zip-top plastic bag, and pour remaining vinaigrette over chicken, turning to coat. Seal and marinate in refrigerator for 30 minutes. Turn bag over after 15 minutes.
- Meanwhile, prepare Couscous: Melt butter with 1 1/2 tsp. oil in a medium saucepan over medium-high heat. Add couscous; cook, stirring constantly, 3 minutes or until toasted. Stir in broth. Bring mixture to a boil; cover, reduce heat to low, and cook, stirring occasionally, 15 minutes or until liquid is absorbed. Uncover and fluff. Stir in 1/4 tsp. each salt and pepper and reserved 2 Tbsp. vinaigrette.
- Preheat oven to 400°. Remove chicken from bag; discard marinade. Place chicken on a wire rack in an aluminum foil-lined jelly-roll pan. Sprinkle with 3/4 tsp. each salt and pepper.
- Bake at 400° for 12 to 15 minutes or until a meat thermometer inserted in thickest portion of chicken registers 165°. Let chicken stand at room temperature 5 minutes.
- Prepare Salad: Cook beans in boiling salted water 3 minutes or until crisp-tender; drain. Halve beans, lengthwise; toss with arugula, next 4 ingredients, and remaining 1/3 cup vinaigrette.
- Divide couscous among 4 plates; top each with a chicken breast, and serve with salad.

42. Chicken Pasta Primavera

Serving: 2 servings (serving size: 3 1/2 cups) | Prep: 5mins | Cook: 15mins | Ready in: 20mins

Ingredients

- 1/2 cup uncooked whole-grain rotini
- 2 teaspoons olive oil
- 1/2 cup (4 ounces) cooked skinless, boneless chicken breast, sliced into 1/2-inch strips
- 1 onion, vertically sliced
- 3 garlic cloves, minced
- 1 teaspoon dried oregano
- 1/8 teaspoon salt
- 1/8 teaspoon pepper
- 2 cups chopped tomato
- 1 zucchini, sliced lengthwise into ribbons
- 2 tablespoons grated Parmesan cheese

Direction

- Cook pasta according to package directions, omitting salt and fat. Drain.
- Heat oil in a nonstick skillet over medium heat. Add chicken; cook 5 minutes.

- Add onion, garlic, oregano, salt, pepper, and tomato to pan; cook 8 to 10 minutes.
- Combine chicken mixture, pasta, and zucchini ribbons; toss gently. Top with Parmesan cheese.

Nutrition Information

- Calories: 410
- Fiber: 12 g
- Total Carbohydrate: 61 g
- Cholesterol: 40 mg
- Sodium: 480 mg
- Protein: 28 g
- Saturated Fat: 2 g
- Total Fat: 9 g

43. Chicken Portobello Lasagna

Serving: Makes 6 servings | Prep: 20mins | Cook: 10mins | Ready in:

Ingredients

- 1 (10-oz.) package frozen chopped spinach, thawed
- 1 tablespoon butter
- 3 (6-oz.) PILGRIM'S PRIDE EatWellStayHealthy Boneless, Skinless Chicken Breasts, diced
- 1 (8-oz.) package sliced fresh baby portobello mushrooms
- 1 (10 3/4-oz.) can reduced-fat cream of mushroom soup
- 1 (8-oz.) container reduced-fat sour cream
- 1/2 teaspoon pepper
- 1/4 teaspoon salt
- 1 (8-oz.) block 2% reduced-fat sharp Cheddar cheese, shredded
- 6 no-boil lasagna noodles
- 3 tablespoons grated Parmesan cheese

Direction

- Preheat oven to 350°. Drain spinach well, pressing between paper towels.
- Melt butter in a large Dutch oven over medium-high heat; add chicken and mushrooms, and sauté 10 minutes or until chicken is done and mushrooms are tender. Remove from heat. Stir in spinach, soup, and next 3 ingredients; fold in cheese.
- Spoon one-fourth of chicken mixture in a lightly greased 8- x 8-inch baking dish. Arrange 2 noodles on top of mixture. Repeat layers twice; top with remaining chicken mixture. Sprinkle with Parmesan cheese.
- Bake, covered, at 350° for 45 minutes; uncover and bake 15 minutes or until bubbly. Let stand 10 minutes before serving.
- Note: To make ahead, prepare recipe as directed through Step Cover and chill at least 8 hours or up to 24 hours. Let stand at room temperature 30 minutes; proceed with recipe as directed.

44. Chicken Puttanesca With Angel Hair Pasta

Serving: 4 servings | Prep: | Cook: | Ready in:

Ingredients

- 8 ounces uncooked angel hair pasta
- 2 teaspoons olive oil
- 4 (6-ounce) skinless, boneless chicken breast halves
- 1/2 teaspoon salt
- 2 cups tomato-basil pasta sauce (such as Muir Glen Organic)
- 1/4 cup pitted and coarsely chopped kalamata olives
- 1 tablespoon capers
- 1/4 teaspoon crushed red pepper
- 1/4 cup (1 ounce) preshredded Parmesan cheese
- Chopped fresh basil or basil sprigs (optional)

Direction

- Cook pasta according to package directions, omitting salt and fat. Drain and keep warm.
- Heat oil in a large nonstick skillet over medium-high heat. Cut chicken into 1-inch pieces. Add chicken to pan; sprinkle evenly with salt. Cook chicken 5 minutes or until lightly browned, stirring occasionally. Stir in pasta sauce, olives, capers, and pepper; bring to a simmer. Cook 5 minutes or until chicken is done, stirring frequently. Arrange 1 cup pasta on each of 4 plates; top with 1 1/2 cups chicken mixture. Sprinkle each serving with 1 tablespoon cheese. Garnish with chopped basil or basil sprigs, if desired.

Nutrition Information

- Calories: 530
- Protein: 51.8 g
- Cholesterol: 104 mg
- Fiber: 2.1 g
- Saturated Fat: 2.8 g
- Sodium: 971 mg
- Total Carbohydrate: 55 g
- Total Fat: 12.4 g

45. Chicken Tetrazzini

Serving: Serves 12 (serving size: about 1 1/3 cups; 6 servings per casserole) | Prep: | Cook: | Ready in:

Ingredients

- 1 tablespoon unsalted butter
- Cooking spray
- 1 cup finely chopped onion
- 2/3 cup finely chopped celery
- 3/4 teaspoon freshly ground black pepper
- 1/4 teaspoon salt
- 3 (8-ounce) packages presliced mushrooms
- 1/2 cup dry sherry
- 3 ounces all-purpose flour (about 2/3 cup)
- 3 (14.5-ounce) cans fat-free, less-sodium chicken broth
- 2 1/4 cups (9 ounces) grated fresh Parmesan cheese, divided
- 1/2 cup (4 ounces) 1/3-less-fat cream cheese
- 7 cups hot cooked vermicelli (about 1 pound uncooked pasta)
- 4 cups chopped cooked chicken breast (about 1 1/2 pounds)
- 1 (1-ounce) slice white bread

Direction

- Preheat oven to 350°.
- Melt butter in a large stockpot over medium-high heat. Add onion, celery, black pepper, salt, and mushrooms; sauté 4 minutes or until mushrooms are tender. Add sherry; cook 1 minute.
- Weigh or lightly spoon flour into dry measuring cups; level with a knife. Gradually add flour to pan; cook 3 minutes, stirring constantly (mixture will be thick) with a whisk. Gradually add broth, stirring constantly. Bring to a boil. Reduce heat; simmer 5 minutes, stirring frequently. Remove from heat.
- Add 1 ¾ cups Parmesan cheese and cream cheese, stirring with a whisk until cream cheese melts. Add pasta and chicken; stir until blended. Divide pasta mixture between 2 (8-inch-square) glass or ceramic baking dishes coated with cooking spray.
- Place bread in food processor; pulse 10 times or until coarse crumbs form. Combine breadcrumbs and ½ cup Parmesan cheese; sprinkle evenly over pasta.
- Bake at 350° for 30 minutes or until lightly browned and bubbly. Remove casserole from oven; let stand 15 minutes.
- To freeze unbaked casserole: Prepare through Step Cool completely in refrigerator. Cover with plastic wrap, pressing to remove as much air as possible. Wrap with heavy-duty foil. Store in freezer for up to 2 months.
- To prepare frozen unbaked casserole: Thaw casserole completely in refrigerator (about 24

hours). Preheat oven to 350°. Remove foil; reserve foil. Remove plastic wrap; discard wrap. Cover casserole with reserved foil; bake at 350° for 30 minutes. Uncover and bake an additional 1 hour or until golden and bubbly. Let stand 15 minutes.

Nutrition Information

- Calories: 422
- Fiber: 2.3 g
- Protein: 35 g
- Saturated Fat: 6.5 g
- Sodium: 702 mg
- Total Carbohydrate: 39.6 g
- Total Fat: 12.1 g
- Cholesterol: 76 mg

46. Chicken Tetrazzini With Prosciutto And Peas

Serving: Makes 6 servings | Prep: 10mins | Cook: 3mins | Ready in:

Ingredients

- 3 ounces finely chopped prosciutto
- 2 teaspoons vegetable oil
- 1 (7-oz.) package vermicelli
- 3 cups chopped cooked chicken
- 1 cup (4 oz.) shredded Parmesan cheese
- 1 (10 3/4-oz.) can cream of mushroom soup
- 1 (10-oz.) container refrigerated Alfredo sauce
- 1 (4-oz.) can sliced mushrooms, drained
- 1/2 cup chicken broth
- 1/4 cup dry dry white wine
- 1/4 teaspoon freshly ground pepper
- 1 cup frozen baby English peas, thawed
- 1/2 cup slivered almonds

Direction

- Sauté prosciutto in hot vegetable oil in a small skillet over medium-high heat 2 to 3 minutes or until crisp.
- Preheat oven to 350°. Prepare pasta according to package directions.
- Meanwhile, stir together chicken, 1/2 cup Parmesan cheese, and next 6 ingredients; stir in prosciutto, pasta, and peas. Spoon mixture into 6 lightly greased 8-oz. ramekins or a lightly greased 11- x 7-inch baking dish. Sprinkle with almonds and remaining 1/2 cup Parmesan cheese.
- Bake at 350° for 35 minutes or until bubbly.

47. Chicken Tetrazzini With Broccoli

Serving: 8 servings | Prep: | Cook: | Ready in:

Ingredients

- 4 cups broccoli florets (about 2 bunches)
- 12 ounces uncooked spaghetti
- 2 tablespoons butter or stick margarine
- 3 cups sliced mushrooms (about 8 ounces)
- 1 teaspoon dried oregano
- 1 teaspoon dried basil
- 2 garlic cloves, crushed
- 1/2 cup all-purpose flour
- 3 cups Chicken Stock
- 1 cup 2% reduced-fat milk
- 3/4 cup (3 ounces) shredded sharp provolone or grated fresh Parmesan cheese
- 2 tablespoons dry sherry
- 3/4 teaspoon salt
- 1/8 teaspoon black pepper
- 4 cups chopped cooked chicken
- Cooking spray
- 1/4 cup dry breadcrumbs

Direction

- Cook broccoli in boiling water 5 minutes or until tender; remove broccoli with a slotted spoon, and drain. Return water to a boil; add spaghetti. Cook pasta according to package directions, omitting salt and fat. Drain; set aside.

- Preheat oven to 450°.
- Melt the butter in a large nonstick skillet over medium-high heat. Add the mushrooms, oregano, basil, and garlic; saute 4 minutes. Lightly spoon flour into a dry measuring cup; level with a knife. Stir flour into mushroom mixture. Gradually add Chicken Stock and milk; stir well with a whisk. Bring to a boil, and cook 5 minutes or until thick, stirring occasionally. Add cheese, sherry, salt, and pepper; stir well. Remove from heat, and stir in chicken.
- Arrange 3 cups spaghetti in a 13 x 9-inch baking dish coated with cooking spray. Top with 2 cups broccoli and half of chicken mixture. Repeat layers. Sprinkle with breadcrumbs. Bake at 450° for 15 minutes or until golden brown.

Nutrition Information

- Calories: 422
- Protein: 30.8 g
- Sodium: 604 mg
- Saturated Fat: 5.5 g
- Total Fat: 12.3 g
- Cholesterol: 74 mg
- Fiber: 3.1 g
- Total Carbohydrate: 46.2 g

48. Chicken And Mushroom Stroganoff

Serving: Serves 4 (serving size: about 1 cup) | Prep: | Cook: | Ready in: 195mins

Ingredients

- 1 (4.5-pound) whole chicken
- 3 quarts water (12 cups)
- 2 teaspoons black peppercorns
- 8 garlic cloves, crushed
- 3 celery stalks, cut into 2-inch pieces
- 2 carrots, cut into 2-inch pieces
- 1 medium yellow onion, quartered
- 1 (1-inch) piece fresh ginger, sliced
- 7 ounces uncooked fettuccine
- 2 teaspoons olive oil
- 1/3 cup chopped shallots
- 3/4 teaspoon kosher salt, divided
- 1 (8-ounce) package sliced cremini mushrooms
- 2 teaspoons all-purpose flour
- 1/2 cup dry white wine
- 1/3 cup crème fraîche
- 1 tablespoon chopped fresh tarragon, divided
- 1/4 teaspoon freshly ground black pepper
- Tarragon sprigs

Direction

- Place first 8 ingredients in a large stockpot; bring to a boil. Reduce heat; cover and simmer 45 minutes or until chicken is done. Place chicken on a cutting board; cool. Remove solids with a slotted spoon, reserving liquid; discard solids.
- Remove skin from chicken; discard skin. Remove breast halves and leg and thigh meat; reserve bones. Shred 1 chicken breast half and dark meat chicken; reserve for Shredded Chicken Tortilla Soup and Chicken Salad with Bok Choy, Almonds, and Apricots. Add bones to pan; simmer, uncovered, 1 1/2 hours, skimming surface occasionally. Discard bones. Bring stock to a boil; cook 12 minutes or until reduced to 4 1/2 cups.
- Cook pasta according to package directions, omitting salt and fat. Drain in a colander over a bowl, reserving 1/3 cup cooking liquid.
- Heat a large nonstick skillet over medium-high heat. Add oil; swirl. Add shallots; sauté 1 minute. Add 1/4 teaspoon salt and mush-rooms; cook 4 minutes. Sprinkle flour over pan; cook 1 minute, stirring constantly. Add wine; cook 1 minute. Add 1/2 cup stock (reserve remaining 4 cups for Shredded Chicken Tortilla Soup) and reserved 1/3 cup

pasta cooking liquid; simmer 2 minutes. Cut remaining chicken breast half into 1/2-inch pieces. Stir in chicken pieces, 1/2 teaspoon salt, crème fraîche, chopped tarragon, ground pepper, and pasta. Garnish with tarragon sprigs.

Nutrition Information

- Calories: 408
- Cholesterol: 61 mg
- Protein: 25 g
- Total Fat: 11.9 g
- Fiber: 2 g
- Sodium: 425 mg
- Total Carbohydrate: 42 g
- Saturated Fat: 5.3 g

49. Chicken With Lemon Leek Linguine

Serving: 4 servings (serving size: 1 chicken breast half and 1 cup pasta mixture) | Prep: | Cook: | Ready in: 30mins

Ingredients

- 6 ounces uncooked linguine
- 4 (6-ounce) skinless, boneless chicken breast halves
- 1/2 teaspoon salt, divided
- 1/4 teaspoon black pepper
- 1/4 cup all-purpose flour
- 3 tablespoons butter, divided
- 3 garlic cloves, thinly sliced
- 1 leek, trimmed, cut in half lengthwise, and thinly sliced (1 1/2 cups)
- 1/2 cup fat-free, lower-sodium chicken broth
- 2 tablespoons fresh lemon juice
- 2 tablespoons chopped fresh flat-leaf parsley

Direction

- Cook pasta according to package directions, omitting salt and fat. Drain; keep warm.
- Place chicken between 2 sheets of heavy-duty plastic wrap; pound to an even thickness using a meat mallet or small heavy skillet. Sprinkle chicken with 1/4 teaspoon salt and pepper. Place flour in a shallow dish; dredge chicken in flour, shaking to remove excess.
- Heat 1 tablespoon butter in a large nonstick skillet over medium-high heat. Add chicken; cook 3 minutes on each side or until done. Remove chicken from pan; keep warm.
- Melt 1 tablespoon butter in skillet over medium-high heat. Add garlic, leek, and remaining 1/4 teaspoon salt; sauté 4 minutes. Add broth and juice; cook 2 minutes or until liquid is reduced by half. Remove from heat; stir in remaining 1 tablespoon butter. Add pasta to leek mixture; toss well to combine. Serve chicken over pasta mixture; sprinkle with parsley.

Nutrition Information

- Calories: 474
- Sodium: 592 mg
- Cholesterol: 121 mg
- Saturated Fat: 6.2 g
- Total Carbohydrate: 44 g
- Protein: 46.8 g
- Total Fat: 11.5 g
- Fiber: 2.3 g

50. Chicken, Corn, And Green Onion Rotini

Serving: 6 servings (serving size: 1 1/3 cups) | Prep: | Cook: | Ready in:

Ingredients

- 8 ounces uncooked rotini (corkscrew pasta; about 4 cups)
- 2 cups chopped roasted skinless, boneless chicken breasts (about 2 breasts)
- 2 cups fresh corn kernels

- 1 1/4 cups thinly sliced green onions
- 1 cup chopped plum tomato
- 1/2 cup (2 ounces) grated fresh Parmesan cheese
- 2 tablespoons balsamic vinegar
- 2 tablespoons extravirgin olive oil
- 1/2 teaspoon salt
- 1 serrano chile, seeded and minced

Direction

- Cook pasta according to package directions, omitting salt and fat. Drain pasta; return to pan. Add chicken and remaining ingredients; toss well.

Nutrition Information

- Calories: 338
- Saturated Fat: 2.9 g
- Total Carbohydrate: 42.6 g
- Fiber: 3.8 g
- Total Fat: 9.4 g
- Sodium: 637 mg
- Protein: 22.7 g
- Cholesterol: 39 mg

51. Chicken, Spinach, And Mushroom Lasagna

Serving: Serves 12 | Prep: | Cook: | Ready in: 105mins

Ingredients

- 3 cups unsalted chicken stock (such as Swanson)
- 1 1/2 pounds skinless, boneless chicken thighs, trimmed
- 2 1/2 tablespoons olive oil
- 1 1/2 cups chopped onion
- 3 tablespoons minced garlic
- 1 1/2 teaspoons kosher salt, divided
- 1/2 teaspoon chopped fresh thyme
- 1/2 teaspoon crushed red pepper
- 10 ounce sliced cremini mushrooms
- 3 (6-ounce) packages fresh spinach
- Cooking spray
- 1 1/2 cups 2% reduced-fat milk
- 1/2 cup all-purpose flour
- 1/4 teaspoon ground nutmeg
- 2 ounces Parmigiano-Reggiano cheese, grated (about 1/2 cup)
- 12 no-boil lasagna noodles
- 5 ounces part-skim mozzarella cheese, shredded (about 1 1/4 cups)

Direction

- Bring stock to a boil in a large saucepan over medium-high heat. Add chicken; reduce heat, and simmer 18 to 20 minutes or until -chicken is done. Remove chicken from pan; reserve stock. When cool enough to handle, shred with 2 forks.
- Heat a large skillet over medium-high heat. Add oil; swirl to coat. Add onion, garlic, 1/2 teaspoon salt, thyme, pepper, and mushrooms; sauté 8 minutes. Stir in spinach, 1 package at a time, cooking 2 minutes after each addition or until spinach wilts before adding more. Remove pan from heat; stir in chicken.
- Preheat oven to 375°.
- Coat 2 (8-inch) square baking dishes with cooking spray. Combine milk, flour, and nutmeg, stirring with a whisk until smooth. Bring reserved stock to a boil over medium-high heat. Gradually add milk mixture to stock mixture, stirring constantly with a whisk. Stir in remaining 1 teaspoon salt. Cook 5 minutes or until thickened, stirring occasionally. Remove pan from heat; stir in Parmigiano-Reggiano. Pour 1/2 cup sauce into bottom of each baking dish. Top each with 2 noodles, 1 1/2 cups chicken mixture, 3/4 cup sauce, and 1/4 cup mozzarella, making sure noodles are covered with sauce. Repeat layers once with noodles, chicken mixture, and sauce. Top dishes evenly with remaining 4 noodles, remaining 1/2 cup sauce, and remaining 3/4 cup mozzarella.

- Cover dishes tightly with foil coated with cooking spray. Bake at 375° for 25 minutes. Uncover and bake at 375° for 10 to 15 minutes or until browned and bubbly, or follow freezing instructions. Let stand 5 minutes before serving.
- How-to Freeze: Cool pan completely. Cover with foil; freeze up to 2 months. Thaw: In metal pan: Thaw overnight in -refrigerator. In glass or ceramic: Uncover and microwave at HIGH 15 minutes or until thawed. Reheat: Cover; bake at 375° for 25 minutes. Uncover and bake 5 minutes.

Nutrition Information

- Calories: 286
- Cholesterol: 67 mg
- Total Fat: 10.2 g
- Saturated Fat: 3.5 g
- Sugar: 4 g
- Protein: 23 g
- Fiber: 2 g
- Total Carbohydrate: 25 g
- Sodium: 523 mg

52. Chicken Ham Lasagna

Serving: 8 servings | Prep: | Cook: | Ready in:

Ingredients

- 2 cups fat-free, less-sodium chicken broth
- 1/2 teaspoon freshly ground black pepper, divided
- 1 pound skinless, boneless chicken breast, cut into bite-sized pieces, divided
- 3 cups 1% low-fat milk
- 1/3 cup all-purpose flour (about 1 1/2 ounces)
- 1 1/2 cups (6 ounces) freshly grated Parmesan cheese, divided
- 1/4 cup chopped fresh parsley
- Cooking spray
- 12 no-cook lasagna noodles (8 ounces), divided
- 8 ounces thinly sliced 96% fat-free deli ham, chopped, divided
- Chopped fresh parsley (optional)

Direction

- Preheat oven to 350°.
- Place broth and 1/4 teaspoon pepper in a large skillet over medium-high heat, and bring to a boil. Add chicken; cover, reduce heat, and simmer 10 minutes or until chicken is done. Remove chicken from pan with a slotted spoon; set aside.
- Combine milk, flour, and remaining 1/4 teaspoon pepper in a bowl; stir well with a whisk until smooth. Add milk mixture to broth in pan. Bring mixture to a boil over medium-high heat, stirring constantly. Cook 1 minute or until mixture thickens, stirring constantly. Remove from heat. Add 1 cup cheese and parsley, stirring until cheese melts.
- Spread 1 cup sauce over bottom of a 13 x 9-inch baking dish coated with cooking spray. Arrange 3 lasagna noodles over sauce. Spoon 3/4 cup sauce evenly over noodles. Top evenly with one-third ham and one-third chicken. Repeat layers twice, ending with noodles. Top with remaining sauce. Sprinkle evenly with remaining 1/2 cup cheese.
- Cover with foil very lightly coated with cooking spray; bake at 350° for 30 minutes. Remove and discard foil; bake 10 minutes or until the cheese lightly browns. Sprinkle with parsley, if desired.
- Wine note: With a cue from the dish's overall unfussy character, the ideal wine needs to be inexpensive and uncomplicated. One of my favorite "comfort wines" to go with a comfort food like this is Australian shiraz. Annie's Lane Shiraz 2002 from Australia's Clare Valley ($15) is a simple blast of berriness with a soft texture. -Karen MacNeil

Nutrition Information

- Calories: 260
- Fiber: 0.8 g
- Sodium: 740 mg
- Cholesterol: 57 mg
- Saturated Fat: 3.7 g
- Total Fat: 7 g
- Protein: 28.9 g
- Total Carbohydrate: 18 g

53. Chicken And Prosciutto Tortelloni Soup

Serving: Makes 2 qt. | Prep: | Cook: | Ready in: 20mins

Ingredients

- 1 (8-oz.) package fresh chopped onions, peppers, and celery
- 1 tablespoon olive oil
- 1/2 teaspoon Italian seasoning
- 1 (14.5-oz.) can diced tomatoes with roasted garlic
- 5 cups reduced-sodium chicken broth
- 1/4 teaspoon table salt
- 1/2 teaspoon ground black pepper
- 1 (9-oz.) package refrigerated chicken-and-prosciutto tortelloni
- 1 (6-oz.) package fresh baby spinach

Direction

- Sauté onions, peppers, and celery in hot oil in a Dutch oven over medium-high heat 3 minutes; add Italian seasoning, and sauté 1 minute. Stir in tomatoes and next 3 ingredients. Increase heat to high; bring to a boil. Stir in tortelloni, and return to a boil. Reduce heat to low, and simmer 8 minutes or until tortelloni are tender. Remove from heat, and stir in spinach.

54. Chili Mac

Serving: Serves 8 (serving size: about 1 1/2 cups) | Prep: | Cook: | Ready in: 55mins

Ingredients

- 12 ounces uncooked rotini, spiral macaroni, or wagon wheel pasta
- 2 cups canned red kidney beans, rinsed and drained
- 2 tablespoons olive oil
- 2 cups chopped onion
- 2 tablespoons minced fresh garlic
- 1 pound cremini mushrooms, finely chopped
- 20 ounces ground turkey breast
- 2 cups chopped green bell pepper
- 4 teaspoons ground cumin
- 2 teaspoons dried oregano
- 1 teaspoon kosher salt
- 1 teaspoon smoked paprika
- 1 teaspoon ancho chile powder
- 1 teaspoon freshly ground black pepper
- 1/4 to 1 teaspoon ground red pepper
- 4 cups lower-sodium marinara sauce
- Cooking spray
- 4 ounces extra-sharp cheddar cheese, shredded (about 1 cup)

Direction

- Preheat oven to 350°.
- Cook pasta in boiling water until almost al dente. Drain. Combine pasta and beans in a large bowl.
- Heat a large skillet over medium heat. Add oil to pan; swirl to coat. Add onion, garlic, and mushrooms to pan; cook 11 minutes or until liquid almost evaporates. Add turkey; cook 5 minutes or until done, stirring to crumble. Add bell pepper and next 7 ingredients (through red pepper); cook 1 minute. Stir in marinara sauce; bring to a boil. Add marinara mixture to pasta mixture; toss to coat. Divide mixture evenly between 2 (2-quart) glass baking dishes coated with cooking spray. Top evenly with cheese. Bake at 350° for 10

minutes or until cheese melts, or follow freezing instructions.

- TO FREEZE: Spoon half of unbaked mixture into a 2-quart glass baking dish (such as a Ziploc VersaGlass large square container). Cover with lid; freeze up to 2 months.
- TO THAW: Remove lid; place casserole in microwave. Microwave at 30% power 30 to 40 minutes (or on defrost setting for 75 pounds).
- TO REHEAT: Cover casserole with foil; bake at 400° for 20 minutes or until a thermometer inserted in center registers 160°.

Nutrition Information

- Calories: 497
- Sodium: 650 mg
- Total Carbohydrate: 60.1 g
- Cholesterol: 44 mg
- Total Fat: 14.5 g
- Fiber: 10.6 g
- Protein: 33.8 g
- Saturated Fat: 5.2 g

55. Chili Cheeseburger Mac And Cheese

Serving: Makes 4 servings | Prep: 10mins | Cook: 18mins | Ready in:

Ingredients

- 1 (12-oz.) box shells and cheese
- 1 pound ground beef
- 1 teaspoon chili powder
- 1/4 teaspoon cumin
- 1/4 teaspoon salt
- 1 (15-oz.) can kidney beans, rinsed and drained
- 1 (14.5-oz.) can diced tomatoes with mild green chiles
- 2 tablespoons chopped fresh parsley

Direction

- Prepare shells and cheese according to package directions.
- Meanwhile, brown beef in a 12-inch (2 1/2-inch-deep) nonstick skillet or Dutch oven over medium-high heat, stirring often, 8 minutes or until no longer pink; drain and rinse under hot running water. Return beef to skillet; stir in chili powder, cumin, and salt. Cook 2 minutes. Add beans, tomatoes, and 1/4 cup water. Cook 5 to 8 minutes or until most of liquid has evaporated.
- Stir prepared pasta into beef mixture, and sprinkle with chopped fresh parsley. Serve immediately.
- Note: For testing purposes only, we used Velveeta Shells & Cheese Original and Delmonte Diced Tomatoes with Zesty Mild Green Chilies.

56. Chocolate Fettuccine

Serving: Serves 6 | Prep: | Cook: | Ready in: 60mins

Ingredients

- 2 3/4 cups, plus 1 tablespoon all-purpose flour
- 1/4 cup unsweetened cocoa powder
- 1/2 teaspoon kosher salt
- 3 large eggs, at room temperature and lightly beaten
- 1 teaspoon vanilla extract

Direction

- Place the flour, cocoa powder, powdered sugar, and salt in the bowl of a food processor; pulse to combine. Add the eggs and vanilla extract. Process for 30 to 60 seconds or until the dough comes together in a shaggy ball.
- Transfer the dough to a lightly floured work surface and knead for 1 to 2 minutes or until the surface of the dough is smooth. Shape dough into a disc; wrap with plastic wrap and let rest in the refrigerator for 30 minutes.

- Remove dough from the refrigerator and cut into four equal pieces. Working with one piece at a time (keeping the others covered in plastic), flatten the dough and run through the widest setting of your pasta roller. Fold one of the one end of the dough lengthwise into the center. Then, fold the other end over the first folded end, forming a letter shape. Run the folded dough through the widest setting of your pasta roller, repeating the folding and rolling process two more times.
- Run the pasta sheet through each successively smaller setting, twice for each setting, until it reaches your desired thinness (we stopped at setting 4 on our KitchenAid attachment).
- Lightly flour both sides of the dough, cut in half and place on a floured baking sheet. Repeat this process with the 3 remaining portions of dough.
- Run each piece of dough through the fettuccine attachment (or cut by hand into 1/2-inch ribbons) and lightly dust with flour to keep the pasta from sticking together.
- Bring a large pot of lightly salted water to a boil. Add pasta to pan and cook for 2 to 3 minutes, or until desired tenderness. Drain. Divide pasta among serving bowls. Top as desired.

57. Chocolate Pasta With Mascarpone Vanilla Cream And Strawberries

Serving: Serves 6 | Prep: | Cook: | Ready in: 30mins

Ingredients

- FOR THE STRAWBERRIES:
- 1 cup hulled, sliced strawberries
- 2 teaspoons sugar
- FOR THE MASCARPONE-VANILLA CREAM:
- 1/2 cup heavy whipping cream
- 1/2 cup mascarpone
- 1/4 cup sugar
- 1 teaspoon vanilla extract
- TO FINISH THE DISH:
- Chocolate Fettuccine
- 2 tablespoons toasted sliced almonds
- Mint leaves, olive oil, and flaky salt, for garnish

Direction

- For the strawberries: In a small bowl, toss together the strawberries and sugar. Let macerate while you prepare the rest of the recipe.
- For the Mascarpone-Vanilla Cream: In a medium-sized mixing bowl, whip the heavy whipping cream, mascarpone, and sugar either by hand or using a mixer just until stiff peaks form. Add vanilla and mix until just blended. Use immediately or store in the fridge, covered, for up to two days, bringing to room temperature before using.
- Cook the pasta as per the recipe's or box's directions.
- To finish the dish, plate the pasta and top with a heaping spoonful of Mascarpone-Vanilla cream and the macerated strawberries and their juices. Sprinkle with the toasted almonds, a few leaves of fresh mint, and a pinch of flakey salt. Drizzle with olive oil and serve.

58. Chorizo And Shrimp With Toasted Pasta

Serving: Serves 4 to 6 | Prep: | Cook: | Ready in: 45mins

Ingredients

- About 2 tbsp. olive oil
- 1 medium onion, chopped fine
- 4 ounces angel hair pasta or coiled fideos, broken into about 2-in. lengths
- 3 garlic cloves, minced
- 1 large pinch saffron threads (optional)

- 1 can (15 oz.) crushed tomatoes
- 1 tablespoon tomato paste
- 1 pound Spanish chorizo or andouille sausages, halved lengthwise and sliced thickly
- 2 1/2 cups reduced-sodium chicken broth
- 1/2 pound medium shrimp (36 to 42 per lb.), deveined; or shelled clams
- Salt
- 1/4 cup chopped flat-leafed parsley

Direction

- Heat 2 tbsp. oil in a large wide pot over medium-low heat. Add onion and cook, covered, until starting to soften, 5 minutes. Add pasta and more oil if it looks dry, then toast over medium-high heat, turning constantly with tongs, until golden. Add garlic and saffron (if using), tomatoes and tomato paste, sausages, and broth.
- Boil pasta in soup, uncovered, until noodles are tender, about 5 minutes.
- Add shrimp and cook just until pink and curled, about 1 minute. Season with salt to taste and stir in parsley.
- Note: Nutritional analysis is per serving.

Nutrition Information

- Calories: 534
- Sodium: 1252 mg
- Fiber: 2 g
- Saturated Fat: 12 g
- Total Carbohydrate: 23 g
- Total Fat: 35 g
- Protein: 30 g
- Cholesterol: 133 mg

59. Chorizo Mussel Noodle Bowl

Serving: 4 servings (serving size: about 1 1/2 cups mussel mixture and 3/4 cup pasta) | Prep: | Cook: | Ready in:

Ingredients

- 6 ounces uncooked linguine
- Cooking spray
- 1 cup chopped onion
- 1/2 cup chopped green bell pepper
- 4 ounces Spanish chorizo sausage or turkey kielbasa, cut into (1/2-inch-thick) slices
- 3 garlic cloves, minced
- 1/4 teaspoon saffron threads, crushed
- 2 cups chopped plum tomatoes
- 1/2 cup dry white wine
- 1/4 teaspoon freshly ground black pepper
- 1 (14-ounce) can fat-free, less-sodium chicken broth
- 2 pounds mussels, scrubbed and debearded (about 60 mussels)
- 1/3 cup chopped fresh parsley

Direction

- Cook pasta according to package directions, omitting salt and fat. Drain.
- While pasta cooks, heat a large nonstick skillet over medium-high heat. Coat pan with cooking spray. Add onion, bell pepper, sausage, and garlic to pan; sauté 3 minutes. Add the saffron, and sauté 4 minutes or until sausage is browned. Stir in tomatoes; cook 2 minutes. Add wine, black pepper, and broth; bring to a boil. Add mussels; cover and cook 4 minutes or until mussels open. Remove from heat; discard any unopened shells. Stir in parsley. Serve mussel mixture over pasta.

Nutrition Information

- Calories: 482
- Protein: 32.4 g
- Cholesterol: 65 mg
- Sodium: 936 mg
- Saturated Fat: 5 g
- Fiber: 3.9 g
- Total Carbohydrate: 49.1 g
- Total Fat: 15.2 g

60. Cincinnati Chili

Serving: Serves 6 (serving size: about 1 1/4 cups chili, 2 tablespoons noodles, 2 tablespoons cheese, and 2 tablespoons onion) | Prep: | Cook: | Ready in: 160mins

Ingredients

- 2 cups water
- 14 ounces 90% lean ground sirloin
- 6 ounces 80% lean ground chuck
- 1 1/2 cups finely chopped sweet onion
- 2 teaspoons cider vinegar, divided
- 1 1/2 teaspoons Worcestershire sauce
- 1 1/2 tablespoons smoked sweet paprika
- 1 1/2 teaspoons ground cumin
- 1 1/2 teaspoons ground cinnamon
- 1 1/2 teaspoons ground allspice
- 1 1/4 teaspoons kosher salt
- 1/2 teaspoon ground red pepper
- 1/2 ounce bittersweet chocolate, finely chopped
- 3 garlic cloves, crushed
- 1 (15-ounce) can unsalted tomato sauce (such as Muir Glen)
- 1 (15-ounce) can unsalted kidney beans, rinsed and drained
- 1 cup cooked bucatini pasta or spaghetti (about 2 ounces uncooked)
- 1/4 cup water
- 1/2 teaspoon canola oil
- 3 ounces reduced-fat cheddar cheese, finely shredded (about 3/4 cup)
- 3/4 cup finely chopped white onion

Direction

- Bring 2 cups water to a boil in a large Dutch oven. Reduce heat to a simmer. Add beef, stirring to crumble. Stir in sweet onion, 1 teaspoon vinegar, Worcestershire sauce, and next 9 ingredients (through tomato sauce). Return to a simmer. Partially cover, and cook 2 hours, stirring occasionally. Stir in kidney beans; cook 5 minutes. Remove from heat; stir in remaining 1 teaspoon vinegar.
- Combine cooked pasta, 1/4 cup water, and oil in a large nonstick skillet over medium-high heat. Cook until water evaporates and pasta is lightly browned, stirring occasionally (about 12 minutes). Coarsely chop noodles. Serve chili with pasta, cheese, and white onion.

Nutrition Information

- Calories: 352
- Cholesterol: 66 mg
- Total Fat: 15.2 g
- Saturated Fat: 6.2 g
- Sodium: 581 mg
- Total Carbohydrate: 27 g
- Fiber: 7 g
- Protein: 27 g

61. Classic Baked Macaroni And Cheese

Serving: Makes 2 to 3 main-dish or 4 to 6 side-dish servings | Prep: 15mins | Cook: 7mins | Ready in:

Ingredients

- 1 (8-oz.) package elbow macaroni
- 2 tablespoons butter
- 2 tablespoons all-purpose flour
- 2 cups milk
- 1/2 teaspoon salt
- 1/2 teaspoon fresh ground black pepper
- 1/4 teaspoon ground red pepper
- 1 (8-oz.) block sharp Cheddar cheese, shredded and divided

Direction

- Prepare pasta according to package directions. Keep warm.
- Melt butter in a large saucepan or Dutch oven over medium-low heat; whisk in flour until smooth. Cook, whisking constantly, 2 minutes. Gradually whisk in milk, and cook, whisking

constantly, 5 minutes or until thickened. Remove from heat. Stir in salt, black and red pepper, 1 cup shredded cheese, and cooked pasta.

- Spoon pasta mixture into a lightly greased 2-qt. baking dish; top with remaining 1 cup cheese.
- Bake at 400° for 20 minutes or until bubbly. Let stand 10 minutes before serving.
- Note: For testing purposes only, we used Kraft Sharp Cheddar Cheese. To lighten, 2% reduced-fat milk and reduced-fat cheese may be substituted.
- One-Pot Macaroni and Cheese: Prepare recipe as directed, stirring all grated Cheddar cheese into thickened milk mixture until melted. Add cooked pasta, and serve immediately. Prep: 10 min., Cook: 7 min.

62. Classic Chicken Tetrazzini

Serving: Makes 8 to 10 servings | Prep: | Cook: | Ready in: 55mins

Ingredients

- 1 1/2 (8-oz.) packages vermicelli
- 1/2 cup butter
- 1/2 cup all-purpose flour
- 4 cups milk
- 1/2 cup dry white wine
- 2 tablespoons chicken bouillon granules
- 1 teaspoon seasoned pepper
- 2 cups freshly grated Parmesan cheese, divided
- 4 cups diced cooked chicken
- 1 (6-oz.) jar sliced mushrooms, drained
- 3/4 cup slivered almonds

Direction

- Preheat oven to 350°. Prepare pasta according to package directions.
- Meanwhile, melt butter in a Dutch oven over low heat; whisk in flour until smooth. Cook 1 minute, whisking constantly. Gradually whisk in milk and wine; cook over medium heat, whisking constantly, 8 to 10 minutes or until mixture is thickened and bubbly. Whisk in bouillon granules, seasoned pepper, and 1 cup Parmesan cheese.
- Remove from heat; stir in diced cooked chicken, sliced mushrooms, and hot cooked pasta.
- Spoon mixture into a lightly greased 13- x 9-inch baking dish; sprinkle with slivered almonds and remaining 1 cup Parmesan cheese.
- Bake at 350° for 35 minutes or until bubbly.

63. Classic Lasagna

Serving: Makes 8 to 10 servings | Prep: 20mins | Cook: 120mins | Ready in:

Ingredients

- 2 medium onions, chopped
- 2 tablespoons olive oil, divided
- 4 garlic cloves, minced
- 1 pound lean ground beef
- 1 (14.5-oz.) can basil, garlic, and oregano diced tomatoes
- 2 (6-oz.) cans tomato paste
- 1 (8-oz.) can basil, garlic, and oregano tomato sauce
- 1 bay leaf
- 1 teaspoon Italian seasoning
- 1 1/4 teaspoons salt, divided
- 3/4 teaspoon pepper, divided
- 12 lasagna noodles, uncooked
- 8 cups boiling water
- 1 (16-oz.) container ricotta cheese
- 2 large eggs, lightly beaten
- 1/4 cup grated Parmesan cheese
- 2 (6-oz.) packages part-skim mozzarella cheese slices
- Garnish: chopped fresh parsley

Direction

- Sauté onion in 1 Tbsp. hot oil in a large skillet over medium-high heat 5 minutes or until tender. Add garlic, and sauté 1 minute. Add beef, and cook, stirring occasionally, 10 minutes or until beef crumbles and is no longer pink. Drain beef mixture, and return to skillet. Stir in diced tomatoes, next 4 ingredients, 1 tsp. salt, and 1/2 tsp. pepper; bring to a boil. Reduce heat, cover, and simmer, stirring occasionally, 30 minutes. Remove and discard bay leaf; set meat sauce aside.
- Place lasagna noodles in a 13- x- 9-inch pan. Carefully pour 8 cups boiling water and remaining 1 Tbsp. olive oil over noodles. Let stand 15 minutes.
- Stir together ricotta cheese, eggs, Parmesan cheese, remaining 1/4 tsp. salt, and remaining 1/4 tsp. pepper until blended.
- Spoon half of the meat sauce mixture in a lightly greased 13- x 9-inch baking dish. Shake excess water from noodles, and arrange 6 noodles over meat sauce; top with half of ricotta mixture and 1 package mozzarella cheese slices. Repeat layers once.
- Bake, covered, at 350° for 55 minutes. Uncover and bake 10 to 15 more minutes or until bubbly. Let lasagna stand 10 minutes before serving. Garnish, if desired.

64. Classic Lasagna With Meat Sauce

Serving: Serves 6 (serving size: 1 piece) | Prep: | Cook: | Ready in: 66mins

Ingredients

- 1 1/2 cups fat-free ricotta cheese
- 6 ounces part-skim mozzarella cheese, shredded (about 1 1/2 cups)
- 1/4 cup fresh flat-leaf parsley leaves, divided
- 1 1/2 tablespoons unsalted butter, melted
- 1 tablespoon finely chopped fresh oregano
- 5 garlic cloves, minced and divided
- 1 large egg, lightly beaten
- 12 ounces extra-lean ground beef (93% lean)
- 1/2 teaspoon freshly ground black pepper
- 1/4 teaspoon crushed red pepper
- 1 (25-ounce) jar lower-sodium marinara sauce (such as Dell'Amore)
- Cooking spray
- 6 lasagna noodles, cooked
- 1 ounce Parmigiano-Reggiano cheese, grated (about 1/4 cup)

Direction

- Preheat oven to 375°.
- Combine ricotta, 2 ounces (about 1/2 cup) mozzarella, 2 tablespoons parsley, butter, oregano, 1 garlic clove, and egg; set aside.
- Place ground beef in a large non-stick skillet over medium-high heat; sprinkle with peppers and remaining 4 garlic cloves. Cook for 9 minutes or until beef is browned, stirring to crumble; drain. Return beef mixture to pan; stir in marinara sauce, and remove from heat.
- Spread 1/2 cup meat sauce in bottom of a broiler-safe 11 x 7-inch glass or ceramic baking dish coated with cooking spray. Cut bottom third off each noodle to form 6 long and 6 short noodles; cut short noodles in half to form 12 pieces. Arrange 2 long noodles along outside edges of dish; arrange 4 short noodle pieces along center of dish.
- Top noodles with 1 cup meat sauce. Top with 2 long noodles and 4 short noodle pieces, all of ricotta mixture, and 1 cup meat sauce. Arrange remaining 2 long noodles and 4 short noodle pieces on top. Spread remaining meat sauce over top noodles. Sprinkle evenly with remaining 4 ounces (1 cup) mozzarella cheese and Parmigiano-Reggiano cheese. Cover with foil coated with cooking spray.
- Bake at 375° for 30 minutes. Uncover and bake for an additional 10 minutes or until bubbly.
- Preheat broiler to high. (Keep lasagna in oven.)
- Broil lasagna for 1 to 2 minutes or until cheese is golden brown and sauce is bubbly. Remove

from oven; let stand 10 minutes. Sprinkle with remaining 2 tablespoons parsley; cut into 6 pieces.

Nutrition Information

- Calories: 378
- Total Fat: 15.3 g
- Protein: 27 g
- Sodium: 591 mg
- Total Carbohydrate: 30 g
- Cholesterol: 92 mg
- Saturated Fat: 6.8 g
- Fiber: 3 g

65. Cold Peanut Sesame Noodles

Serving: 6 servings | Prep: | Cook: | Ready in: 90mins

Ingredients

- 1 tablespoon fresh ginger, minced
- 1/3 cup soy sauce
- 3 tablespoons toasted sesame oil
- 3 tablespoons natural, unsweetened, salted peanut butter
- 3 tablespoons sugar
- 3 tablespoons rice vinegar
- 2 tablespoons rice wine or sake
- 1 clove (small) garlic, minced
- 3 tablespoons Chinese sesame paste or tahini
- 1 (small) shallot, minced
- 5 tablespoons roasted peanut oil (see Note)
- 1 pound dried Chinese egg noodles
- 1/2 (large) seedless cucumber, peeled, halved lengthwise, seeded and cut into fine matchsticks
- 4 scallions, thinly sliced
- Ma La Oil

Direction

- In a blender, combine the ginger, soy sauce, sesame oil, peanut butter, sugar, vinegar, rice wine, garlic, sesame paste, shallot and 3 tablespoons of the peanut oil and puree until smooth. Transfer the sauce to a bowl and refrigerate for 45 minutes.
- In a large pot of boiling water, cook the noodles until al dente. Drain and rinse under cold running water until chilled. Shake out the excess water and blot dry; transfer the noodles to a bowl and toss with the remaining 2 tablespoons of peanut oil. Add the peanut-sesame sauce and toss well to coat. Garnish with the cucumber and scallions and drizzle with Ma La Oil, leaving the solid spices behind.

66. Cold Noodle Salad With Sesame Crab

Serving: Serves 2 (serving size: 1 cup salad) | Prep: | Cook: | Ready in: 30mins

Ingredients

- 3 cups water
- 1/2 cup reduced-sodium soy sauce
- 1/2 cup mirin
- 1 teaspoon sesame oil
- 4 ounces uncooked dried udon noodles (thick, round Japanese wheat noodles)
- 1/2 cup fresh or frozen English peas
- 1/2 cup fresh lump crabmeat, picked and drained
- 2 teaspoons thinly sliced green onions
- 1/2 teaspoon grated lemon rind
- 4 cilantro sprigs
- 1 jalapeno, seeded and thinly sliced
- Hot chili oil (optional)

Direction

- Combine first 4 ingredients in a medium saucepan; bring to a simmer over medium-high heat. Add noodles; cook until al dente, about 3 minutes. Place noodles and broth in a small bowl. Set bowl in a larger bowl of ice water; cool noodles completely, about 10 minutes. Drain noodles. Discard broth.

- Bring a small saucepan of water to a boil. Add peas; cook 1 minute. Drain and plunge peas into ice water. Drain well.
- Divide noodles between 2 bowls. Top each with half of crabmeat; stir gently. Divide peas between bowls. Top with onions, rind, cilantro, and jalapeño. Drizzle with chili oil, if desired.

Nutrition Information

- Calories: 206
- Protein: 14 g
- Total Carbohydrate: 22 g
- Sugar: 4 g
- Cholesterol: 45 mg
- Saturated Fat: 0.7 g
- Total Fat: 5.7 g
- Fiber: 3 g
- Sodium: 542 mg

67. Confetti Macaroni Salad

Serving: Serves 8 | Prep: 45mins | Cook: 11mins | Ready in: 56mins

Ingredients

- 1 tablespoon cider vinegar
- 1 cup buttermilk
- 1 tablespoon lemon juice
- 2 tablespoons olive oil
- 1 clove garlic, minced
- 1 teaspoon Dijon mustard
- 1 tablespoon chopped fresh parsley
- 1 tablespoon chopped fresh dill
- Salt and pepper
- 1 pound box elbow macaroni
- 1/2 cup fresh or frozen peas
- 1/2 small red bell pepper, seeded, cut into 1/4-inch dice
- 1/2 small orange bell pepper, seeded, cut into 1/4-inch dice
- 1/2 small green bell pepper, seeded, cut into 1/4-inch dice
- 1/2 small sweet onion, cut into 1/4-inch dice
- 2 ribs celery, finely chopped
- 1/2 English cucumber, cut into 1/4-inch dice
- 1 small yellow squash, cut into 1/4-inch dice
- 1/2 cup finely chopped radish

Direction

- Make dressing: In a bowl, whisk together vinegar, buttermilk, lemon juice, oil, garlic, mustard, parsley and dill. Season with salt and pepper.
- Bring a large pot of salted water to a boil. Cook macaroni for about 10 minutes, or as package label directs. Stir in peas 2 minutes before end of cooking time. Drain; rinse under cold water until cool. In a large bowl, toss macaroni, vegetables and dressing.

Nutrition Information

- Calories: 280
- Total Fat: 5 g
- Fiber: 3 g
- Protein: 9 g
- Sodium: 197 mg
- Total Carbohydrate: 48 g
- Cholesterol: 2 mg
- Saturated Fat: 1 g

68. Couscous Salad With Roasted Chicken

Serving: 4 servings (serving size: about 1 cup) | Prep: 8mins | Cook: 2mins | Ready in:

Ingredients

- 1/3 cup uncooked couscous
- 1 1/2 cups chopped roasted chicken breast

- 1 cup chopped English cucumber
- 1 cup halved grape tomatoes
- 1 cup chopped fresh parsley
- 1/4 cup chopped fresh mint
- 4 green onions, chopped
- 1 garlic clove, minced
- 1/4 cup fresh lemon juice
- 2 tablespoons olive oil
- 1/4 teaspoon salt

Direction

- Prepare couscous according to package directions, omitting salt and fat. Fluff couscous with a fork.
- Combine couscous, chicken, and next 6 ingredients in a large bowl. Set aside.
- Combine lemon juice, olive oil, and salt in a small bowl; stir well with a whisk. Pour dressing over couscous mixture; toss gently.
- Serve with: Greek Pita Chips

Nutrition Information

- Calories: 230
- Protein: 19.7 g
- Fiber: 2.8 g
- Sodium: 356 mg
- Cholesterol: 45 mg
- Total Fat: 9.3 g
- Total Carbohydrate: 17.7 g
- Saturated Fat: 1.6 g

69. Couscous With Chicken And Root Vegetables

Serving: Serves 6 (serving size: 1 cup) | Prep: | Cook: | Ready in: 32mins

Ingredients

- 1 tablespoon olive oil
- 2 cups chopped onion
- 2 garlic cloves, coarsely chopped
- 1/2 teaspoon salt
- 1 1/2 teaspoons curry powder
- 1 1/2 teaspoons ground cumin
- 1 teaspoon turmeric
- 1/2 teaspoon freshly ground black pepper
- 2 (3-inch) cinnamon sticks
- 1 tablespoon tomato paste
- 2 cups fat-free, lower-sodium chicken broth
- 1 (14.5-ounce) can diced tomatoes, drained
- 2 (6-ounce) skinless, boneless chicken breast halves, cut into 1-inch pieces
- 1 1/4 cups diced peeled turnips (about 2 small)
- 1 cup chopped carrot (about 3 medium)
- 1/4 cup diced parsnip
- 1 cup raisins
- 3 cups hot cooked couscous
- 2 tablespoons chopped fresh flat-leaf parsley

Direction

- Heat a large nonstick skillet over medium-high heat. Add oil; swirl to coat. Add onion to pan; sauté 5 minutes or until tender. Add garlic; sauté 1 minute. Stir in salt and next 5 ingredients (through cinnamon sticks); cook 30 seconds. Stir in tomato paste. Stir in chicken broth and tomatoes; bring to a boil. Stir in chicken and next 3 ingredients (through parsnip). Bring to a boil. Reduce heat; simmer, uncovered, 5 minutes. Stir in raisins, and cook 5 minutes or until vegetables are tender and chicken is done. Discard cinnamon sticks.
- Spoon 1/2 cup couscous into each of 6 bowls. Ladle 1 cup stew evenly over couscous. Sprinkle with parsley.
- Tip: Do yourself a favor and prep all your ingredients first. It saves so much time and makes the recipe come together in a snap.

Nutrition Information

- Calories: 310
- Protein: 19.1 g
- Sodium: 555 mg
- Saturated Fat: 0.6 g

- Total Carbohydrate: 52 g
- Fiber: 5.9 g
- Cholesterol: 33 mg
- Total Fat: 3.6 g

70. Crab And Spinach Gnocchi

Serving: Serves 4 | Prep: | Cook: | Ready in: 120mins

Ingredients

- GNOCCHI
- 1 tablespoon olive oil, divided
- 2 pounds spinach, rinsed well and large stems trimmed
- About 3/4 tsp. kosher salt, divided
- About 3/4 tsp. pepper, divided
- 1 pound shelled cooked Dungeness crab, large pieces broken up
- 1 large egg plus 1 large egg yolk
- 1/2 teaspoon red chile flakes*
- 1/2 cup flour
- BUTTER SAUCE AND SERVING
- 1/3 cup dry white wine, such as Pinot Grigio
- 1/4 cup minced shallot (about 1 medium)
- 2 garlic cloves, minced
- 3 tablespoons whipping cream
- 1/2 cup cold unsalted butter, cut into cubes
- Large pinch kosher salt
- Large pinch pepper
- 1 1/2 teaspoons Vietnamese fish sauce or colatura (Italian fish sauce)*
- Hunk of parmesan cheese

Direction

- Make gnocchi: Heat 1/2 tbsp. oil in a large pot over medium-high heat. Add half of spinach and a pinch each salt and pepper. Cook, tossing often, until barely wilted and still bright green, 2 to 3 minutes. Drain in a colander. Repeat with another 1/2 tbsp. oil, remaining spinach, and a pinch more of salt and pepper. Let cool in colander.
- Gently squeeze excess liquid from cooled spinach. Chop 1/3 cup finely and set the rest aside.
- Mix crab, chopped spinach, whole egg and yolk, chile flakes, and 1/4 tsp. each salt and pepper in a medium bowl. Add flour and mix thoroughly until it holds together like a soft dough.
- Dip 2 small spoons (soup spoons are too big) in very hot water. Scoop 1 scant tbsp. dough with one spoon. Set second spoon upside down over dough and press firmly, then scoop underneath dough and onto second spoon. Repeat motion with first spoon. Scoop back and forth until you have a compact quenelle of dough. Alterna-tively, using wet hands to keep dough from sticking, and firmly roll it into scant 1-tbsp. balls. Set quenelles or balls on a baking sheet as you work, then chill while you make sauce.
- Bring a large pot of lightly salted water to a boil. Meanwhile, make butter sauce: Cook wine, shallot, and garlic in a large frying pan over medium-low heat until wine has almost evaporated and shallot is softened, 3 to 5 minutes. Add cream and cook until simmering. Whisk in butter, a few cubes at a time, until melted and creamy. Whisk in salt, pepper, and fish sauce. Remove from heat to a warm spot. Let sit, whisking occasionally, until ready to serve, up to 30 minutes.
- Reduce heat under boiling water to an active simmer. Drop in gnocchi and cook until they float, 3 to 4 minutes. With a slotted spoon, transfer to a plate. Meanwhile, reheat reserved spinach in a microwave.
- Divide spinach among four plates. Top each with 6 to 8 gnocchi and drizzle generously with butter sauce. Serve with cheese hunk and a grater.
- *Campbell likes smoky Controne hot pepper (find at markethallfoods.com) and salty, intense colatura (amazon.com).
- Make ahead: Formed gnocchi, up to 1 day, chilled, or up to 2 months, frozen. (Freeze on baking sheet, then pop off and seal in a resealable plastic bag. Boil directly from the

freezer, 5 to 6 minutes.) Spinach, up to 1 day, chilled. Butter sauce, up to 1 day, reheated in a bowl set over steaming water, whisking often.

Nutrition Information

- Calories: 535
- Fiber: 4.2 g
- Sodium: 1077 mg
- Protein: 35 g
- Total Carbohydrate: 23 g
- Total Fat: 37 g
- Saturated Fat: 19 g
- Cholesterol: 268 mg

71. Creamy Chipotle Manicotti

Serving: 4 servings | Prep: | Cook: | Ready in:

Ingredients

- 8 manicotti shells
- 1 (15-ounce) container part-skim ricotta cheese
- 2 green onions, chopped
- 2 tablespoons chopped fresh cilantro
- 1 cup (4 ounces) shredded part-skim mozzarella cheese
- 1/4 cup egg substitute
- Vegetable cooking spray
- 2 cups chipotle salsa, divided*
- 1 cup (4 ounces) shredded Monterey Jack cheese with peppers

Direction

- Cook pasta according to package directions, omitting salt and oil. Rinse with cold water; drain and set aside.
- Stir together ricotta cheese and next 4 ingredients.
- Coat an 11- x 7-inch baking dish with cooking spray, and pour 1/2 cup salsa in bottom of dish. Spoon cheese mixture evenly into shells, and arrange in dish. Pour remaining salsa over shells.
- Bake at 350° for 20 minutes. Sprinkle with Monterey Jack cheese. Bake 10 more minutes or until thoroughly heated and cheese melts. Let stand 10 minutes before serving.
- Note: For testing purposes only, we used D. L. Jardine's Holy Chipotle Salsa.
- * 1 or 2 canned chipotle peppers in adobo stirred into 2 cups reglar mild salsa may be substituted for chipotle salsa. Canned Chipotle peppers may be found in the Mexica section of supermarket. Store remaining peppers in a zip-top plastic bag in refrigerator up to 2 weeks or in freezer up to 2 months.

Nutrition Information

- Calories: 507
- Cholesterol: 74 mg
- Fiber: 4.8 g
- Sodium: 1277 mg
- Total Carbohydrate: 40 g
- Total Fat: 23 g
- Protein: 35 g
- Saturated Fat: 14 g

72. Creamy Four Cheese Macaroni

Serving: 8 servings (serving size: 1 cup) | Prep: | Cook: | Ready in:

Ingredients

- 1.5 ounces all-purpose flour (about 1/3 cup)
- 2 2/3 cups 1% low-fat milk
- 2 ounces shredded fontina cheese (about 1/2 cup)
- 2 ounces grated Parmesan cheese (about 1/2 cup)
- 2 ounces shredded extra-sharp cheddar cheese (about 1/2 cup)
- 3 ounces light processed cheese (such as light Velveeta)

- 6 cups cooked elbow macaroni (about 3 cups uncooked)
- 1/2 teaspoon salt
- 1/4 teaspoon freshly ground black pepper
- Cooking spray
- 1/3 cup crushed melba toasts (about 12 pieces)
- 1 tablespoon canola oil
- 1 garlic clove, minced

Direction

- Preheat oven to 375°.
- Weigh or lightly spoon flour into a dry measuring cup; level with a knife. Place flour in a large saucepan. Gradually add milk, stirring with a whisk until blended. Cook over medium heat until thick (about 8 minutes), stirring constantly with a whisk. Remove from heat; let stand 4 minutes or until sauce cools to 155°. Add cheeses, and stir until the cheeses melt. Stir in cooked macaroni, salt, and black pepper.
- Spoon mixture into a 2-quart glass or ceramic baking dish coated with cooking spray. Combine crushed toasts, oil, and garlic in small bowl; stir until well blended. Sprinkle over macaroni mixture. Bake at 375° for 30 minutes or until bubbly.

Nutrition Information

- Calories: 347
- Sodium: 607 mg
- Total Fat: 11.5 g
- Saturated Fat: 5.9 g
- Fiber: 1.9 g
- Protein: 17.4 g
- Total Carbohydrate: 43.8 g
- Cholesterol: 29 mg

73. Creamy Gruyère And Shrimp Pasta

Serving: 6 servings | Prep: | Cook: | Ready in:

Ingredients

- 8 ounces uncooked cavatelli or orecchiette pasta (
- 1/4 cup all-purpose flour
- 1/2 teaspoon salt
- 2 cups 2% reduced-fat milk
- 1 1/4 cups (5 ounces) shredded Gruyère cheese, divided
- 1 tablespoon butter
- 1 1/2 pounds large shrimp, peeled and deveined
- 3 garlic cloves, minced
- 2 tablespoons dry white wine
- 1/4 teaspoon ground red pepper
- 2 cups frozen green peas, thawed
- Cooking spray
- Parsley sprigs (optional)

Direction

- Preheat oven to 375°.
- Cook pasta according to package directions, omitting salt and fat. Drain well.
- Combine the flour and salt in a Dutch oven over medium heat. Gradually add milk, stirring constantly with a whisk; bring to a boil. Cook 1 minute or until slightly thick, stirring constantly with a whisk. Remove from heat. Stir in 3/4 cup cheese, stirring until melted.
- Heat butter in a large nonstick skillet over medium-high heat. Add shrimp and garlic; sauté 3 minutes. Stir in wine and pepper, and cook 1 minute or until shrimp is done.
- Add pasta, shrimp mixture, and peas to cheese mixture, tossing well to combine. Spoon the pasta mixture into a 13 x 9-inch baking dish lightly coated with cooking spray; sprinkle evenly with remaining 1/2 cup cheese. Bake at 375° for 20 minutes or until cheese melts and begins to brown. Garnish with the parsley, if desired. Serve immediately.

Nutrition Information

- Calories: 459

- Protein: 39.6 g
- Fiber: 2.5 g
- Cholesterol: 210 mg
- Saturated Fat: 7.1 g
- Sodium: 535 mg
- Total Carbohydrate: 41.2 g
- Total Fat: 13.8 g

74. Creamy Mascarpone And Spinach Linguine

Serving: Serves 4 (serving size: about 2 cups pasta and 1 1/2 teaspoons cheese) | Prep: | Cook: | Ready in: 21mins

Ingredients

- 1 (9-ounce) package refrigerated fresh linguine
- 3 tablespoons 1/3-less-fat cream cheese
- 1 1/2 tablespoons mascarpone cheese
- 1/2 teaspoon grated lemon rind
- 2 teaspoons fresh lemon juice
- 1/2 teaspoon salt
- 1/8 teaspoon freshly ground black pepper
- 1/8 teaspoon freshly grated nutmeg
- 4 cups baby spinach leaves
- 1 pint cherry tomatoes, halved
- 1/4 cup sliced fresh basil
- 2 tablespoons grated Parmigiano-Reggiano cheese

Direction

- Cook pasta according to package directions, omitting salt and fat. Drain pasta in a colander over a bowl, reserving 1 cup cooking liquid.
- Add cream cheese and mascarpone cheese to bowl, stirring with a whisk until smooth. Stir in lemon rind and the next 4 ingredients (through nutmeg).
- Heat saucepan over medium-high heat. Add pasta and cream cheese mixture to pan; cook 1 minute, stirring constantly. Stir in spinach and tomatoes; cook 2 minutes or until spinach wilts, stirring frequently. Remove pan from heat; stir in basil. Sprinkle evenly with cheese; serve immediately.

Nutrition Information

- Calories: 292
- Total Carbohydrate: 41 g
- Total Fat: 10.2 g
- Cholesterol: 61 mg
- Saturated Fat: 5.6 g
- Sodium: 454 mg
- Fiber: 4 g
- Protein: 12 g

75. Creamy Mushroom Fettuccine

Serving: Serves 4 (serving size: 1 1/2 cups) | Prep: | Cook: | Ready in:

Ingredients

- 1 (9-ounce) package refrigerated fresh fettuccine
- 1 tablespoon extra-virgin olive oil
- 1/2 cup chopped onion
- 12 ounces presliced cremini mushrooms
- 2 garlic cloves, minced
- 3/4 teaspoon salt, divided
- 1/4 teaspoon freshly ground black pepper
- 1/4 cup white wine
- 1 teaspoon chopped fresh thyme
- 1/2 cup half-and-half
- 1 ounce Parmesan cheese, grated (about 1/4 cup)
- 1/4 cup chopped fresh parsley

Direction

- Cook pasta according to package directions, omitting salt and fat. Drain.
- Heat a large nonstick skillet over medium-high heat. Add oil; swirl to coat. Add onion, mushrooms, garlic, 1/4 teaspoon salt, and pepper; sauté 10 minutes or until mushrooms

are browned and have released their liquid. Add wine and thyme; cook 2 minutes or until liquid evaporates, stirring occasionally. Remove pan from heat. Add hot cooked pasta, remaining 1/2 teaspoon salt, half-and-half, and Parmesan cheese to pan, tossing to combine. Sprinkle with chopped parsley. Serve immediately.

Nutrition Information

- Calories: 323
- Saturated Fat: 4.6 g
- Protein: 13.7 g
- Sodium: 587 mg
- Cholesterol: 55 mg
- Total Fat: 10.9 g
- Fiber: 2.6 g
- Total Carbohydrate: 42.2 g

76. Creamy Rigatoni With Gruyère And Brie

Serving: 6 servings (serving size: 1 cup) | Prep: | Cook: | Ready in:

Ingredients

- 3 1/2 teaspoons salt, divided
- 12 ounces rigatoni pasta
- 3 tablespoons all-purpose flour
- 2 cups 2% reduced-fat milk, divided
- 1 tablespoon butter
- 1 1/4 cups (5 ounces) finely shredded Gruyère cheese
- 3 ounces soft-ripened Brie cheese, rind removed
- 1/2 teaspoon freshly ground black pepper
- Fresh flat-leaf parsley leaves (optional)

Direction

- Bring 6 quarts water to a boil in a large saucepan. Add 1 tablespoon salt and pasta; cook 6 minutes or until al dente. Drain.
- Place flour in a medium saucepan over medium heat; add 1/2 cup milk, stirring with a whisk until smooth. Gradually add remaining 1 1/2 cups milk to pan, stirring with a whisk; bring to a boil, stirring constantly with a whisk. Cook 2 minutes or until slightly thick, stirring constantly; stir in butter. Remove from heat; let stand 4 minutes or until sauce cools to 155°. Add cheeses; stir until smooth. Stir in remaining 1/2 teaspoon salt, pepper, and pasta. Garnish with parsley, if desired.

Nutrition Information

- Calories: 424
- Fiber: 1.9 g
- Saturated Fat: 9.2 g
- Total Carbohydrate: 49.9 g
- Total Fat: 15.6 g
- Protein: 21 g
- Sodium: 544 mg
- Cholesterol: 51 mg

77. Creamy Spinach Lasagna

Serving: 8 servings (serving size: 1 piece) | Prep: | Cook: | Ready in:

Ingredients

- 1 tablespoon olive oil
- 2 1/4 cups chopped onion (about 2 medium)
- 2 garlic cloves, minced
- 1 (16-ounce) package frozen chopped spinach, thawed, drained, and squeezed dry
- 1/3 cup all-purpose flour (about 1 1/2 ounces)
- 3 cups 2% reduced-fat milk
- 1/2 teaspoon salt
- 1/4 teaspoon freshly ground black pepper
- 1/4 teaspoon ground red pepper

- 1 (26-ounce) jar marinara sauce, divided
- Cooking spray
- 12 cooked whole wheat lasagna noodles, divided
- 1 1/2 cups (6 ounces) shredded part-skim mozzarella cheese, divided
- Parsley sprigs (optional)

Direction

- Preheat oven to 375°.
- Heat oil in a large skillet over medium heat. Add onion; cook 10 minutes or until onion is browned, stirring occasionally. Stir in garlic and spinach. Reduce heat, cover, and cook 3 minutes or until spinach is tender. Set aside.
- Lightly spoon flour into a dry measuring cup; level with a knife. Combine flour, milk, salt, black pepper, and red pepper in a small saucepan, stirring with a whisk. Bring to a boil over medium-high heat, stirring frequently. Reduce heat and simmer 1 minute, stirring frequently. Add 2 cups milk mixture to spinach mixture. Cover remaining milk mixture, and set aside.
- Spread 1/2 cup marinara sauce in bottom of a 13 x 9-inch baking dish coated with cooking spray. Arrange 3 lasagna noodles over sauce; top with half of spinach mixture. Top with 3 lasagna noodles, 1 cup marinara sauce, and 3/4 cup cheese. Layer 3 more lasagna noodles, remaining spinach mixture, and remaining 3 lasagna noodles. Top with remaining marinara sauce. Pour reserved milk mixture over the top, and sprinkle with remaining 3/4 cup cheese. Bake at 375° for 50 minutes or until lasagna is browned on top. Garnish with parsley sprigs, if desired.

Nutrition Information

- Calories: 328
- Cholesterol: 19 mg
- Total Fat: 9.3 g
- Fiber: 6.9 g
- Saturated Fat: 3.8 g
- Total Carbohydrate: 45.6 g
- Protein: 17.3 g
- Sodium: 726 mg

78. Creamy Stove Top Macaroni And Cheese

Serving: 6 servings (serving size: 1 1/2 cups) | Prep: | Cook: | Ready in:

Ingredients

- 4 cups uncooked medium elbow macaroni
- 3 tablespoons all-purpose flour
- 1 teaspoon salt
- 1/4 teaspoon black pepper
- 2 1/4 cups fat-free milk
- 1/4 cup (2 ounces) 1/3-less-fat cream cheese, softened
- 2 teaspoons Dijon mustard
- 2 teaspoons Worcestershire sauce
- 1/2 teaspoon bottled minced garlic
- 1 1/4 cups (5 ounces) shredded reduced-fat cheddar cheese

Direction

- Cook pasta according to package directions, omitting salt and fat. Drain and set aside.
- While pasta cooks, place flour, salt, and pepper in a large saucepan. Add milk, stirring with a whisk until well blended. Drop cream cheese by teaspoonfuls into milk mixture; bring to a boil over medium-high heat, stirring constantly. Reduce heat; simmer 2 minutes or until thick and cream cheese melts, stirring occasionally. Stir in mustard, Worcestershire, and garlic; simmer 1 minute. Remove from heat. Add cheddar cheese, stirring until cheese melts. Combine pasta and cheese sauce in a large bowl; toss well.

Nutrition Information

- Calories: 252

- Cholesterol: 27 mg
- Total Fat: 8.2 g
- Fiber: 1.1 g
- Sodium: 536 mg
- Protein: 14.5 g
- Saturated Fat: 5.1 g
- Total Carbohydrate: 30.9 g

79. Creamy Tuna Noodle Casserole With Peas And Breadcrumbs

Serving: Serves 4 (serving size: about 1 1/2 cups) | Prep: | Cook: | Ready in:

Ingredients

- 6 ounces uncooked no-yolk egg noodles
- 1 tablespoon olive oil
- 1 tablespoon unsalted butter
- 1 cup finely chopped onion
- 1 cup thinly sliced celery
- 3 tablespoons all-purpose flour
- 2 1/4 cups 1% low-fat milk
- 1/2 cup frozen green peas, thawed
- 1 1/2 tablespoons chopped fresh dill
- 1 teaspoon finely grated lemon rind
- 1 tablespoon fresh lemon juice
- 1 teaspoon dry mustard (such as Colman's)
- 1/2 teaspoon kosher salt
- 1/4 teaspoon black pepper
- 1 (5-ounce) can solid white albacore tuna packed in water, drained and broken into chunks
- 1/4 cup whole-wheat panko (Japanese breadcrumbs)
- 1.5 ounces Parmesan cheese, grated (about 1/3 cup)

Direction

- Preheat broiler to low.
- Fill a large saucepan with water; bring to a boil. Add noodles; cook 3 minutes or until al dente. Drain. Heat a 10-inch ovenproof skillet over medium heat. Add oil and butter; swirl until butter melts. Add onion and celery; sauté 6 minutes or until tender. Sprinkle flour over pan; cook 45 seconds. Add milk, stirring constantly. Stir in peas and next 7 ingredients (through tuna). Remove pan from heat; gently stir in noodles. Sprinkle breadcrumbs and cheese over top. Broil 2 minutes or until topping is lightly browned.

Nutrition Information

- Calories: 436
- Total Fat: 11.9 g
- Protein: 27 g
- Sodium: 550 mg
- Saturated Fat: 5.2 g
- Fiber: 5 g
- Total Carbohydrate: 54 g
- Cholesterol: 34 mg

80. Creamy Tuna And Mushroom Linguine

Serving: Serves 4 | Prep: 15mins | Cook: 25mins | Ready in:

Ingredients

- Salt and pepper
- 12 ounces linguine
- 2 tablespoons unsalted butter
- 2 tablespoons all-purpose flour
- 1 1/4 cups milk, warmed
- 1 tablespoon vegetable oil
- 3 cloves garlic, minced
- 5 ounces mushrooms, sliced (about 1 1/2 cups)
- 1 medium onion, chopped
- 2 ribs celery, thinly sliced
- Pinch of crushed red pepper
- 1 5-oz. can water-packed tuna, drained
- Fresh parsley, optional

Direction

- Bring a pot of salted water to a boil. Cook linguine until al dente, about 9 minutes, or as package directs. Reserve 1/2 cup of cooking water; drain pasta.
- Melt butter in a small pan over medium-low heat. Sprinkle in flour and cook, stirring, until thickened but not browned, about 2 minutes. Whisk in milk and continue to whisk until sauce is thick enough to coat the back of a spoon, about 3 minutes. Season with salt and pepper. Remove from heat.
- Warm oil in a large skillet over medium-high heat. Add garlic and cook, stirring, until golden, about 1 minute. Add mushrooms and sauté until they release their liquid and begin to turn golden, about 5 minutes. Add onion, celery and crushed red pepper and cook, stirring, until vegetables are tender, about 5 minutes longer.
- Stir sauce and reserved pasta water into vegetable mixture and cook, stirring, until heated through, about 5 minutes. Reduce heat to medium-low, add tuna, breaking it up, and cook until warmed through, about 2 minutes. Season with salt and pepper. Toss linguine with sauce, sprinkle with parsley, if desired, and serve hot.

Nutrition Information

- Calories: 521
- Sodium: 559 mg
- Total Carbohydrate: 77 g
- Protein: 23 g
- Total Fat: 14 g
- Fiber: 3 g
- Saturated Fat: 5 g
- Cholesterol: 42 mg

81. Crunchy Couscous Salad With Currants And Mint

Serving: Serves 6 (serving size: about 1/3 cup) | Prep: | Cook: | Ready in: 12mins

Ingredients

- 1 cup water
- 1 cup uncooked couscous
- 1/4 cup fresh lemon juice
- 1 teaspoon Dijon mustard
- 1/2 teaspoon kosher salt
- 1/4 teaspoon freshly ground black pepper
- 1/4 cup canola oil
- 1/4 cup currants
- 1/2 cup diced carrot
- 1/3 cup pine nuts, toasted
- 1/3 cup sliced green onions
- 3 tablespoons chopped fresh mint

Direction

- Bring 1 cup water to a boil in a medium saucepan. While water comes to a boil, place couscous in a large skillet. Cook, stirring constantly, over medium-high heat 3 minutes or until lightly toasted and fragrant. Stir couscous into boiling water. Cover and let stand 5 minutes; fluff with a fork.
- While couscous stands, combine lemon juice and next 3 ingredients (through pepper) in a large bowl, stirring with a whisk. Gradually add oil, stirring constantly with a whisk. Add couscous, currants, and remaining ingredients; fluff with a fork. Serve warm, or cover and cool to room temperature.

Nutrition Information

- Calories: 269
- Fiber: 2.7 g
- Total Carbohydrate: 30.5 g
- Sodium: 193 mg
- Protein: 5.1 g
- Total Fat: 14.7 g
- Saturated Fat: 1.1 g

- Cholesterol: 0.0 mg

82. Easy Beef Lasagna

Serving: Makes 6 to 8 servings | Prep: 15mins | Cook: | Ready in:

Ingredients

- 3 cups cooked lean ground beef
- 1 (26-oz.) jar fire-roasted tomato-and-garlic pasta sauce
- 1 (15-oz.) container ricotta cheese
- 1/2 cup shredded Parmesan cheese
- 6 no-cook lasagna noodles
- 2 cups (8 oz.) shredded mozzarella cheese

Direction

- Stir together ground beef and pasta sauce. Stir together ricotta cheese and Parmesan cheese.
- Spread one-third of meat sauce in a lightly greased 11- x 7-inch baking dish; layer with 3 lasagna noodles and half each of ricotta cheese mixture and shredded mozzarella cheese. Repeat procedure once. Spread remaining one-third of meat sauce over mozzarella cheese.
- Bake, covered, at 375° for 1 hour; uncover and bake 15 more minutes. Let stand 10 minutes before serving.
- Note: For testing purposes only, we used Classico Fire Roasted Tomato & Garlic pasta sauce and Barilla Oven Ready Lasagne.
- Easy Turkey Lasagna: Substitute 3 cups cooked ground turkey for 3 cups cooked lean ground beef, and proceed as directed.
- Freeze Frame: If using frozen cooked ingredients, add 15 minutes to your bake time. If the recipe is covered during the first part of baking, then you'll add the 15 minutes to the covered baking time.

83. Easy Lasagna

Serving: Makes 6 to 8 servings | Prep: 15mins | Cook: 55mins | Ready in:

Ingredients

- 1 pound mild Italian sausage
- 1 (15-oz.) container part-skim ricotta cheese
- 1/4 cup refrigerated ready-made pesto
- 1 large egg, lightly beaten
- 2 (26-oz.) jars pasta sauce
- 9 no-boil lasagna noodles
- 4 cups (16 oz.) shredded Italian three-cheese blend or mozzarella cheese

Direction

- Remove and discard casings from sausage. Cook sausage in a large skillet over medium heat, stirring until meat crumbles and is no longer pink; drain.
- Stir together ricotta cheese, pesto, and egg.
- Spread half of 1 jar pasta sauce evenly in a lightly greased 13- x 9-inch baking dish. Layer with 3 lasagna noodles (noodles should not touch each other or sides of dish), half of ricotta mixture, half of sausage, 1 cup three-cheese blend, and remaining half of 1 jar pasta sauce. Repeat layers using 3 lasagna noodles, remaining ricotta mixture, remaining sausage, 1 cup three-cheese blend. Top with remaining 3 noodles and second jar of pasta sauce, covering noodles completely. Sprinkle evenly with remaining 2 cups three-cheese blend.
- Bake, covered, at 350° for 40 minutes. Uncover and bake 15 more minutes or until cheese is melted and edges are lightly browned and bubbly. Let stand 15 minutes.
- Note: For testing purposes only, we used Classico Tomato & Basil spaghetti sauce and Barilla Lasagne Oven-Ready noodles.

84. Easy Meatless Manicotti

Serving: 7 servings (serving size: 2 manicotti) | Prep: | Cook: | Ready in:

Ingredients

- 2 cups (8 ounces) shredded part-skim mozzarella cheese, divided
- 1 (16-ounce) carton fat-free cottage cheese
- 1 (10-ounce) package frozen chopped spinach, thawed, drained, and squeezed dry
- 1/4 cup (1 ounce) grated fresh Parmesan cheese
- 1 1/2 teaspoons dried oregano
- 1/4 teaspoon salt
- 1/4 teaspoon black pepper
- 1 (8-ounce) package manicotti (14 shells)
- 1 (26-ounce) jar fat-free tomato-basil pasta sauce
- Cooking spray
- 1 cup water

Direction

- Preheat oven to 375°.
- Combine 1 1/2 cups mozzarella, cottage cheese, and the next 5 ingredients (through black pepper) in a medium bowl. Spoon about 3 tablespoons cheese mixture into each uncooked manicotti. Pour half of tomato-basil pasta sauce into a 13 x 9-inch baking dish coated with cooking spray. Arrange stuffed shells in a single layer over sauce, and top with the remaining sauce. Pour 1 cup water into dish. Sprinkle the remaining 1/2 cup mozzarella evenly over sauce. Cover tightly with foil. Bake at 375° for 1 hour or until shells are tender. Let stand 10 minutes before serving.

Nutrition Information

- Calories: 328
- Total Carbohydrate: 38.3 g
- Fiber: 3.9 g
- Protein: 23.8 g
- Sodium: 891 mg
- Cholesterol: 23 mg
- Total Fat: 9 g
- Saturated Fat: 4.8 g

85. Easy Ravioli Lasagna

Serving: Serves 6 | Prep: | Cook: | Ready in: 53mins

Ingredients

- Cooking spray
- 4 ounces hot pork Italian sausage
- 4 ounces 90% lean ground sirloin
- 4 garlic cloves, minced
- 2 cups lower-sodium marinara sauce (such as Dell'Amore)
- 1/8 teaspoon kosher salt
- 1/4 teaspoon crushed red pepper
- 1 (22-ounce) bag frozen whole-wheat spinach and cheese ravioli (such as Whole Foods 365 Everyday Value)
- 3 ounces part-skim mozzarella cheese, shredded (about 3/4 cup)
- 1 ounce Parmigiano-Reggiano cheese, grated (about 1/4 cup)

Direction

- Preheat oven to 375°.
- Heat a large skillet over medium-high heat. Coat pan with cooking spray. Add sausage, beef, and garlic; cook 4 minutes or until meat is browned, stirring frequently to crumble. Stir in marinara sauce, salt, and pepper; bring just to a simmer. Remove from heat. Stir in frozen ravioli; toss to combine.
- Coat an 8-inch square broiler-safe glass or ceramic baking dish with cooking spray. Spoon ravioli mixture into pan; top evenly with mozzarella cheese. Cover dish tightly with foil coated with cooking spray. Bake at 375° for 40 minutes. Uncover and sprinkle evenly with Parmigiano-Reggiano cheese.

- Preheat broiler (leave dish in oven). Broil 3 minutes or until cheese is bubbly and lightly browned.

Nutrition Information

- Calories: 397
- Protein: 22 g
- Saturated Fat: 5.7 g
- Total Carbohydrate: 42.6 g
- Cholesterol: 46 mg
- Total Fat: 14.7 g
- Fiber: 7.4 g
- Sodium: 666 mg

86. Easy Thai Steak Noodle Bowl

Serving: Serves 4 (serving size: 1 bowl) | Prep: | Cook: | Ready in: 21mins

Ingredients

- 2 1/2 cups very thinly sliced green cabbage
- 1 tablespoon fresh lime juice, divided
- 2 teaspoons sugar, divided
- 1 teaspoon kosher salt, divided
- 8 ounces uncooked flat brown rice noodles (pad Thai noodles, such as Annie Chun's)
- 12 ounces top sirloin steak, trimmed and thinly sliced
- 1 1/2 teaspoons canola oil
- 1/2 cup water
- 2 tablespoons red curry paste (such as Thai Kitchen)
- 1 (13.5-ounce) can light coconut milk
- 4 lime wedges (optional)

Direction

- Combine cabbage, 1 teaspoon lime juice, 1/2 teaspoon sugar, and 1/4 teaspoon salt; toss well to combine. Set aside at room temperature for 15 minutes.
- Prepare rice noodles according to package directions. Drain and rinse with cold water; drain.
- Toss steak with 1/2 teaspoon sugar. Heat a large skillet over high heat. Add oil; swirl to coat. Add steak to pan; cook 2 minutes. Turn steak over; cook an additional 30 seconds or just until browned. Remove from pan; keep warm.
- Add 1/2 cup water to pan, scraping pan to loosen browned bits. Add curry paste and coconut milk, stirring well to combine; bring to a simmer. Reduce heat to low; simmer for 5 minutes. Stir in remaining 2 teaspoons lime juice, remaining 1 teaspoon sugar, and 1/2 teaspoon salt. Arrange about 1 cup noodles in each of 4 bowls; divide steak evenly over servings. Ladle about 1/2 cup broth over each serving; top each with about 1/2 cup cabbage mixture. Sprinkle remaining 1/4 teaspoon salt evenly over servings. Serve with lime wedges, if desired.

Nutrition Information

- Calories: 395
- Sodium: 690 mg
- Sugar: 4 g
- Total Carbohydrate: 54 g
- Cholesterol: 45 mg
- Fiber: 5 g
- Total Fat: 10.6 g
- Protein: 22 g
- Saturated Fat: 6.1 g

87. Easy Turkey Lasagna

Serving: Makes 6 to 8 servings | Prep: 15mins | Cook: | Ready in:

Ingredients

- 3 cups cooked ground turkey

- 1 (26-oz.) jar fire-roasted tomato-and-garlic pasta sauce
- 1 (15-oz.) container ricotta cheese
- 1/2 cup shredded Parmesan cheese
- 6 no-cook lasagna noodles
- 2 cups (8 oz.) shredded mozzarella cheese

Direction

- Stir together ground turkey and pasta sauce. Stir together ricotta cheese and Parmesan cheese.
- Spread one-third of meat sauce in a lightly greased 11- x 7-inch baking dish; layer with 3 lasagna noodles and half each of ricotta cheese mixture and shredded mozzarella cheese. Repeat procedure once. Spread remaining one-third of meat sauce over mozzarella cheese.
- Bake, covered, at 375° for 1 hour; uncover and bake 15 more minutes. Let stand 10 minutes before serving.
- Note: For testing purposes only, we used Classico Fire Roasted Tomato & Garlic pasta sauce and Barilla Oven Ready Lasagne.
- Freeze Frame: If using frozen cooked ingredients, add 15 minutes to your bake time. If the recipe is covered during the first part of baking, then you'll add the 15 minutes to the covered baking time.

88. Egg Noodle Stir Fry With Broccoli

Serving: Serves 4 | Prep: | Cook: | Ready in: 35mins

Ingredients

- 2 tablespoons dark sesame oil, divided
- 1 (3.5-ounce) package shiitake mushrooms
- 1/2 cup diagonally cut carrot (about 2 ounces)
- 4 Thai red chile peppers, halved
- 3 garlic cloves, minced
- 1 (1-inch) piece fresh ginger, thinly sliced
- 2 cups chicken stock (reserved from Dinner 3)
- 2 1/2 tablespoons lower-sodium soy sauce
- 2 teaspoons honey
- 7 ounces broccoli florets (about 3 cups)
- 4 baby bok choy, quartered (about 10 ounces)
- 1 (16-ounce) package refrigerated cooked Chinese egg noodles (such as Twin Marquis)
- 2 teaspoons canola oil
- 4 large eggs
- 1 tablespoon rice vinegar

Direction

- Heat a medium saucepan over medium-high heat. Add 1 tablespoon sesame oil to pan; swirl to coat. Thinly slice mushroom caps. Add mushrooms and carrot to pan; sauté 5 minutes or until tender. Add peppers, garlic, and ginger; cook 30 seconds, stirring constantly. Add stock; bring to a boil, scraping pan to loosen browned bits. Cover and simmer 10 minutes. Remove from heat; stir in soy sauce and honey. Keep warm.
- Heat a wok or large skillet over high heat. Add remaining 1 tablespoon sesame oil to pan; swirl to coat. Add broccoli; stir-fry 3 minutes. Add bok choy; stir-fry 1 minute.
- Place noodles in a colander; rinse under hot water to separate noodles. Drain; divide noodles evenly among 4 bowls. Top evenly with broccoli, bok choy, and stock mixture.
- Heat a large nonstick skillet over medium heat. Add canola oil to pan; swirl to coat. Crack eggs into pan; cook 4 minutes or until whites are just set. Top each bowl with 1 egg. Drizzle servings evenly with rice vinegar.

Nutrition Information

- Calories: 471
- Saturated Fat: 3.2 g
- Sodium: 785 mg
- Fiber: 4 g
- Total Carbohydrate: 52 g
- Total Fat: 22 g
- Protein: 19 g
- Cholesterol: 214 mg

89. Egg Noodles In Cream Sauce With Asiago

Serving: Makes 4 servings | Prep: 8mins | Cook: 15mins | Ready in:

Ingredients

- 3 quart water
- 1 tablespoon chicken bouillon granules
- 1 (8-oz.) package wide egg noodles
- 2 1/2 cups whipping cream
- 1/4 cup dry white wine or chicken broth
- 1/2 teaspoon salt
- 4 ounces sliced shiitake mushrooms
- 3/4 cup frozen sweet peas
- 2 tablespoons olive oil
- 1 tablespoon grated Parmesan cheese
- 1/2 cup grated Asiago cheese
- 1/4 teaspoon ground white pepper

Direction

- Combine water and chicken bouillon granules in a Dutch oven; bring to a boil. Add noodles, and cook according to package directions. Drain and return to Dutch oven.
- Meanwhile, combine whipping cream, wine, and salt in a large saucepan; cook over medium-high heat 5 minutes or until reduced to 2 cups.
- Sauté mushrooms and peas in hot olive oil in a large skillet over medium-high heat 5 minutes or until mushrooms are tender.
- Pour cream mixture over noodles; toss to coat. To serve, divide noodle mixture evenly among 4 serving plates. For plain servings, top 2 portions with Parmesan cheese. For grown-up servings, top remaining 2 portions with mushroom mixture, Asiago cheese, and white pepper. Stir gently to blend.
- MENU IDEA FOR 4 * Egg Noodles in Cream Sauce with Asiago * Spinach salad
- GROCERIES NEEDED Check staples: chicken bouillon granules, salt, olive oil, grated Parmesan cheese, white pepper, salad dressing * 1 (8-oz.) package wide egg noodles * 1 qt. whipping cream * 1 bottle dry white wine or 1 (14-oz.) can chicken broth * 4 oz. shiitake mushrooms * 1 package frozen sweet peas * 1/2 cup grated Asiago cheese * 1 (12-oz.) package fresh spinach
- NOTE: Nutritional analysis is for grown-up entrée servings. For plain servings, nutritional analysis is as follows: CALORIES 703 (69% from fat); FAT 6g (sat 31g, mono 16g, poly 8g); PROTEIN 3g; CARB 3g; FIBER 7g; CHOL 242mg; IRON 1mg; SODIUM 794mg; CALC 146mg

Nutrition Information

- Calories: 976
- Saturated Fat: 37.3 g
- Sodium: 915 mg
- Total Carbohydrate: 56.8 g
- Cholesterol: 265 mg
- Total Fat: 73.8 g
- Protein: 17.6 g
- Fiber: 4.6 g

90. Egg Noodles With Chicken And Escarole

Serving: 4 servings (serving size: about 1 3/4 cups) | Prep: | Cook: | Ready in:

Ingredients

- 3 1/2 cups uncooked wide egg noodles (about 6 ounces)
- 1 pound skinless, boneless chicken thighs, cut into bite-sized pieces
- 2 bacon slices, chopped
- 1/2 teaspoon crushed red pepper
- 1 1/2 teaspoons bottled minced garlic
- 1 cup fat-free, less-sodium chicken broth
- 1/2 teaspoon salt
- 1 small head of escarole, cut into large pieces (about 3/4 pound)

Direction

- Cook noodles according to package directions, omitting salt and fat.
- While noodles cook, heat a large nonstick skillet over medium-high heat. Add chicken and bacon to pan; cook for 5 minutes or until chicken is done, stirring frequently. Add red pepper and garlic; sauté 30 seconds. Add broth, salt, and escarole. Cover and cook 3 minutes or until escarole wilts, stirring occasionally. Combine the chicken mixture and noodles.

Nutrition Information

- Calories: 374
- Saturated Fat: 3.2 g
- Sodium: 684 mg
- Cholesterol: 143 mg
- Protein: 33.1 g
- Total Carbohydrate: 33.9 g
- Total Fat: 11.1 g
- Fiber: 3.9 g

91. Egg Noodles With Peas And Brown Butter

Serving: 8 servings (serving size: 2/3 cup) | Prep: 3mins | Cook: 18mins | Ready in:

Ingredients

- 1 (8-ounce) package uncooked medium egg noodles
- 2 1/2 tablespoons light stick butter
- 2 tablespoons minced garlic
- 1 cup frozen petite green peas
- 1/2 cup grated Parmesan cheese
- 2 tablespoons lemon juice
- 1/2 teaspoon salt
- 1/2 teaspoon black pepper

Direction

- Cook pasta according to package directions, omitting salt and fat; drain and set aside.
- Melt butter in a large nonstick skillet over medium heat. Add garlic; sauté 2 minutes or until garlic is lightly browned. Add cooked pasta, peas, and remaining ingredients; cook 2 to 3 minutes or until thoroughly heated.

Nutrition Information

- Calories: 158
- Total Fat: 5.2 g
- Fiber: 1.8 g
- Sodium: 267 mg
- Total Carbohydrate: 21.5 g
- Cholesterol: 29 mg
- Protein: 6 g
- Saturated Fat: 2.3 g

92. Egg Noodles With Turkey, Bacon, And Rosemary

Serving: 4 | Prep: | Cook: | Ready in:

Ingredients

- 1/4 pound sliced bacon, cut crosswise into 1/2-inch strips
- 1 pound turkey cutlets, cut into 1/2-by-1 1/2-inch strips
- 3/4 teaspoon salt
- 1/2 teaspoon fresh-ground black pepper
- 10 ounce prewashed spinach
- 1/2 cup canned low-sodium chicken broth or homemade stock
- 3/4 teaspoon dried rosemary, crumbled
- 1/2 pound wide egg noodles
- 1 tablespoon butter, at room temperature

Direction

- In a large frying pan, cook the bacon, stirring occasionally, until golden brown and just crisp, about 5 minutes. Remove and drain on paper towels. Pour off all but 2 tablespoons of the fat from the pan.

- Heat the remaining bacon fat over moderately high heat. Sprinkle the turkey with 1/4 teaspoon each of the salt and pepper. Add the turkey to the pan, in two batches if necessary, and cook, stirring frequently, until golden brown and just cooked through, about 3 minutes. Transfer to a plate.
- Remove any tough stems from the spinach. Add the broth, rosemary, and the remaining 1/2 teaspoon salt to the pan and bring to a simmer, stirring to dislodge any brown bits that cling to the bottom of the pan. Add the spinach and cook, stirring, just until wilted, 1 to 2 minutes.
- In a large pot of boiling, salted water, cook the noodles until just done, about 3 minutes. Drain. Add the noodles, butter, and the remaining 1/4 teaspoon pepper to the frying pan and stir until the butter melts. Stir in the turkey with any accumulated juices and the bacon.
- Wine Recommendation: The rosemary in this dish will go well with a light French red wine, such as a Côtes-du-Rhône. Or try a moderately priced California cabernet sauvignon.

93. Egg Ravioli

Serving: Serves 8 (serving size: 1 ravioli) | Prep: | Cook: | Ready in: 32mins

Ingredients

- 1/2 cup fat-free ricotta cheese
- 2 1/2 tablespoons chopped fresh basil
- 4 teaspoons extra-virgin olive oil
- 2 teaspoons grated lemon rind
- 1/2 teaspoon freshly ground black pepper
- 1/4 teaspoon kosher salt
- 2/3 ounce Parmesan cheese, grated
- 16 round gyoza skins (pot sticker wrappers)
- 8 unbroken egg yolks
- 1 large egg white, lightly beaten
- 4 teaspoons chopped fresh chives
- Grated lemon rind (optional)

Direction

- Combine first 7 ingredients in a small bowl.
- Roll each gyoza skin to 4 inches in diameter; set aside 8 wrappers.
- Divide ricotta mixture into 8 portions (about 1 tablespoon each). Place 1 portion in the center of each of 8 skins. Make a well about 1 1/2 inches wide (about the diameter of a large egg yolk) in the center of each portion using the back of a tablespoon. Place 1 yolk (without breaking) in each well. Brush the edge of each gyoza skin with egg white. Cover each with 1 reserved gyoza skin, pressing edges firmly between your thumb and forefinger to seal ravioli tightly.
- Bring a large pot of water to a gentle boil; carefully drop each ravioli into water. Cook 2 1/2 minutes or until dough is cooked and yolk is cooked but still runny. Remove each ravioli with a slotted spoon to a small plate. Sprinkle with chives and additional lemon rind, if desired. Serve immediately.

Nutrition Information

- Calories: 121
- Saturated Fat: 2.2 g
- Sugar: 1 g
- Cholesterol: 191 mg
- Total Carbohydrate: 8 g
- Fiber: 0.0 g
- Protein: 6 g
- Total Fat: 6.4 g
- Sodium: 198 mg

94. Extra Easy Lasagna

Serving: 6 to 8 servings | Prep: | Cook: | Ready in:

Ingredients

- 1 pound lean ground beef
- 4 cups tomato-basil pasta sauce
- 6 uncooked lasagna noodles
- 1 (15-ounce) container ricotta cheese
- 2 1/2 cups (10 ounces) shredded mozzarella cheese
- 1/4 cup hot water

Direction

- Cook beef in a large skillet over medium heat, stirring until it crumbles and is no longer pink; drain. Stir in pasta sauce.
- Spread one-third of meat sauce in a lightly greased 11- x 7-inch baking dish; layer with 3 noodles and half each of ricotta cheese and mozzarella cheese. (The ricotta cheese layers will be thin.) Repeat procedure; spread remaining one-third of meat sauce over mozzarella cheese. Slowly pour 1/4 cup hot water around inside edge of dish. Tightly cover baking dish with 2 layers of heavy-duty aluminum foil.
- Bake at 375° for 45 minutes; uncover and bake 10 more minutes. Let stand 10 minutes before serving.
- Note: For testing purposes only, we used Classico Tomato & Basil pasta sauce.

95. Family Style Chicken Spaghetti

Serving: Serves 4 (serving size: 2 cups) | Prep: | Cook: | Ready in:

Ingredients

- 8 ounces uncooked whole-wheat spaghetti
- 2 teaspoons olive oil
- 3 garlic cloves, smashed
- 2 pt. cherry tomatoes
- 1 medium onion, cut into 1-in. wedges
- 1/4 cup fresh basil leaves, divided
- 2 tablespoons unsalted tomato paste
- 1/2 teaspoon kosher salt
- 1/2 teaspoon freshly ground black pepper
- 8 ounces shredded skinless, boneless rotisserie chicken breast (about 2 cups)
- 3 tablespoons shaved Parmesan cheese

Direction

- Preheat broiler. Line a jelly-roll pan with foil.
- Cook pasta according to package directions, omitting salt and fat.
- While pasta cooks, combine oil, garlic, tomatoes, and onion on prepared pan; toss. Broil 4 to 6 minutes. Transfer mixture and any liquid from pan to a blender. Add 2 tablespoons basil and tomato paste; secure blender lid on blender. Remove center piece of blender lid; cover with a kitchen towel. Blend until smooth.
- Drain pasta; return to pan. Stir in tomato sauce, salt, pepper, and chicken. Cook over medium heat until heated. Place spaghetti mixture on a serving platter. Chop remaining 2 tablespoons basil leaves. Sprinkle basil and Parmesan evenly over spaghetti.

Nutrition Information

- Calories: 404
- Protein: 34 g
- Total Carbohydrate: 55 g
- Cholesterol: 70 mg
- Fiber: 10 g
- Sodium: 603 mg
- Saturated Fat: 2.1 g
- Sugar: 9 g
- Total Fat: 7.5 g

96. Fettuccine Alfredo With Asparagus

Serving: Serves 4 (serving size: about 2 cups) | Prep: | Cook: | Ready in: 23mins

Ingredients

- 8 ounces uncooked fettuccine
- 1 teaspoon olive oil
- 1 pound fresh asparagus spears, trimmed and cut into 2-inch pieces
- 3/4 teaspoon kosher salt, divided
- 1/2 teaspoon black pepper, divided
- 1 teaspoon grated lemon rind
- 2 teaspoons fresh lemon juice
- 1 tablespoon butter
- 1 tablespoon vodka or water
- 4 garlic cloves, minced
- 2 ounces 1/3-less-fat cream cheese
- 1/4 cup fat-free milk
- 1.5 ounces vegetarian Parmesan cheese, grated (about 6 tablespoons)
- 1 tablespoon chopped fresh chives

Direction

- Cook pasta according to package directions. Drain in a colander over a bowl. Reserve 1/4 cup pasta water.
- Heat a large skillet over medium-high heat. Add oil to pan; swirl to coat. Add asparagus, 1/4 teaspoon salt, and 1/4 teaspoon pepper; sauté 6 minutes or until crisp-tender. Remove from heat. Add rind and juice; toss. Keep warm.
- Melt butter in a medium saucepan over medium heat. Add vodka and garlic; cook 1 minute. Add cream cheese, stirring until smooth. Stir in milk, Parmesan cheese, remaining 1/2 teaspoon salt, and remaining 1/4 teaspoon pepper. Stir in reserved pasta water, pasta, and asparagus; toss to coat noodles. Sprinkle with chives.

Nutrition Information

- Calories: 365
- Fiber: 4 g
- Saturated Fat: 5.9 g
- Cholesterol: 28 mg
- Total Carbohydrate: 50 g
- Total Fat: 11.2 g
- Sodium: 609 mg
- Protein: 16 g

97. Fettuccine With Edamame, Mint, And Pecorino

Serving: Serves 4 (serving size: 1 3/4 cups) | Prep: | Cook: | Ready in: 27mins

Ingredients

- 8 ounces uncooked fettuccine
- 2 tablespoons extra-virgin olive oil
- 2 medium onions, halved vertically and thinly sliced
- 5 garlic cloves, thinly sliced
- 2 cups frozen shelled edamame (green soybeans)
- 1 cup frozen peas
- 1 tablespoon grated lemon rind
- 2 tablespoons fresh lemon juice
- 1 tablespoon unsalted butter
- 6 tablespoons grated fresh pecorino Romano cheese
- 3 tablespoons chopped fresh mint
- 1/4 teaspoon salt
- 1/4 teaspoon freshly ground black pepper

Direction

- Cook pasta according to package directions, omitting salt and fat. Drain in a colander over a bowl, reserving 2/3 cup cooking liquid.
- Heat a large nonstick skillet over medium-high heat. Add oil; swirl to coat. Add onion; cook 9 minutes or until lightly browned, stirring occasionally. Stir in garlic; cook 2 minutes or until garlic is lightly browned, stirring occasionally. Stir in edamame and peas; cook 2 minutes or until thoroughly heated. Add pasta, rind, juice, and butter; stir until butter melts. Remove pan from heat; stir in pecorino Romano cheese, mint, salt, and pepper. Stir in reserved 2/3 cup cooking liquid. Serve immediately.

Nutrition Information

- Calories: 443
- Protein: 18 g
- Saturated Fat: 4.5 g
- Cholesterol: 15 mg
- Fiber: 7.5 g
- Total Carbohydrate: 59.3 g
- Sodium: 329 mg
- Total Fat: 15.7 g

98. Fettuccine With Pistachio Mint Pesto And Tomatoes

Serving: Serves 4 (serving size: 1 cup) | Prep: | Cook: | Ready in:

Ingredients

- 1/2 cup fresh mint leaves
- 1/2 cup fresh flat-leaf parsley leaves
- 1/4 cup plus 4 teaspoons unsalted, shelled dry-roasted pistachios, divided
- 3 tablespoons extra-virgin olive oil
- 5/8 teaspoon kosher salt
- 1/4 teaspoon freshly ground black pepper
- 1 large garlic clove
- 1 (9-ounce) package refrigerated fettuccine
- 12 cherry tomatoes, halved
- 1 ounce fresh pecorino Romano cheese, shaved (about 1/4 cup)

Direction

- Combine mint leaves, parsley leaves, 1/4 cup pistachios, olive oil, kosher salt, ground black pepper, and garlic in a mini food processor; pulse mixture until coarsely chopped.
- Cook fettuccine according to the package directions, omitting salt and fat. Drain fettuccine over a bowl, reserving 1/4 cup of the cooking liquid. Combine pesto mixture and reserved cooking liquid in a large bowl, stirring with a whisk. Add pasta to bowl; toss well to coat. Gently fold in cherry tomatoes. Coarsely chop remaining 4 teaspoons pistachios. Top pasta evenly with pecorino Romano cheese and chopped pistachios.

Nutrition Information

- Calories: 371
- Total Fat: 19.1 g
- Total Carbohydrate: 40.1 g
- Cholesterol: 45 mg
- Protein: 12.3 g
- Saturated Fat: 4.5 g
- Fiber: 3.7 g
- Sodium: 463 mg

99. Fettuccine With Seared Tomatoes, Spinach, And Burrata

Serving: Serves 4 | Prep: | Cook: | Ready in: 25mins

Ingredients

- 8 ounces uncooked fettuccine
- Cooking spray
- 2/3 cup grape tomatoes, halved (about 10 large)
- 3 tablespoons extra-virgin olive oil
- 1/4 teaspoon crushed red pepper
- 4 garlic cloves, thinly sliced
- 1 (14.5-ounce) can unsalted diced tomatoes, undrained
- 3/4 teaspoon salt
- 3 ounces fresh baby spinach (about 3 cups)
- 4 ounces burrata cheese
- Freshly ground black pepper

Direction

- Cook pasta according to package directions, omitting salt and fat; drain.
- While pasta cooks, heat a large skillet over medium-high heat. Coat pan with cooking spray. Arrange tomato halves, cut sides down,

in pan; cook 1 1/2 minutes or until seared. Stir tomatoes; cook 30 seconds. Remove tomatoes from pan; set aside.

- Reduce heat to low. Add oil to pan; swirl to coat. Add red pepper and garlic; cook 2 minutes or until fragrant, stirring occasionally. Place canned tomatoes in a mini chopper or food processor; process until almost smooth. Add pureed tomatoes and salt to oil mixture; cook 8 minutes, stirring occasionally.
- Remove skillet from heat. Add spinach and cooked pasta; toss well until spinach wilts slightly. Arrange about 1 1/3 cups pasta mixture in each of 4 shallow bowls. Divide the seared grape tomato halves evenly among the servings. Dollop about 2 table-spoons burrata cheese over each serving, and sprinkle with freshly ground black pepper.

Nutrition Information

- Calories: 415
- Sodium: 593 mg
- Cholesterol: 20 mg
- Total Fat: 17.1 g
- Fiber: 4.8 g
- Protein: 13.5 g
- Saturated Fat: 5.7 g
- Total Carbohydrate: 51.4 g

100. Fettuccine With Squash Ribbons

Serving: Serves 4 (serving size: about 1 3/4 cups) | Prep: | Cook: | Ready in: 21mins

Ingredients

- 8 ounces uncooked fettuccine
- 2 small zucchini
- 1 large yellow squash
- 3 tablespoons olive oil, divided
- 1 cup grape tomatoes
- 1/2 teaspoon kosher salt
- 1/2 teaspoon crushed red pepper
- 6 garlic cloves, thinly sliced
- 1 ounce Parmesan cheese, shaved (about 1/4 cup)
- 3 tablespoons torn fresh mint

Direction

- Cook pasta according to package directions, omitting salt and fat. Drain in a colander over a bowl, reserving 3/4 cup cooking liquid. Shave zucchini and squash into thin ribbons using a vegetable peeler; discard seeds. Place ribbons in a large bowl.
- Heat a large skillet over medium heat. Add 1 tablespoon oil to pan; swirl to coat. Add tomatoes, salt, and pepper to pan; cook 8 minutes or until tomatoes begin to break down, stirring occasionally. Remove tomatoes from pan using a slotted spoon; add to squash ribbons. Add garlic to pan; cook 1 minute or until fragrant, stirring constantly. Stir in reserved 3/4 cup cooking liquid; bring to a boil. Gradually add remaining 2 tablespoons oil to pan, stirring constantly with a whisk.
- Add pasta to pan; cook 1 minute, tossing to coat. Remove pan from heat. Add pasta mixture to squash mixture; toss. Sprinkle with Parmesan cheese and mint.

Nutrition Information

- Calories: 364
- Protein: 13 g
- Fiber: 4 g
- Total Carbohydrate: 50 g
- Cholesterol: 6 mg
- Saturated Fat: 3 g
- Sodium: 361 mg
- Total Fat: 13.4 g

101. Flemish Beef And Beer Stew

Serving: Serves 6 | Prep: | Cook: | Ready in: 100mins

Ingredients

- 4 center-cut bacon slices
- 2 pounds boneless chuck roast, trimmed and cut into 1-inch pieces
- 1 1/4 teaspoons kosher salt, divided
- 1/2 teaspoon freshly ground black pepper, divided
- 1 teaspoon olive oil
- 2 cups sliced yellow onion
- 1/2 teaspoon dried thyme
- 3 garlic cloves, minced
- 1.5 ounces all-purpose flour (about 1/3 cup)
- 2 cups unsalted beef stock
- 2 tablespoons brown sugar
- 2 tablespoons cider vinegar
- 2 bay leaves
- 1 (12-ounce) bottle Belgian-style brown ale (such as Petrus Oud Bruin or Leffe)
- 4 cups hot cooked medium egg noodles (about 3 cups pasta)
- 2 tablespoons chopped fresh parsley

Direction

- Heat a large Dutch oven over medium heat. Add bacon to pan; cook 5 minutes or until crisp. Place bacon on paper towels; let stand 3 minutes. Chop.
- Sprinkle beef with 3/4 teaspoon salt and 1/4 teaspoon pepper. Add oil to pan. Add half of beef; cook 6 minutes or until browned, turning occasionally. Place browned beef on a plate. Repeat with remaining beef.
- Add onion, thyme, and garlic to pan; cook 8 minutes or until lightly browned, stirring occasionally. Weigh or lightly spoon flour into a dry measuring cup. Sprinkle flour evenly over onion mixture; cook 1 minute, stirring constantly. Stir in stock, sugar, vinegar, bay leaves, beer, and bacon; bring to a simmer. Add beef, remaining 1/2 teaspoon salt, and 1/4 teaspoon pepper; cover, reduce heat, and simmer 1 hour or until beef is tender. Discard bay leaves.
- Place about 2/3 cup noodles in each of 6 bowls. Top each serving with about 1 cup stew; sprinkle each with 1 teaspoon parsley.
- Petrus Oud Bruin ABV 5%
- Aged for two years in oak barrels, this Flemish-style oud bruin (old brown ale) walks the line between sweet and sour, and tastes like a combination of brown ale and burgundy wine. Add to that its hints of plum, black cherry, and brown sugar, and it's the perfect base--and accompaniment--for this hearty beef stew.

Nutrition Information

- Calories: 403
- Saturated Fat: 3.3 g
- Total Carbohydrate: 36 g
- Protein: 41 g
- Cholesterol: 135 mg
- Sodium: 632 mg
- Total Fat: 9.6 g
- Fiber: 2 g

102. Four Cheese Stuffed Shells With Smoky Marinara

Serving: 2 casseroles, 5 servings per dish (serving size: about 4 stuffed shells and about 1/2 cup smoky marinara) | Prep: | Cook: | Ready in:

Ingredients

- 1 pound jumbo shell pasta (40 shells)
- Cooking spray
- 1 (12-ounce) carton 1% low-fat cottage cheese
- 1 (15-ounce) carton ricotta cheese
- 1 cup (4 ounces) shredded Asiago cheese
- 3/4 cup (3 ounces) grated fresh Parmesan cheese
- 2 tablespoons chopped fresh chives

- 2 tablespoons chopped fresh parsley
- 1/4 teaspoon black pepper
- 1/4 teaspoon salt
- 1 (10-ounce) package frozen chopped spinach, thawed and drained
- 6 cups Smoky Marinara
- 1 cup (4 ounces) shredded part-skim mozzarella cheese, divided

Direction

- Cook pasta according to package directions, omitting salt and fat. Drain and set aside.
- Preheat oven to 375°.
- Coat 2 (13 x 9-inch) baking dishes with cooking spray; set aside.
- Place cottage cheese and ricotta cheese in a food processor; process until smooth. Combine cottage cheese mixture, Asiago, and next 6 ingredients (Asiago through spinach).
- Spoon or pipe 1 tablespoon cheese mixture into each shell. Arrange half of stuffed shells, seam sides up, in one prepared dish. Pour 3 cups Smoky Marinara over stuffed shells. Sprinkle with 1/2 cup mozzarella. Repeat procedure with remaining stuffed shells, Smoky Marinara, and mozzarella in remaining prepared dish.
- Cover with foil. Bake at 375° for 30 minutes or until thoroughly heated.
- To freeze unbaked casserole: Prepare through Step Cover with plastic wrap, pressing to remove as much air as possible. Wrap with heavy-duty foil. Store in freezer for up to 2 months.
- To prepare frozen unbaked casserole: Preheat oven to 375°. Remove foil; reserve foil. Remove plastic wrap; discard wrap. Cover frozen casserole with reserved foil; bake at 375° for 1 hour and 10 minutes or until the shells are thoroughly heated.

Nutrition Information

- Calories: 470
- Total Carbohydrate: 52.7 g
- Fiber: 5.3 g
- Total Fat: 15.7 g
- Sodium: 916 mg
- Cholesterol: 47 mg
- Protein: 28.3 g
- Saturated Fat: 8.8 g

103. Free Form Lasagna

Serving: Serves 6 | Prep: 15mins | Cook: 40mins | Ready in:

Ingredients

- Salt
- 8 ounces sweet or hot Italian sausage, removed from casing
- 1 28-oz. can crushed tomatoes
- 1/2 teaspoon dried oregano
- 2 cups ricotta (not nonfat)
- 1 cup grated Parmesan
- 2 tablespoons finely chopped fresh basil
- 12 lasagna noodles, each broken in half

Direction

- Bring a large pot of salted water to boil.
- Cook sausage in a skillet over medium-high heat, breaking up large pieces, until it loses its pink color, about 5 minutes. Stir in tomatoes, oregano and 1/2 tsp. salt, reduce heat to medium-low and simmer until thick, stirring occasionally, about 20 minutes.
- Combine ricotta, Parmesan and basil in a medium microwave-safe bowl.
- Add noodles to boiling water; cook until just tender, 10 minutes or as package label directs. Just before noodles are done, microwave ricotta mixture on high for 30 seconds, stirring once. Drain noodles well.
- Spread 1 1/2 Tbsp. sauce on each of 4 dinner plates. Place a noodle on top and spread with 1 1/2 Tbsp. cheese mixture. Top with 1 1/2 Tbsp. sauce. Repeat with noodles, cheese mixture and sauce, ending with a layer of

sauce. Sprinkle Parmesan on top. Serve, passing additional Parmesan.

Nutrition Information

- Calories: 567
- Total Fat: 28 g
- Protein: 30 g
- Sodium: 1194 mg
- Fiber: 3 g
- Total Carbohydrate: 48 g
- Cholesterol: 77 mg
- Saturated Fat: 14 g

104. Fresh Thai Noodle Bowl

Serving: Serves 4 (serving size: 1 bowl) | Prep: | Cook: | Ready in:

Ingredients

- 1 (8-ounce) package rice vermicelli noodles
- 1 teaspoon canola oil
- 1 tablespoon minced peeled fresh ginger
- 4 garlic cloves, minced
- 3 1/2 cups unsalted vegetable stock (such as Kitchen Basics)
- 2 1/2 tablespoons lower-sodium soy sauce
- 1 cup matchstick-cut carrots
- 1 red bell pepper, thinly sliced
- 1 small English cucumber, halved lengthwise and thinly sliced
- 5 tablespoons chopped fresh mixed herbs (such as basil, mint, and cilantro)
- 6 tablespoons chopped unsalted, dry-roasted peanuts
- 2 teaspoons chili oil

Direction

- Cook noodles according to package directions; drain.
- Heat a medium saucepan over medium heat. Add oil to pan; swirl to coat. Add ginger and garlic; cook 1 minute, stirring constantly. Add stock and soy sauce; bring to a boil. Simmer 10 minutes.
- Place carrots, bell pepper, and cucumber in a bowl; toss to combine. Divide noodles evenly among 4 serving bowls; top each serving with one-fourth of vegetable mixture. Pour about 3/4 cup warm stock mixture into each bowl. Sprinkle evenly with herbs and peanuts; drizzle chili oil over top.

Nutrition Information

- Calories: 488
- Protein: 11 g
- Sodium: 567 mg
- Total Carbohydrate: 59 g
- Fiber: 4 g
- Cholesterol: 0.0 mg
- Saturated Fat: 1.4 g
- Total Fat: 11.9 g

105. Garlicky Angel Hair With Roasted Broccoli

Serving: Serves: 6 | Prep: 15mins | Cook: 15mins | Ready in:

Ingredients

- 1 12-oz. package fresh broccoli florets
- 6 tablespoons olive oil
- 1 tablespoon Italian seasoning
- Salt
- 8 ounces angel hair pasta
- 10 cloves garlic, thinly sliced
- 1/2 teaspoon crushed red pepper
- 1 cup grated Parmesan
- 2 tablespoons chopped fresh basil

Direction

- Preheat oven to 450°F; line a large, rimmed baking sheet with foil. Combine broccoli, 1

Tbsp. olive oil and Italian seasoning in a large bowl; toss to coat. Place broccoli in a single layer on baking sheet. Roast, stirring once or twice, until broccoli is crisp-tender and beginning to lightly brown, about 15 minutes.
- Bring a pot of salted water to a boil. Cook pasta until al dente, about 4 minutes or as package label directs. Drain, reserving 1 1/2 cups pasta cooking water.
- Warm 3 Tbsp. olive oil in a Dutch oven over medium heat. Sauté garlic until just golden brown, about 2 minutes. Remove from heat; stir in crushed red pepper, 1 tsp. salt, 1 1/4 cups reserved pasta water and remaining olive oil. Add pasta and 1/2 cup cheese; simmer over medium heat, tossing gently, until sauce thoroughly coats pasta (add remaining 1/4 cup pasta water if needed), 2 to 3 minutes. Remove from heat and toss in broccoli, remaining cheese and basil. Serve immediately.

Nutrition Information

- Calories: 357
- Total Carbohydrate: 33 g
- Total Fat: 19 g
- Protein: 13 g
- Cholesterol: 15 mg
- Saturated Fat: 5 g
- Fiber: 3 g
- Sodium: 657 mg

106. Giant Butternut Squash Ravioli

Serving: Serves 8 (makes 24 to 30) | Prep: | Cook: | Ready in:

Ingredients

- FILLING
- 1 butternut squash* (about 3 1/2 lbs.), peeled, seeded, and cut into 2-in. chunks
- 1 tablespoon extra-virgin olive oil
- Salt and freshly ground black pepper
- 3/4 cup ground toasted almonds
- 1 tablespoon minced fresh sage
- 4 ounces freshly grated parmesan cheese (1 3/4 cups)
- 1/2 teaspoon freshly grated nutmeg
- ASSEMBLING & SERVING
- Fine semolina*
- Fresh Pasta Dough, rolled into sheets as directed, or 2 lbs. purchased fresh ravioli or lasagna sheets*
- 1 qt. reduced-sodium chicken broth or homemade chicken broth*
- 2 tablespoons butter
- 2 teaspoons extra-virgin olive oil
- 1 tablespoon minced flat-leaf parsley
- Freshly grated parmesan cheese

Direction

- Make filling: Preheat oven to 425°. Put squash chunks in a rimmed baking pan, drizzle with olive oil, and season generously with salt and pepper. Toss to coat. Bake, stirring squash every 20 minutes, until very tender, 35 to 45 minutes. Carefully spoon hot squash into a food processor and whirl until very smooth.
- Scrape squash into a large bowl and let cool. Stir in almonds, sage, parmesan, and nutmeg. Add salt and pepper to taste.
- Assemble ravioli: Line a rimmed baking pan with parchment paper and sprinkle with semolina; set aside. Lay 1 pasta sheet on a work surface. Starting 2 in. away from a short end, spoon a 2-tbsp. mound of filling onto the middle of pasta sheet; repeat at 4-in. intervals. Around mounds of filling, brush pasta with water. Place a second pasta sheet over the first, starting at a short end and easing pasta over filling, gently pressing out air and sealing pasta around each mound of filling as you go.
- Trim long sides of pasta sheet with a pastry wheel or knife so sheet is 4 in. wide. Cut ravioli between filling to make 4-in. squares. Transfer ravioli to parchment-lined pan and cover with plastic wrap; also gather and wrap

pasta scraps. Continue shaping ravioli, rerolling scraps according to directions for Fresh Pasta Dough and stacking one more layer of parchment over first (add another pan if needed), until you've used all the filling; you should have 24 to 30 ravioli and may have leftover pasta dough. (If dough scraps become too dry to reroll, crumble into food processor and pulse with 1 tsp. water at a time until moistened.)

- To serve: In a saucepan, boil broth until reduced by a third. Add butter; keep warm.
- Preheat oven to 150° and set 8 wide soup plates or rimmed dinner plates in oven to warm. Bring 2 large pots (8 to 10 qt. each) of generously salted water to a rolling boil and add 1 tsp. olive oil to each. Divide ravioli between pots, reduce heat so water boils gently, and cook ravioli, occasionally pushing down into the water, just until al dente (test a corner of one to check), 5 to 7 minutes.
- Set out soup plates. Using a slotted spoon, transfer 3 ravioli from water to each plate. Ladle broth over ravioli, sprinkle with parsley, and serve with parmesan.
- *Shortcuts: Buy 2 3/4 lbs. peeled chunks of butternut squash instead of a whole squash. Buy semolina in the baking aisle of well-stocked markets. Instead of making pasta, buy about 2 lbs. fresh ravioli or lasagna sheets from a well-stocked grocery store or Italian deli, or from freshpasta.com ($79 for 16 oz.; 5-lb. minimum order). You may need to cut the ravioli in slightly different dimensions to make at least 24, and you may have leftover filling. For a recipe for chicken broth, see sunset.com/chickenbroth.
- Make ahead: Make filling (through step 2) and chill overnight. Fill ravioli (through step 4) and chill them as long as 1 day, or freeze on pans until firm, transfer to bags, and freeze up to 3 weeks.
- Note: Nutritional analysis is per serving.

Nutrition Information

- Calories: 572
- Sodium: 877 mg
- Total Carbohydrate: 75 g
- Saturated Fat: 6.4 g
- Cholesterol: 123 mg
- Fiber: 7 g
- Protein: 22 g
- Total Fat: 22 g

107. Glass Noodles With Green Papaya, Peanuts, And Chili Vinaigrette

Serving: Serves 8 (serving size: about 3/4 cup) | Prep: | Cook: | Ready in: 29mins

Ingredients

- 1/4 cup champagne vinegar
- 3 tablespoons sugar
- 2 tablespoons red wine vinegar
- 5 1/2 teaspoons fish sauce
- 1 Fresno chile, minced
- 1 shallot, minced
- 2 garlic cloves, minced
- 4 1/2 ounces uncooked bean threads (cellophane noodles)
- 2 cups julienne-cut green papaya
- 2 cups julienne-cut chayote
- 1 cup chopped fresh mint
- 1 cup chopped fresh basil
- 1 cup chopped fresh cilantro
- 1 cup roasted, unsalted peanuts

Direction

- Combine first 7 ingredients in a small saucepan over medium heat; bring to a boil. Simmer 5 minutes; remove from heat. Cool.
- Cook threads according to directions. Drain; cool. Combine threads, papaya, chayote, mint, basil, and cilantro; drizzle with vinegar mixture. Toss well; sprinkle with peanuts.

Nutrition Information

- Calories: 214
- Fiber: 3 g
- Protein: 5 g
- Total Fat: 9.3 g
- Sodium: 331 mg
- Total Carbohydrate: 30 g
- Saturated Fat: 1.3 g
- Sugar: 9 g
- Cholesterol: 0.0 mg

108. Gnocchi Primavera

Serving: Serves: 4 | Prep: 15mins | Cook: 20mins | Ready in:

Ingredients

- Salt and pepper
- 1 pound asparagus, tough ends removed, cut into 1-inch pieces
- 1 tablespoon unsalted butter
- 1 tablespoon olive oil
- 10 ounce button mushrooms, sliced
- 2 cloves garlic, finely chopped
- 3 plum tomatoes, seeded and diced (about 1 1/2 cups)
- 1 cup frozen peas
- 1/2 cup heavy cream, warmed
- 1/2 cup low-sodium vegetable broth, warmed
- 1 pound frozen or shelf-stable gnocchi
- 2/3 cup grated Parmesan
- 2 tablespoons chopped fresh basil

Direction

- Bring a pot of salted water to boil. Place asparagus in a bowl with 2 Tbsp. water; microwave on high until tender, 3 to 4 minutes.
- Melt butter with oil in a large skillet over medium heat. Add mushrooms, garlic and 1/2 tsp. salt and sauté until mushrooms have given off most of their liquid, about 8 minutes. Add tomatoes and sauté until softened, about 3 minutes longer. Stir in peas, cream and broth, bring to a simmer, and cook until slightly thickened, about 5 minutes.
- Cook gnocchi in boiling water until they float, about 5 minutes for frozen and 2 minutes for shelf-stable, or as package label directs. Drain and add to vegetable mixture, along with asparagus. Stir in Parmesan and toss to coat. Season with salt and pepper, sprinkle with basil and serve immediately.

Nutrition Information

- Calories: 580
- Total Fat: 28 g
- Saturated Fat: 12 g
- Sodium: 773 mg
- Cholesterol: 63 mg
- Protein: 22 g
- Total Carbohydrate: 74 g
- Fiber: 7 g

109. Gnocchi With Shrimp, Asparagus, And Pesto

Serving: 4 servings (serving size: 2 cups) | Prep: | Cook: | Ready in:

Ingredients

- 2 quarts plus 1 tablespoon water, divided
- 1 (16-ounce) package vacuum-packed gnocchi (such as Vigo)
- 4 cups (1-inch) slices asparagus (about 1 pound)
- 1 pound peeled and deveined large shrimp, coarsely chopped
- 1 cup basil leaves
- 2 tablespoons pine nuts, toasted
- 2 tablespoons preshredded Parmesan cheese
- 2 teaspoons fresh lemon juice
- 2 teaspoons bottled minced garlic
- 4 teaspoons extravirgin olive oil

- 1/4 teaspoon salt

Direction

- Bring 2 quarts water to a boil in a Dutch oven. Add gnocchi to pan; cook 4 minutes or until done (gnocchi will rise to surface). Remove gnocchi with a slotted spoon; place in a large bowl. Add asparagus and shrimp to pan; cook 5 minutes or until shrimp are done. Drain. Add shrimp mixture to gnocchi.
- Combine remaining 1 tablespoon water, basil, and next 4 ingredients (through garlic) in a food processor; process until smooth, scraping sides. Drizzle oil through food chute with food processor on; process until well blended. Add salt and basil mixture to shrimp mixture; toss to coat. Serve immediately.

Nutrition Information

- Calories: 355
- Saturated Fat: 1.6 g
- Total Fat: 9.3 g
- Protein: 26.5 g
- Sodium: 894 mg
- Total Carbohydrate: 42.7 g
- Cholesterol: 170 mg
- Fiber: 3 g

110. Gnocchi With Turkey Ragù

Serving: 4 servings | Prep: | Cook: | Ready in:

Ingredients

- 1 (16-ounce) package gnocchi
- Cooking spray
- 8 ounces ground turkey breast
- 1 cup chopped onion
- 3/4 cup chopped red bell pepper
- 1 tablespoon bottled minced garlic
- 1 teaspoon dried basil
- 1/4 teaspoon fennel seeds
- 1/2 cup dry white wine
- 3 tablespoons tomato paste
- 1 (14.5-ounce) can diced tomatoes with basil, garlic, and oregano
- 1 tablespoon finely grated fresh Romano cheese
- 1/2 teaspoon black pepper
- Basil sprigs (optional)

Direction

- Cook gnocchi according to package directions, omitting salt and fat. Drain.
- Heat a large nonstick skillet over medium-high heat. Coat pan with cooking spray. Add turkey to pan; cook 3 minutes or until browned, stirring to crumble. Drain. Add onion and next 4 ingredients (through fennel seeds); sauté 2 minutes. Return turkey to pan. Stir in wine; cook 2 minutes. Stir in tomato paste and tomatoes; cook 4 minutes, stirring occasionally. Remove from heat; stir in cheese and black pepper. Place about 1 cup gnocchi in each of 4 shallow bowls; top each serving with about 1/2 cup sauce. Garnish with basil, if desired.

Nutrition Information

- Calories: 317
- Sodium: 651 mg
- Total Carbohydrate: 38 g
- Protein: 18.7 g
- Saturated Fat: 5.5 g
- Fiber: 3.7 g
- Cholesterol: 45 mg
- Total Fat: 9.7 g

111. Golden Macaroni And Cheese

Serving: Makes 8 servings | Prep: | Cook: | Ready in:

Ingredients

- 1 (8-ounce) package elbow macaroni (about 2 cups uncooked macaroni)
- 2 cups milk
- 1/4 cup all-purpose flour
- 1 teaspoon onion salt
- 2 (10-ounce) blocks sharp Cheddar cheese, shredded (about 4 1/2 cups) and divided*
- 1 cup soft breadcrumbs (4 slices, crusts removed)
- 1/4 cup butter or margarine, melted

Direction

- Cook macaroni according to package directions; drain well. Set aside.
- Place milk, flour, and onion salt in a quart jar; cover tightly, and shake vigorously 1 minute.
- Stir together flour mixture, 3 1/2 cups cheese, and macaroni.
- Pour macaroni mixture into a lightly greased 13- x 9-inch baking dish or 2 (11-inch) oval baking dishes. Sprinkle evenly with breadcrumbs and remaining 1 cup cheese; drizzle evenly with melted butter.
- Bake at 350° for 45 minutes or until golden brown.
- *20 ounces loaf pasteurized prepared cheese product, shredded or cut into small cubes, may be substituted. Omit breadcrumbs if using prepared cheese product.
- Note: For testing purposes only, we used Kraft Cracker Barrel Sharp Cheddar Cheese.

112. Greek Baked Ziti

Serving: Makes 6 to 8 servings | Prep: | Cook: | Ready in: 80mins

Ingredients

- 12 ounces ziti pasta
- 1 small yellow onion, chopped
- 1 tablespoon olive oil
- 2 garlic cloves, minced
- 1 1/2 pounds lean ground beef
- 2 (15-oz.) cans tomato sauce
- 1 tablespoon fresh lemon juice
- 1 1/2 teaspoons dried oregano
- 1 teaspoon sugar
- 1/2 teaspoon ground cinnamon
- 1 1/2 teaspoons kosher salt, divided
- 3 tablespoons butter
- 3 tablespoons all-purpose flour
- 3 cups milk
- 1 cup grated Parmesan cheese
- 1/2 teaspoon freshly ground black pepper
- Vegetable cooking spray
- 1 (8-oz.) package shredded mozzarella cheese
- 1/3 cup fine, dry breadcrumbs

Direction

- Preheat oven to 350°. Cook pasta in a Dutch oven according to package directions.
- Meanwhile, sauté onion in hot oil in large skillet over medium-high heat 4 to 5 minutes or until tender. Add garlic; sauté 30 seconds. Add beef; cook, stirring occasionally, 5 minutes or until crumbled and no longer pink. Drain mixture, and return to skillet.
- Stir tomato sauce, next 4 ingredients, and 1 tsp. salt into meat mixture. Bring to a simmer over medium-high heat, and cook, stirring occasionally, 2 minutes. Remove from heat.
- Melt butter in a large saucepan over low heat. Whisk in flour, and cook, whisking constantly, 2 minutes. Gradually whisk in milk. Increase heat to medium, and cook, whisking constantly, 5 to 7 minutes or until thickened and bubbly. Stir in Parmesan cheese, pepper, and remaining 1/2 tsp. salt. Add sauce to pasta, stirring to coat.
- Transfer pasta mixture to a lightly greased (with cooking spray) 13- x 9-inch baking dish. Top with beef mixture, mozzarella cheese, and breadcrumbs.
- Bake at 350° for 20 to 25 minutes or until mixture is bubbly and cheese is melted. Let stand 10 minutes before serving.

- MAKE IT AHEAD Fix and freeze this dish (unbaked) for a hands-off dinner. Let it stand 30 minutes before baking, and add 15 to 20 minutes in the oven.

113. Greek Baked Ziti (Pastitsio)

Serving: Serves 10 (serving size: 1/10 of casserole) | Prep: | Cook: | Ready in: 115mins

Ingredients

- 1 tablespoon olive oil
- 1 3/4 cups chopped onion
- 1 large garlic clove, minced
- 1/2 pound lean ground lamb
- 1/2 pound ground sirloin
- 3 (14.5-ounce) cans unsalted diced tomatoes, undrained
- 1 teaspoon dried oregano
- 1 teaspoon salt, divided
- 1/2 teaspoon ground cinnamon
- 2 tablespoons butter
- 1/4 cup all-purpose flour
- 3 cups 2% reduced-fat milk, divided
- 3 large eggs, lightly beaten
- 3/4 cup crumbled feta cheese, divided
- 10 ounce uncooked ziti (short tube-shaped pasta)
- Cooking spray
- 1/4 cup dry breadcrumbs
- Fresh oregano leaves (optional)

Direction

- Heat a large skillet over medium heat. Add oil to pan; swirl to coat. Add onion; sauté 5 minutes or until tender. Add garlic; sauté 1 minute. Add lamb and beef; cook 4 minutes or until browned, stirring to crumble. Add tomatoes, oregano, 1/2 teaspoon salt, and cinnamon; bring to a simmer over medium-high heat. Reduce heat to low, and cook 20 minutes, stirring occasionally and mashing with a spatula or flat side of a wooden spoon. Remove from heat; set aside.
- While sauce cooks, melt butter in medium saucepan over medium heat. Add flour, stirring with a whisk. Cook 1 minute, stirring constantly. Add 1/2 cup milk, stirring with a whisk until smooth. Gradually add remaining 2 1/2 cups milk and remaining 1/2 teaspoon salt, stirring until smooth. Bring to boil over medium-high heat, and cook 1 minute or until slightly thick. Remove from heat. Gradually add hot milk to eggs, stirring constantly with a whisk. Stir in 1/2 cup cheese. Keep warm.
- Preheat oven to 350°.
- Cook pasta in boiling water 9 minutes or until al dente, omitting salt and fat. Drain. Stir 3 cups pasta into tomato sauce; stir remaining 3 cups pasta into white sauce.
- Spoon tomato-sauced pasta into a 13 x 9-inch glass or ceramic baking dish coated with cooking spray. Top with white-sauced pasta, spreading evenly. Sprinkle with remaining 1/4 cup cheese and breadcrumbs. Bake at 350° for 30 minutes or until bubbly. Let stand 5 minutes; sprinkle with oregano leaves, if desired.

Nutrition Information

- Calories: 383
- Protein: 19.8 g
- Fiber: 3.7 g
- Sodium: 532 mg
- Cholesterol: 108 mg
- Total Fat: 16.8 g
- Saturated Fat: 7.9 g
- Total Carbohydrate: 38 g

114. Greek Chicken With Angel Hair Pasta

Serving: 8 servings (serving size: 1/2 chicken breast, about 1/2 cup tomato mixture, and about 1 cup pasta) | Prep: | Cook: | Ready in:

Ingredients

- 1 pound uncooked angel hair pasta
- 1 tablespoon olive oil
- 4 (6-ounce) skinless, boneless chicken breasts, halved
- 2 cups chopped red onion
- 1 cup chopped yellow bell pepper
- 6 tablespoons fresh lemon juice
- 1 teaspoon dried basil
- 1/2 teaspoon dried oregano
- 2 (14.5-ounce) cans diced tomatoes with basil, garlic, and oregano
- 3/4 cup (3 ounces) feta cheese, crumbled

Direction

- Cook pasta according to package directions, omitting salt and fat.
- Heat oil in a large nonstick skillet over medium-high heat. Add chicken to pan; sauté 3 minutes on each side. Add onion and next 5 ingredients (through tomatoes) to pan; stir well. Cover, reduce heat, and simmer 25 minutes or until chicken is done. Remove from heat; sprinkle with cheese. Serve with pasta.

Nutrition Information

- Calories: 400
- Sodium: 694 mg
- Total Fat: 7.3 g
- Total Carbohydrate: 54.3 g
- Protein: 30 g
- Cholesterol: 60 mg
- Fiber: 3.1 g
- Saturated Fat: 2.7 g

115. Greek Lamb And Feta Lasagna

Serving: Serves 9 | Prep: | Cook: | Ready in: 90mins

Ingredients

- 2 teaspoons olive oil
- 1 1/2 cups chopped onion
- 1 1/2 tablespoons minced garlic
- 1 tablespoon chopped fresh rosemary
- 9 ounces lean ground lamb
- 9 ounces extra-lean ground beef
- 1 1/4 cups unsalted chicken stock (such as Swanson)
- 3/4 teaspoon kosher salt
- 3/4 teaspoon freshly ground black pepper
- 1 (28-ounce) can crushed tomatoes, undrained
- 1 (14-ounce) can crushed tomatoes, undrained
- 1 1/4 cups part-skim ricotta cheese
- 1/2 teaspoon grated lemon rind
- 9 no-boil lasagna noodles
- Cooking spray
- 3 ounces feta cheese, crumbled (about 3/4 cup)
- 3 tablespoons chopped fresh flat-leaf parsley

Direction

- Preheat oven to 375°.
- Heat a large skillet over medium heat. Add oil to pan; swirl to coat. Add onion and next 4 ingredients (through beef); cook 14 minutes or until lamb and beef are browned, stirring to crumble. Add stock to pan; cook 3 minutes. Stir in salt, pepper, and tomatoes. Bring to a boil; reduce heat, and simmer 4 minutes, scraping pan to loosen browned bits.
- Combine ricotta and rind in a small bowl. Spread 1 tablespoon ricotta mixture over one side of each lasagna noodle.
- Spread 2 cups tomato mixture in bottom of an 11 x 7-inch glass or ceramic baking dish coated with cooking spray. Arrange 3 lasagna noodles, ricotta side up, over tomato mixture; top with 2 cups tomato mixture. Repeat layers twice, ending with 2 cups tomato mixture.

Sprinkle evenly with feta cheese. Cover with foil; bake at 375° for 40 minutes. Remove foil; let stand 10 minutes. Sprinkle with parsley.

Nutrition Information

- Calories: 321
- Protein: 23.8 g
- Total Fat: 13.3 g
- Fiber: 3.8 g
- Total Carbohydrate: 28.5 g
- Cholesterol: 62 mg
- Sodium: 543 mg
- Saturated Fat: 6 g

116. Greek Style Couscous

Serving: Serves 4 (serving size: 3/4 cup) | Prep: | Cook: | Ready in:

Ingredients

- 3/4 cup unsalted chicken stock
- 3/4 cup uncooked couscous
- 1/2 teaspoon kosher salt, divided
- 2 tablespoons extra-virgin olive oil
- 1 tablespoon red wine vinegar
- 1/4 teaspoon freshly ground black pepper
- 1 cup (1/4-inch) diced English cucumber
- 1 cup (1/4-inch) diced tomato
- 3 tablespoons fresh oregano leaves
- 1 ounce crumbled feta cheese (about 1/4 cup)

Direction

- Bring stock to a boil in a small saucepan over high heat. Place couscous and 1/4 teaspoon salt in a small baking dish. Pour stock over couscous; stir to combine. Cover tightly with plastic wrap; let stand 8 minutes. Fluff with a fork.
- Combine remaining 1/4 teaspoon salt, oil, vinegar, and pepper in a large bowl, stirring with a whisk. Add cucumber, tomato, and oregano; toss to coat. Add cooked couscous; stir to combine. Sprinkle with feta.
- Orange and Fennel Couscous: Prepare couscous as directed in step 1 of base recipe. Combine 2 tablespoons extra-virgin olive oil, 1 tablespoon fresh lemon juice, 1/4 teaspoon kosher salt, and 1/4 teaspoon crushed red pepper in a bowl, stirring with a whisk. Add 3/4 cup rinsed and drained unsalted canned chickpeas, 3/4 cup thinly sliced fennel bulb, 3/4 cup orange sections, and 1/3 cup chopped fresh flat-leaf parsley; toss. Stir in couscous.
- SERVES 4 (serving size: about 1 cup)
- Calories 251; Fat 1g (sat 1g, mono 2g, poly 4g); Protein 8g; Carb 38g; Fiber 3g; Chol 0g; Iron 1mg; Sodium 340mg; calc 54mg
- Cabbage and Radish Couscous: Prepare couscous as directed in step 1 of base recipe. Combine 1 cup very thinly sliced green cabbage, 3/4 cup very thinly sliced radishes, 1/2 cup prepared refrigerated salsa fresca, 2 tablespoons extra-virgin olive oil, 1 tablespoon fresh lime juice, and 1/4 teaspoon freshly ground black pepper in a large bowl. Stir in couscous. Sprinkle with 5 ounces queso fresco.
- SERVES 4 (serving size: 1 cup)
- Calories 242; FatT 8g (sat 4g, mono 1g, poly 9g); Protein 7g; Carb 29g; Fiber 3g; Chol 7g; Iron 1mg; Sodium 315mg; Calc 87mg
- Celery and Cashew Couscous: Prepare couscous as directed in step 1 of base recipe. Combine 2 tablespoons extra-virgin olive oil, 1 tablespoon fresh lemon juice, 1 tablespoon lower-sodium soy sauce, and 1/2 teaspoon brown sugar in a bowl, stirring. Add 1 cup sliced celery and 1 cup mung bean sprouts; toss. Stir in couscous. Sprinkle with 3 1/2 tablespoons chopped unsalted cashews and 2 tablespoons fresh cilantro.
- SERVES 4 (serving size: 3/4 cup)
- Calories 248; Fat 8g (sat 7g, mono 5g, poly 3g); Protein 7g; Carb 31g; Fiber 3g; Chol 0g; Iron 1mg; Sodium 296mg; Calc 26mg

Nutrition Information

- Calories: 223
- Total Fat: 8.9 g
- Total Carbohydrate: 28 g
- Saturated Fat: 2.1 g
- Cholesterol: 6 mg
- Protein: 7 g
- Sodium: 350 mg
- Fiber: 2 g

117. Green Bean Alfredo With Cheese Ravioli

Serving: Makes 6 servings | Prep: 20mins | Cook: 23mins | Ready in:

Ingredients

- 1 (1-pound) package frozen cheese-filled ravioli
- 3 tablespoons butter or margarine
- 1 pound fresh green beans
- 2 garlic cloves, pressed
- 1/2 teaspoon chopped fresh rosemary
- 1 1/2 cups whipping cream
- 3/4 cup dry white wine or chicken broth
- 3/4 teaspoon freshly ground pepper
- 1/4 cup shredded Parmesan cheese
- Garnish: fresh rosemary sprigs

Direction

- Cook pasta according to package directions; keep warm.
- Melt butter in a large nonstick skillet over medium-high heat; add green beans, garlic, and rosemary, and sauté 6 minutes or until beans are crisp-tender. Remove mixture, and set aside.
- Add whipping cream to skillet, and bring to a boil, stirring constantly. Cook, stirring constantly, 10 minutes.
- Return green bean mixture to skillet; add wine and pepper, and cook 5 minutes. Stir in 2 tablespoons cheese. Serve over ravioli, and sprinkle evenly with remaining 2 tablespoons cheese. Garnish, if desired.

118. Grilled Chicken And Soba Noodles With Miso Vinaigrette

Serving: Serves 4 (serving size: 1 chicken cutlet and 3/4 cup noodle mixture) | Prep: | Cook: | Ready in: 22mins

Ingredients

- 3 ounces uncooked soba noodles
- 1/2 cup shredded carrot
- 2 tablespoons canola oil
- 1 tablespoon white/yellow miso (soybean paste)
- 1 tablespoon rice wine vinegar
- 1 tablespoon lower-sodium soy sauce
- 2 teaspoons dark sesame oil
- 1 1/2 teaspoons minced peeled fresh ginger
- 1 teaspoon honey
- 1 1/2 cups thinly sliced red cabbage
- 1/2 cup diagonally sliced green onions
- 1 teaspoon black sesame seeds
- 2 (8-ounce) skinless, boneless chicken breast halves, halved horizontally to form 4 (4-ounce) cutlets
- 1/2 teaspoon freshly ground black pepper
- 1/4 teaspoon kosher salt
- Cooking spray

Direction

- Prepare soba noodles according to package directions. Add carrot during last minute of cooking. Drain; rinse with cold water. Drain.
- Combine oil and next 6 ingredients (through honey) in a large bowl, stirring with a whisk. Place 2 tablespoons miso mixture in a medium bowl. Add noodle mixture, cabbage, and green onions to remaining miso mixture; toss to coat. Sprinkle with sesame seeds.
- Sprinkle chicken with pepper and salt. Add chicken to reserved 2 tablespoons miso mixture, turning to coat. Heat a grill pan over

medium-high heat. Coat pan with cooking spray. Add chicken to pan; cook 3 minutes on each side or until done. Serve with noodle mixture.

Nutrition Information

- Calories: 329
- Fiber: 2 g
- Protein: 30 g
- Total Fat: 12.9 g
- Sodium: 586 mg
- Cholesterol: 73 mg
- Saturated Fat: 1.6 g
- Total Carbohydrate: 25 g

119. Grilled Chicken And Toasted Couscous Salad With Lemon Buttermilk Dressing

Serving: Serves 4 (serving size: 1 chicken cutlet and about 1 cup salad) | Prep: | Cook: | Ready in: 80mins

Ingredients

- MARINADE
- 3 tablespoons olive oil
- 2 garlic cloves, minced
- 1 tablespoon lemon zest plus 2 tsp. fresh lemon juice
- 3 teaspoons chopped fresh thyme
- 1/2 teaspoon kosher salt
- 1/2 teaspoon black pepper
- 4 (5- to 6-oz.) chicken cutlets
- DRESSING
- 3/4 cup buttermilk
- 1/2 cup mayonnaise
- 3 tablespoons finely chopped chives
- 1 tablespoon fresh lemon juice
- 1 garlic clove, pressed
- 1/2 teaspoon finely chopped fresh thyme
- 1/2 teaspoon kosher salt
- 1/2 teaspoon black pepper
- COUSCOUS
- 1 cup uncooked pearl couscous
- 2 (1- x 3-in.) lemon peel strips
- 1 tablespoon olive oil
- 2 cups water
- 1/4 teaspoon kosher salt
- VEGETABLES
- l pound fresh asparagus, trimmed
- 2 tablespoons olive oil, divided
- 1/2 teaspoon kosher salt
- 1/4 teaspoon black pepper
- 3 (1/2-inch-thick) red onion slices

Direction

- Marinade: Whisk together olive oil, garlic cloves, lemon zest and juice, chopped thyme, salt, and black pepper in a small bowl. Place chicken cutlets in a 1-gallon zip-top plastic freezer bag, and add marinade. Seal bag, and turn to coat. Chill 30 minutes to 1 hour, turning occasionally. Remove chicken from bag and marinade; discard marinade.
- Dressing: Whisk together buttermilk, mayonnaise, chives, lemon juice, pressed garlic clove, thyme, salt, and black pepper in a small bowl; cover and chill.
- Couscous: Cook couscous and lemon peel strips in heated olive oil in a medium saucepan over medium, stirring often, until mostly golden, 7 to 8 minutes. Add water and salt; bring to a boil. Cover, reduce heat to low, and simmer until barely tender, 8 to 10 minutes. Drain and discard lemon peel strips.
- Chicken and vegetables: Coat cold cooking grate of grill with cooking spray, and place on grill. Preheat grill to medium (350° to 400°). Toss asparagus with 1 tablespoon olive oil, and sprinkle with salt and black pepper. Brush both sides of onion slices with remaining olive oil. Grill chicken, asparagus, and onions until chicken is done and vegetables are tender and charred, about 3 minutes on each side.
- Slice chicken; cut asparagus into 2-inch pieces, and roughly chop onions. Toss together couscous, chicken, asparagus, onions, and 1/2

cup dressing. Serve salad with remaining dressing.

120. Grilled Chicken And Veggie Tortellini

Serving: Makes 4 servings | Prep: | Cook: | Ready in: 32mins

Ingredients

- 4 small zucchini, cut in half lengthwise (about 1 1/4 lb.)
- 2 skinned and boned chicken breasts (13 oz.)
- 1 tablespoon freshly ground Italian herb seasoning
- 1 (19-oz.) package frozen cheese-filled tortellini
- 1 (7-oz.) container refrigerated reduced-fat pesto
- 2 large tomatoes, seeded and chopped
- Garnish: grated Parmesan cheese

Direction

- Preheat grill to 300° to 350° (medium) heat. Sprinkle zucchini and chicken with seasoning.
- Grill zucchini and chicken at the same time, covered with grill lid. Grill zucchini 6 to 8 minutes on each side or until tender. Grill chicken 5 to 6 minutes on each side or until done. Remove from grill; let stand 10 minutes.
- Meanwhile, prepare tortellini according to package directions.
- Coarsely chop chicken and zucchini. Toss tortellini with pesto, tomatoes, chicken, and zucchini. Serve immediately. Garnish, if desired.
- Note: We tested with McCormick Italian Herb Seasoning Grinder.

121. Grilled Seafood Paella

Serving: 6 | Prep: | Cook: | Ready in:

Ingredients

- BROTH:
- 2 tablespoons vegetable oil
- Reserved shrimp shells (see below)
- 1 medium onion, thinly sliced
- 1 small carrot, thinly sliced
- 3 tablespoons tomato paste
- 1/4 cup dry sherry
- 2 quarts of water
- 6 large garlic cloves, chopped
- 4 thyme sprigs
- 2 bay leaves
- 1 large chipotle chile in adobo
- Large pinch of saffron threads
- Salt
- PAELLA:
- 2 tablespoons extra-virgin olive oil
- 4 scallions, cut into 1-inch lengths
- 1 small onion, finely chopped
- 1 large poblano chile-stemmed, seeded and cut into 1/2-inch dice
- 1 3/4 cups short-grain Spanish rice, such as Valencia or Bomba
- 2 medium tomatoes, chopped
- 1 cup fresh corn kernels
- 1/2 pound green beans, preferably flat Romano, cut into 1-inch lengths
- 1 teaspoon kosher salt
- Large handful of woody herb sprigs, such as rosemary or thyme
- 1 1/2 pounds medium shrimp, shelled and deveined, shells reserved
- 1 1/2 pounds small mussels, scrubbed and debearded

Direction

- MAKE THE BROTH: In a large saucepan, heat the oil. Add the shrimp shells and cook over moderate heat, stirring, until browned, about 5 minutes. Add the onion and carrot and cook, stirring, until the onion begins to brown, 5 minutes longer. Stir in the tomato paste and cook for 2 minutes, stirring. Add the sherry and boil for 1 minute, then add the water and return to a boil. Stir in the garlic, thyme, bay leaves, chipotle and saffron and simmer over low heat for 25 minutes.

- Strain the broth into a saucepan, pressing hard on the solids; you should have 6 cups. Season with salt. Cover and keep warm over low heat.
- MAKE THE PAELLA: Light a grill. If using charcoal, build a large fire that will last at least 30 minutes. Start more coals in a chimney starter to feed the fire. If using a gas grill, set the center burner on high heat and the side or front and back burners on low.
- Place a 14- to 16-inch paella pan or a 14-inch stainless steel roasting pan over a medium-hot fire. Add the olive oil and heat until sizzling. Add the scallions, onion and poblano. If using charcoal, move the pan over to the cooler side of the grill; if using gas, reduce the heat to low. Cook, stirring with a large wooden paddle or spoon, until the vegetables soften, about 5 minutes. Add the rice and cook, stirring, for 2 minutes. Stir in the tomatoes, corn, green beans and salt.
- Add the hot broth to the rice; shake the pan to distribute the rice evenly. Move the pan to the hotter part of a charcoal grill or increase the heat to moderately low on a gas grill. If using charcoal, scatter the herbs over the coals. If using a gas grill, place the herbs in the smoker box or scatter over the heat bars. Cover the grill and let the paella cook, shaking the pan once or twice, until the broth has been absorbed and the rice is almost tender, about 20 minutes. The rice should cook at a steady simmer; add hot coals to the fire if it starts to fade.
- Scatter the shrimp over the rice and nestle the mussels in the paella, hinge side down. Cover the grill; cook until the shrimp are pink and the mussels open, about 5 minutes. Discard any mussels that do not open. Using a large wooden paddle or spoon, transfer the seafood paella to plates, scraping up the crusty rice from the bottom of the pan, and serve.
- Wine Recommendation: A Portuguese Vinho Verde is a refreshing match for the smoky chiles here. Look for a Nonvintage Quinta da Aveleda or the 2000 Grinalda.

122. Grilled Summer Vegetable Lasagna

Serving: 8 servings (serving size: 1 piece) | Prep: | Cook: | Ready in:

Ingredients

- Grilled vegetables:
- 3 large red or yellow bell peppers, seeded and each cut lengthwise into quarters
- Cooking spray
- 3 medium yellow squash, each cut lengthwise into 1/4-inch slices
- 1 large red onion, cut into 1/4-inch slices
- Tomato puree
- 4 pounds tomatoes, cut lengthwise into quarters
- 1/3 cup vodka
- 1 1/2 teaspoons salt
- White sauce:
- 2 1/2 tablespoons all-purpose flour
- 1/4 teaspoon salt
- 1/4 teaspoon ground nutmeg
- 2 cups fat-free milk
- Remaining ingredients:
- 4 quarts water
- 12 uncooked lasagna noodles
- 1 cup chopped fresh basil
- 3/4 teaspoon freshly ground black pepper
- 1 cup (4 ounces) finely shredded Gruyère cheese
- 1/2 cup (2 ounces) grated fresh Parmesan cheese

Direction

- Prepare grill.
- To prepare grilled vegetables, place bell peppers, skin sides down, on a grill rack

coated with cooking spray; cook 15 minutes or until blackened. Place in a zip-top plastic bag; seal. Let stand 15 minutes. Peel and cut into strips.

- Place squash and onion on grill; cook 5 minutes on each side or until tender.
- To prepare tomato purée, place tomatoes in a large Dutch oven. Cover and cook over medium heat 30 minutes or until tender, stirring occasionally. Place tomatoes in a blender or food processor; process until smooth. Return to pan. Stir in vodka; bring to a boil. Reduce heat, and simmer 10 minutes, stirring occasionally. Stir in 1 1/2 teaspoons salt. (You will have 5 cups purée.)
- To prepare white sauce, combine flour, 1/4 teaspoon salt, and nutmeg in a medium saucepan; gradually add the milk, stirring with a whisk. Cook over medium-high heat until thick (about 7 minutes), stirring constantly. Set aside.
- Bring water to a boil in a large stockpot. Add noodles; return to a boil. Cook, uncovered, 10 minutes or until noodles are done, stirring occasionally. Drain.
- Preheat oven to 375°.
- Spread 1/3 cup white sauce in bottom of a 13 x 9-inch baking dish coated with cooking spray. Arrange 3 noodles over white sauce; top with one-third of grilled vegetables, 1/3 cup basil, 1/3 cup white sauce, and 1/2 cup tomato purée. Sprinkle with 1/4 teaspoon black pepper, 1/4 cup Gruyère, and 2 tablespoons Parmesan. Repeat layers twice, ending with noodles. Spread remaining white sauce, 1 1/2 cups tomato purée, remaining Gruyère, and remaining Parmesan over noodles. Bake at 375° for 45 minutes or until bubbly and top is browned. Remove from oven; let stand 15 minutes.
- Note: You will have 2 cups of leftover tomato purée. Cover refriderate for 1 week or freeze up to 3 months.

Nutrition Information

- Calories: 347
- Saturated Fat: 4.3 g
- Total Carbohydrate: 51.8 g
- Fiber: 4.7 g
- Sodium: 567 mg
- Cholesterol: 22 mg
- Total Fat: 8.4 g
- Protein: 17.4 g

123. Ham, Collard Greens, And Egg Noodle Bowl

Serving: 6 servings (serving size: about 1 1/4 cups) | Prep: | Cook: | Ready in:

Ingredients

- 3 1/3 cups uncooked wide egg noodles (about 6 ounces)
- 1 tablespoon butter
- 2 cups diced reduced-sodium smoked ham (about 11 ounces)
- 1 cup chopped onion
- 1/2 cup chopped carrot
- 1/2 cup chopped celery
- 1/2 cup chopped red bell pepper
- 1 teaspoon dried oregano
- 1/2 teaspoon dried thyme
- 3 garlic cloves, minced
- 4 cups sliced collard greens, stems removed
- 2 tablespoons cider vinegar
- 3 cups fat-free, less-sodium chicken broth
- 1/4 teaspoon freshly ground black pepper

Direction

- Cook noodles according to package directions, omitting salt and fat. Drain.
- Melt butter in a large Dutch oven over medium-high heat. Add smoked ham; cook 8 minutes or until lightly browned, stirring frequently. Add chopped onion and next 6 ingredients (through garlic); cook 5 minutes or until vegetables are just tender, stirring frequently. Add collard greens; cook 1 minute,

stirring constantly. Stir in vinegar; cook 1 minute. Stir in chicken broth; bring to a boil. Cover, reduce heat, and simmer 12 minutes. Stir in the egg noodles and black pepper, and cook 1 minute or until thoroughly heated.

Nutrition Information

- Calories: 270
- Fiber: 3.5 g
- Total Fat: 8.8 g
- Sodium: 999 mg
- Cholesterol: 76 mg
- Protein: 18.8 g
- Saturated Fat: 2.8 g
- Total Carbohydrate: 29.4 g

124. Heavenly Chicken Lasagna

Serving: Makes 8 to 10 servings | Prep: | Cook: | Ready in:

Ingredients

- 1 tablespoon butter or margarine
- 1/2 large onion
- 1 (10 1/2-ounce) can reduced-fat cream of chicken soup, undiluted
- 1 (10-ounce) container refrigerated reduced-fat Alfredo sauce
- 1 (7-ounce) jar diced pimiento, undrained
- 1 (6-ounce) jar sliced mushrooms, drained
- 1/3 cup dry white wine
- 1/2 teaspoon dried basil
- 1 (10-ounce) package frozen chopped spinach, thawed
- 1 cup cottage cheese
- 1 cup ricotta cheese
- 1/2 cup grated Parmesan cheese
- 1 large egg, lightly beaten
- 9 lasagna noodles, cooked
- 2 1/2 cups chopped cooked chicken
- 3 cups (12 ounces) shredded sharp Cheddar cheese, divided

Direction

- Melt butter in a skillet over medium-high heat. Add onion, and sauté 5 minutes or until tender. Stir in soup and next 5 ingredients. Reserve 1 cup sauce.
- Drain spinach well, pressing between layers of paper towels.
- Stir together spinach, cottage cheese, and next 3 ingredients.
- Place 3 lasagna noodles in a lightly greased 13- x 9-inch baking dish. Layer with half each of sauce, spinach mixture, and chicken. Sprinkle with 1 cup Cheddar cheese. Repeat procedure. Top with remaining 3 noodles and reserved 1 cup sauce. Cover and chill up to 1 day ahead.
- Bake at 350° for 45 minutes. Sprinkle with remaining 1 cup Cheddar cheese, and bake 5 more minutes or until cheese is melted. Let stand 10 minutes before serving.
- NOTE: For testing purposes only, we used Cantadina Light Alfredo Sauce, found in the dairy section of the supermarket.

125. Individual White Lasagnas

Serving: Serves 8 (serving size: 1 lasagna) | Prep: | Cook: | Ready in: 75mins

Ingredients

- 8 uncooked lasagna noodles
- 1 ounce prosciutto, thinly sliced
- 1 teaspoon extra-virgin olive oil
- 1 shallot, chopped
- 1 (12-ounce) package presliced mushrooms
- 1 (9-ounce) package fresh spinach
- 2 cups part-skim ricotta cheese
- 2 ounces Parmesan cheese, grated
- 2 tablespoons fresh thyme, divided
- 1/2 teaspoon kosher salt

- 1/2 teaspoon black pepper
- 1 ounce fontina cheese, shredded
- Cooking spray
- 2 ounces part-skim mozzarella cheese, shredded (about 1/2 cup)

Direction

- Preheat oven to 350°.
- Cook pasta according to directions until al dente, omitting salt and fat; drain. Cut each noodle crosswise into 4 pieces, forming 32 squares.
- Cook prosciutto in a large skillet over medium-high heat until crisp. Remove prosciutto from pan; crumble. Return pan to medium-high heat. Add oil to pan; swirl to coat. Add shallot; sauté 2 minutes. Add mushrooms; cook 8 minutes, stirring occasionally. Stir in spinach; cook 2 minutes or until spinach wilts. Remove from heat. Drain.
- Combine ricotta cheese, Parmesan, 1 1/2 tablespoons thyme, and next 3 ingredients (through fontina) in a large bowl. Add spinach mixture and prosciutto, stirring well to combine.
- Coat 8 (6-ounce) ramekins with cooking spray. Place ramekins on a jelly-roll pan. Arrange 1 pasta square in bottom of each ramekin. Spoon one-third of filling evenly over pasta squares; top filling with 1 pasta square. Repeat layers twice, ending with pasta. Combine remaining 1 1/2 teaspoons thyme and mozzarella cheese. Sprinkle evenly over lasagnas.
- Cover pan loosely with foil coated with cooking spray. Bake at 350° for 20 minutes. Uncover and bake an additional 15 minutes or until bubbly and browned. Let stand 10 minutes before serving.

Nutrition Information

- Calories: 276
- Total Carbohydrate: 26 g
- Sodium: 503 mg
- Cholesterol: 35 mg
- Total Fat: 11.3 g
- Protein: 19 g
- Saturated Fat: 6 g
- Fiber: 2 g

126. Israeli Couscous And Tomato Salad With Arugula Pesto

Serving: 8 | Prep: | Cook: | Ready in: 30mins

Ingredients

- 6 cups (6 ounces) packed arugula, plus whole leaves for garnish
- 2 cups (12 ounces) Israeli couscous
- 1/2 cup extra-virgin olive oil, plus more for drizzling
- 1/4 cup pine nuts
- 4 garlic cloves, chopped
- 1/4 cup freshly grated Parmigiano-Reggiano cheese
- Salt and freshly ground pepper
- 1 1/2 pints red cherry tomatoes, halved
- 4 yellow or orange tomatoes, cut into 1-inch dice

Direction

- Bring a large saucepan of salted water to a boil. Add the 6 cups of arugula and blanch for 10 seconds. With a slotted spoon, transfer the arugula to a colander. Rinse under cold water to stop the cooking, then drain.
- Add the couscous to the boiling water and cook over moderately high heat, stirring occasionally, until al dente, about 10 minutes. Drain the couscous and spread it out on a large baking sheet. Drizzle lightly with olive oil and toss to prevent clumping. Let the couscous cool to room temperature.
- In a small skillet, toast the pine nuts over moderate heat, tossing, until golden brown, about 2 minutes. Let cool.
- Squeeze the excess water from the arugula and coarsely chop it. Transfer the arugula to a food

processor. Add the pine nuts, garlic, cheese and the 1/2 cup of olive oil and process until the pine nuts are finely chopped. Season the pesto with salt and pepper.

- Transfer the couscous to a large serving bowl and stir in the pesto. Gently fold in the tomatoes. Garnish with the arugula leaves and serve.

127. Italian Sausage And Spinach Lasagna

Serving: 8 servings (serving size: 1/8 of lasagna) | Prep: | Cook: | Ready in:

Ingredients

- 6 whole wheat uncooked lasagna noodles
- 8 ounces hot or mild turkey Italian sausage
- 1 (26-ounce) jar no-salt-added spaghetti sauce
- 1 cup shredded carrot
- 1 (15-ounce) carton fat-free ricotta cheese
- 1/4 teaspoon salt
- 1/2 cup hot water
- 1 (10-ounce) package frozen chopped spinach, thawed, drained, and squeezed dry
- 1/4 cup chopped fresh basil
- 2 cups (8 ounces) preshredded part-skim mozzarella cheese, divided

Direction

- Preheat oven to 375°.
- Cook noodles according to package directions, omitting salt and fat. Drain, but do not rinse. Arrange noodles in a single layer on wax paper to prevent sticking.
- Remove casings from sausage. Cook sausage in a large nonstick skillet over medium-high heat until browned, stirring to crumble. Drain well; return to pan. Add spaghetti sauce and carrot; simmer, uncovered, 10 minutes.
- Spoon 3/4 cup sauce mixture in bottom of a 13 x 9-inch baking dish. Arrange 3 noodles over sauce. Combine ricotta cheese, salt, 1/2 cup hot water, spinach, and basil in a large bowl; spoon half of mixture over noodles. Top with 1 cup mozzarella cheese and 1 cup sauce mixture. Repeat layers with remaining ricotta mixture, 3 noodles, and remaining sauce mixture. Cover dish with foil; bake at 375° for 35 minutes. Uncover, sprinkle with remaining 1 cup mozzarella, and bake 30 minutes. Let stand 10-15 minutes before serving.

Nutrition Information

- Calories: 354
- Total Fat: 14 g
- Saturated Fat: 5 g
- Sodium: 439 mg
- Cholesterol: 35 mg
- Total Carbohydrate: 36 g
- Fiber: 7 g
- Protein: 21 g

128. Korean Shrimp BBQ Bowl

Serving: Serves 1 | Prep: | Cook: | Ready in:

Ingredients

- 2 cups fresh spinach
- 1 ounce shiitake mushrooms
- 1/2 teaspoon canola oil
- 2/3 cup cooked brown rice
- 1/3 cup matchstick-cut carrot
- 1/3 cup shredded cabbage
- 2 tablespoons chopped green onions
- 3 ounces pan-seared large shrimp
- 1 fried egg
- Spicy Aioli:
- 2 teaspoons gochujang (Korean chile sauce)
- 1 1/2 teaspoons canola mayonnaise
- 1/4 teaspoon dark sesame oil
- 1 small garlic clove, minced

Direction

- Sauté spinach and mushrooms in canola oil. Top cooked brown rice with wilted spinach mixture, carrot, cabbage, green onions, shrimp, and egg.
- In a small bowl, combine gochujang, mayonnaise, sesame oil, and minced garlic. Drizzle over bowl.

Nutrition Information

- Calories: 400
- Sodium: 595 mg
- Fiber: 6 g
- Total Fat: 14.3 g
- Protein: 27 g
- Sugar: 7 g
- Total Carbohydrate: 43 g
- Cholesterol: 311 mg
- Saturated Fat: 2.2 g

129. Lamb With Couscous And Roasted Eggplant

Serving: 4 servings (serving size: about 2/3 cup lamb mixture and 3/4 cup eggplant slices) | Prep: 5mins | Cook: 8mins | Ready in:

Ingredients

- 1/2 cup uncooked couscous
- 1 pound lean lamb, cut into 1-inch pieces
- 1/4 teaspoon salt
- 1/4 teaspoon freshly ground black pepper
- Cooking spray
- 1 (14.5-ounce) can diced tomatoes with basil, garlic, and oregano, drained
- 1/3 cup crumbled feta cheese
- Fresh rosemary leaves (optional)
- Roasted Eggplant

Direction

- Prepare couscous according to package directions, omitting salt and fat. Keep warm.
- Sprinkle lamb with salt and pepper. Heat a large nonstick skillet over medium-high heat; coat pan with cooking spray. Add lamb; cook 5 minutes or until browned, turning after 3 minutes. Stir in couscous, tomatoes, cheese, and rosemary, if desired; cook 1 additional minute or until thoroughly heated. Serve over Roasted Eggplant.

Nutrition Information

- Calories: 375
- Protein: 30.8 g
- Saturated Fat: 5.2 g
- Cholesterol: 84 mg
- Sodium: 717 mg
- Total Carbohydrate: 33 g
- Fiber: 7.5 g
- Total Fat: 13.4 g

130. Lasagna Rolls With Roasted Red Pepper Sauce

Serving: 4 servings (serving size: 2 rolls) | Prep: | Cook: | Ready in:

Ingredients

- Lasagna:
- 8 uncooked lasagna noodles
- 4 teaspoons olive oil
- 1/2 cup finely chopped onion
- 1 (8-ounce) package presliced mushrooms
- 1 (6-ounce) package fresh baby spinach
- 3 garlic cloves, minced
- 1/2 cup (2 ounces) shredded mozzarella cheese
- 1/2 cup part-skim ricotta cheese
- 1/4 cup minced fresh basil, divided
- 1/2 teaspoon salt
- 1/4 teaspoon crushed red pepper
- Sauce:
- 1 tablespoon red wine vinegar
- 1/4 teaspoon salt

- 1/4 teaspoon freshly ground black pepper
- 2 garlic cloves, minced
- 1 (14.5-ounce) can diced tomatoes, undrained
- 1 (7-ounce) bottle roasted red bell peppers, undrained
- 1/8 teaspoon crushed red pepper

Direction

- To prepare lasagna, cook noodles according to package directions, omitting salt and fat. Drain and rinse under cold water. Drain.
- Heat oil in a large nonstick skillet over medium-high heat. Add onion, mushrooms, spinach, and 3 garlic cloves; sauté 5 minutes or until onion and mushrooms are tender. Remove from heat, and stir in cheeses, 2 tablespoons basil, 1/2 teaspoon salt, and 1/4 teaspoon crushed red pepper.
- To prepare sauce, place vinegar and remaining ingredients in a blender; process until smooth.
- Place cooked noodles on flat surface; spread 1/4 cup cheese mixture over each noodle. Roll up noodles, jelly-roll fashion, starting with short side. Place the rolls, seam sides down, in a shallow 2-quart microwave-safe dish. Pour 1/4 cup sauce over each roll, and cover with heavy-duty plastic wrap. Microwave at high 5 minutes or until thoroughly heated. Sprinkle with 2 tablespoons basil.

Nutrition Information

- Calories: 393
- Total Carbohydrate: 58.3 g
- Cholesterol: 20 mg
- Protein: 19.3 g
- Fiber: 5.9 g
- Sodium: 924 mg
- Saturated Fat: 4.3 g
- Total Fat: 11.7 g

131. Lasagna With Fall Vegetables, Gruyère, And Sage Béchamel

Serving: 9 servings | Prep: | Cook: | Ready in:

Ingredients

- B[SPECIAL_CHAR
- 2/3 cup all-purpose flour
- 6 cups fat-free milk
- 1/2 cup finely chopped onion
- 1/4 cup chopped fresh sage
- 2 tablespoons finely chopped shallots
- 1/2 teaspoon sea salt
- 1 bay leaf
- Filling:
- 1 tablespoon olive oil, divided
- 2 1/2 cups finely chopped onion
- 3 garlic cloves, minced
- 1 teaspoon sea salt, divided
- 1 (10-ounce) package fresh spinach
- 8 cups chopped portobello mushroom caps (about 1 1/2 pounds)
- 6 cups (1/2-inch) cubed peeled sweet potato (about 2 1/2 pounds)
- Cooking spray
- 1 cup (4 ounces) shredded Gruyère cheese
- 3/4 cup (3 ounces) grated fresh Parmesan cheese
- Noodles:
- 12 precooked lasagna noodles
- 2 cups warm water

Direction

- Preheat oven to 450°.
- To prepare béchamel, lightly spoon flour into dry measuring cups; level with a knife. Place flour in a Dutch oven, and gradually add milk, stirring with a whisk. Add 1/2 cup onion, sage, shallots, 1/2 teaspoon salt, and bay leaf. Bring the mixture to a boil; cook 1 minute or until thick. Strain béchamel through a sieve over a bowl, and discard solids. Set the béchamel aside.

- To prepare the filling, heat 1 1/2 teaspoons olive oil in a large nonstick skillet over medium-high heat. Add 2 1/2 cups onion and garlic; sauté 3 minutes. Add 1/2 teaspoon salt and spinach; sauté 2 minutes or until spinach wilts. Set aside.
- Combine 1 1/2 teaspoons oil, 1/2 teaspoon salt, mushroom, and sweet potato on a jelly roll pan coated with cooking spray. Bake at 450° for 15 minutes.
- Combine cheeses; set aside.
- To prepare noodles, soak noodles in warm water in a 13 x 9-inch baking dish 5 minutes. Drain.
- Spread 3/4 cup béchamel in bottom of a 13 x 9-inch baking dish coated with cooking spray. Arrange 3 noodles over béchamel; top with half of mushroom mixture, 1 1/2 cups béchamel, and 1/3 cup cheese mixture. Top with 3 noodles, spinach mixture, 1 1/2 cups béchamel, and 1/3 cup cheese mixture. Top with 3 noodles, remaining mushroom mixture, 1 1/2 cups béchamel, and 3 noodles. Spread remaining béchamel over noodles. Bake at 450° for 20 minutes. Sprinkle with remaining cheese; bake an additional 10 minutes. Let stand 10 minutes before serving.

Nutrition Information

- Calories: 418
- Total Carbohydrate: 62.7 g
- Cholesterol: 24 mg
- Protein: 22.3 g
- Saturated Fat: 4.5 g
- Total Fat: 9.5 g
- Fiber: 6.4 g
- Sodium: 703 mg

132. Lasagna With Sausage Ragu Redux

Serving: Serves 6 to 8 | Prep: | Cook: | Ready in:

Ingredients

- About 2 tbsp. olive oil, divided
- 1/2 cup chopped onion
- 1/2 cup chopped celery
- 1/2 cup chopped carrot
- 1 pound turkey Italian sausage, casings removed
- 1 teaspoon salt, divided
- 1 cup low-fat (1%) milk
- 1/2 cup dry white wine, such as Chardonnay
- 1 can (28 oz.) whole tomatoes, including juices, finely chopped or crushed with your hands
- 1 cup tomato juice
- 1/2 teaspoon freshly ground black pepper, divided
- 2 1/2 cups low-fat (1%) cottage cheese
- 1 large egg
- 1/2 cup freshly grated parmesan cheese, divided
- 1/4 teaspoon freshly grated nutmeg
- 12 ounces lasagna noodles

Direction

- In a large, heavy saucepan, heat 1 tbsp. oil over medium heat. Add onion; sauté until golden, 5 minutes. Stir in celery and carrot; cook 5 more minutes. Add sausage and 1/2 tsp. salt, breaking up meat with a spoon, and cook until it loses its raw color.
- Add milk and cook over medium heat, stirring, until completely evaporated, 10 to 12 minutes. (The mixture will appear quite curdled at this point.) Add wine and cook until reduced by half, about 3 minutes. Add tomatoes and juice, bring to a boil, lower heat, and gently simmer, uncovered. Cook ragù until liquid reduces by a third, about 30 minutes. Season with 1/4 tsp. pepper and remaining 1/2 tsp. salt.
- In a food processor, whirl cottage cheese, egg, 1/4 cup parmesan, remaining 1/4 tsp. pepper, and the nutmeg until smooth.
- Preheat oven to 375°. Cook lasagna noodles according to package directions; don't

overcook. Drain noodles and lay flat on kitchen towels without overlapping. Oil a 9-by 13-in. baking dish and spread with about 1/2 cup ragù. Add a single layer of noodles (for most brands this is 3 sheets per layer). Spread with a third of ragu, then top with another layer of noodles, half the cheese mixture, and another layer of noodles. Repeat layering, giving you 2 alternating layers of sauce and cheese. Cover with remaining third of ragù and sprinkle evenly with remaining parmesan.

- Cover lasagna with oiled foil and bake until hot, 30 minutes. Let stand 15 minutes before serving.
- Note: Nutritional analysis is per serving.

Nutrition Information

- Calories: 407
- Total Fat: 12 g
- Sodium: 1315 mg
- Total Carbohydrate: 47 g
- Fiber: 3.7 g
- Protein: 29 g
- Saturated Fat: 3.6 g
- Cholesterol: 74 mg

133. Lasagna With Sausage Ragù

Serving: Makes 6 to 8 servings | Prep: | Cook: | Ready in: 180mins

Ingredients

- About 7 tbsp. butter
- 1 tablespoon vegetable oil
- 1/2 cup onion, cut into 1/4-in. dice
- 1/2 cup carrots, cut into 1/4-in. dice
- 1/2 cup celery, cut into 1/4-in. dice
- 1 pound bulk sweet Italian sausage (or 1 lb. sausage links removed from their casings)
- About 1 1/2 tsp. salt
- 4 cups whole milk
- 1/2 cup dry white wine
- 1 can (28 oz.) whole tomatoes, including juices, finely chopped or crushed with your hands
- Freshly ground black pepper
- 1/4 cup flour
- 1/4 teaspoon freshly grated nutmeg
- 12 ounces lasagna noodles (see Notes)
- 1 cup good-quality grated parmesan

Direction

- In a large, heavy-bottomed saucepan, melt 2 tbsp. butter in oil over medium heat. Add onion and cook until golden, about 5 minutes. Add carrots and celery and cook 5 more minutes. Add sausage and 1/2 tsp. salt, breaking up meat with a wooden spoon, and cook until meat loses its raw color.
- Add 1 cup milk and cook over medium heat, stirring, until completely absorbed, 10 to 12 minutes. (The milk will appear quite curdled at this point; don't be alarmed.) Add wine and cook until reduced by half, about 3 minutes. Add tomatoes, bring to a boil, lower heat, and gently simmer, uncovered, 2 hours. Season with salt and pepper to taste.
- After the ragù has cooked for 1 1/2 hours, make the béchamel by melting remaining 5 tbsp. butter in a heavy-bottomed saucepan over medium heat. Add flour and cook, stirring constantly, until it turns light golden brown, about 5 minutes. Slowly drizzle in remaining 3 cups milk, whisking constantly. Bring to a simmer and continue to cook, whisking, until thickened, about 10 minutes. Season with remaining 1 tsp. salt, nutmeg, and pepper to taste.
- Preheat oven to 375°. Cook lasagna noodles according to package directions, being careful not to overcook. Drain and lay flat on dish towels, making sure the noodles do not overlap. Butter the bottom of a 9- by 13-in. baking dish and coat with about 1/2 cup of ragù. Add a single layer of noodles (for most brands this is 4 sheets per layer). Spread on

1/3 of the béchamel; top béchamel with 1/4 of the remaining ragù, then 1/4 of the parmesan. Repeat layering two more times, covering final layer with remaining ragù and parmesan.

- Cover lasagna with buttered aluminum foil and bake 20 minutes. Uncover and bake an additional 10 minutes, or until the top browns slightly. Let sit 15 minutes before serving.
- Note: Nutritional analysis is per serving.

Nutrition Information

- Calories: 721
- Protein: 28 g
- Saturated Fat: 20 g
- Total Carbohydrate: 54 g
- Fiber: 2.7 g
- Sodium: 1617 mg
- Total Fat: 44 g
- Cholesterol: 111 mg

134. Lasagna Style Baked Ziti

Serving: Makes 4 servings | Prep: 20mins | Cook: | Ready in:

Ingredients

- 1 pound ziti
- 1 tablespoon olive oil
- 1 large yellow onion, diced
- 3/4 teaspoon kosher salt
- 1/4 teaspoon black pepper
- 1 pound lean ground beef
- 3 cloves garlic, minced
- 1/2 cup chopped fresh oregano (optional)
- 1 26-ounce jar pasta sauce
- 1/2 cup (2 ounces) grated Parmesan
- 1 15-ounce container ricotta
- 1 10-ounce box frozen spinach, thawed and squeezed to remove liquid
- 1 cup grated mozzarella

Direction

- Cook the ziti according to the package instructions.Heat oven to 400° F.In a large pot, over medium-low heat, heat the oil. Add the onion, salt, and pepper. Cover and cook until the onion is softened, 5 to 7 minutes. Add the beef, increase heat to medium-high, and cook until no trace of pink remains, 5 to 8 minutes. Drain any remaining liquid. Add the garlic and oregano (if using) and cook for 2 minutes. Add the pasta sauce and heat for 3 minutes. Remove from heat. Add the cooked pasta and toss to coat. Add the Parmesan, ricotta, and spinach and toss again. Spread the mixture into a 9-by-13-inch baking dish or individual ramekins and sprinkle with the mozzarella. Bake until the mozzarella melts, about 15 minutes.Tip: If you prefer, substitute Italian sausage for the ground beef and chopped broccoli for the spinach.To Freeze: Assemble (but do not bake) the casserole. Cover tightly with two layers of aluminum foil. Store for up to 3 months.To Reheat: Thaw overnight in the refrigerator or thaw partially in the microwave. Cover and heat in a 350° F oven for 1 hour. Uncover and heat until the mozzarella melts, about 10 minutes more.

Nutrition Information

- Calories: 1165.23
- Fiber: 7.12 g
- Total Carbohydrate: 117.18 g
- Protein: 70.1 mg
- Sodium: 1628.12 mg
- Total Fat: 46.43 g
- Saturated Fat: 21.31 g
- Cholesterol: 176.15 mg

135. Latina Lasagna

Serving: Makes 8 servings | Prep: | Cook: | Ready in: 108mins

Ingredients

- 1 1/2 pounds fresh chorizo sausage, casings removed
- 2 (24-oz.) jars tomato-and-basil pasta sauce
- 1 cup chopped fresh cilantro
- 1 (4.5-oz.) can chopped green chiles
- 1 (15-oz.) container ricotta cheese
- 1 cup whipping cream
- 2 large eggs, lightly beaten
- 12 no-boil lasagna noodles
- 1 (16-oz.) package shredded Mexican four-cheese blend

Direction

- Preheat oven to 375°. Cook sausage in a Dutch oven over medium heat 8 to 10 minutes or until meat is no longer pink, breaking sausage into pieces while cooking. Drain; return sausage to Dutch oven. Reduce heat to medium-low. Stir in pasta sauce, cilantro, and chiles; cook, stirring often, 5 minutes.
- Stir together ricotta cheese, whipping cream, and eggs until smooth.
- Spoon 1 cup sauce mixture into a lightly greased 13- x 9-inch pan. Top with 4 lasagna noodles. Top with half of ricotta cheese mixture, one-third of shredded Mexican cheese blend, and one-third of remaining sauce mixture. Repeat layers once, beginning with noodles. Top with remaining 4 noodles, sauce mixture, and shredded cheese blend. Cover with aluminum foil.
- Bake at 375° for 45 minutes. Uncover and bake 15 minutes or until golden and bubbly. Let stand 20 minutes before serving.

136. Lemon Soy Beef Kebabs With Pearl Couscous

Serving: Serves 4 to 6 | Prep: | Cook: | Ready in:

Ingredients

- 1 lemon
- 1/3 cup vegetable oil
- 1 tablespoon minced garlic
- 1 tablespoon soy sauce
- 1 teaspoon kosher salt, divided
- 1 teaspoon pepper, divided
- 1 1/2 pounds beef sirloin steak, cut into 1 1/2-in. cubes
- 1 cup pearl couscous
- 1 tablespoon extra-virgin olive oil
- 2 medium tomatoes, coarsely chopped (about 1 1/2 cups)
- 1/3 cup chopped red onion
- 1/3 cup chopped fresh parsley

Direction

- Zest and juice lemon. Reserve zest, chilled, for couscous. Combine 3 tbsp. lemon juice (save extra for other uses) with the vegetable oil, garlic, soy sauce, and 1/2 tsp. each salt and pepper in a large resealable plastic bag. Add beef, seal bag, and chill at least 30 minutes and up to 24 hours.
- Heat a grill to high (450° to 550°). Thread beef onto 8 soaked wooden skewers and discard marinade.
- Prepare couscous according to package instructions. In a large bowl, combine couscous with reserved lemon zest, remaining 1/2 tsp. each salt and pepper, the olive oil, tomatoes, red onion, and parsley. Chill if you like or serve at room temperature.
- Grill beef, turning once or twice, until grill marks appear and meat is done the way you like (cut to test), about 8 minutes total for medium-rare. Serve beef with couscous.

Nutrition Information

- Calories: 304
- Total Carbohydrate: 23 g
- Saturated Fat: 2.5 g
- Protein: 26 g
- Total Fat: 12 g
- Fiber: 1.8 g
- Sodium: 416 mg
- Cholesterol: 42 mg

137. Linguine Carbonara

Serving: Serves 4 (serving size: about 3/4 cup) | Prep: | Cook: | Ready in: 22mins

Ingredients

- 8 ounces uncooked linguine
- 3 center-cut bacon slices, cut into 1-inch pieces
- 1/4 cup 1% low-fat milk
- 1/4 teaspoon freshly ground black pepper
- 1/4 teaspoon kosher salt
- 3 large eggs
- 2 ounces Parmigiano-Reggiano cheese, grated (about 1/2 cup)
- 1/4 cup fresh flat-leaf parsley leaves

Direction

- Bring a large pot of water to a boil. Cook pasta according to package directions. Reserve 1/4 cup pasta water; drain pasta.
- Cook bacon in a large skillet over medium heat 5 minutes or until crisp. Remove bacon from pan with a slotted spoon, reserving drippings in pan. Remove pan from heat.
- Combine milk, pepper, salt, eggs, and cheese in a medium bowl, stirring with a whisk. Slowly drizzle in reserved 1/4 cup pasta water, stirring constantly with a whisk. Slowly add pasta to egg mixture, stirring constantly. Add egg mixture to bacon drippings. Place pan over low heat; cook 2 minutes or until liquid begins to thicken, stirring constantly. Sprinkle with bacon and parsley; serve immediately.

Nutrition Information

- Calories: 348
- Cholesterol: 158 mg
- Total Fat: 10.1 g
- Protein: 20 g
- Total Carbohydrate: 44 g
- Sodium: 503 mg
- Fiber: 2 g
- Saturated Fat: 4.7 g

138. Linguine And Clam Sauce

Serving: Serves 4 (serving size: 1 cup pasta and about 7 1/2 clams) | Prep: | Cook: | Ready in: 30mins

Ingredients

- 1/4 cup extra-virgin olive oil, divided
- 6 garlic cloves, finely chopped
- 3 1/4 cups water, divided
- 1 cup dry white wine
- 2 1/2 dozen littleneck clams, scrubbed
- 1 cup clam juice
- 8 ounces uncooked whole-wheat linguine or spaghetti (such as Wild Oats)
- 1/2 teaspoon salt
- 6 tablespoons chopped fresh parsley, divided
- 2 tablespoons minced seeded red serrano or Fresno chile
- 4 lemon wedges

Direction

- Place a 12-inch high-sided sauté pan over medium-high heat. Add 1 tablespoon oil; swirl to coat. Stir in garlic; cook 30 seconds, stirring constantly. Add 1/2 cup water, wine, and clams; cover and cook 6 minutes or until clams open. Discard any unopened shells. Remove clams with a slotted spoon to a plate. Place 12 clams on another plate; cover to keep warm. Remove meat from remaining clams; coarsely chop, and add to plate. Re-cover; keep warm.
- Return pan to medium-high heat. Add clam juice, 2 3/4 cups water, and pasta; bring to a boil. Cook 10 minutes or until pasta is done, stirring frequently. Stir in salt, 3 tablespoons oil, parsley, chile, and chopped clams; toss. Divide pasta among 4 bowls; top each with 3 clams in the shell. Serve with lemon wedges.

Nutrition Information

- Calories: 417
- Sodium: 470 mg
- Protein: 18 g
- Sugar: 3 g
- Total Fat: 16.2 g
- Saturated Fat: 2 g
- Fiber: 7 g
- Cholesterol: 22 mg
- Total Carbohydrate: 47 g

139. Linguine With Arugula Pesto

Serving: 6 servings (serving size: 1 1/3 cups pasta and 1 tablespoon cheese) | Prep: | Cook: | Ready in:

Ingredients

- 12 ounces uncooked linguine
- 1 tablespoon pine nuts, toasted
- 1 garlic clove, crushed
- 2 cups loosely packed arugula
- 2 cups loosely packed basil leaves
- 2 tablespoons extra-virgin olive oil
- 2 teaspoons fresh lemon juice
- 3/4 teaspoon salt
- 1/4 teaspoon black pepper
- 6 tablespoons grated fresh pecorino Romano cheese

Direction

- Cook pasta according to package directions, omitting salt and fat. Drain in a colander over a bowl, reserving 1/2 cup cooking liquid. Place pasta in a bowl.
- Place 1 tablespoon pine nuts and garlic in a food processor; process until minced. Add arugula and the next 5 ingredients (through black pepper), and process until well combined.
- Add arugula mixture and reserved cooking liquid to serving bowl; toss well to coat. Serve with cheese.

Nutrition Information

- Calories: 291
- Saturated Fat: 2 g
- Total Fat: 8.3 g
- Fiber: 2.6 g
- Protein: 10.2 g
- Sodium: 376 mg
- Cholesterol: 7 mg
- Total Carbohydrate: 44 g

140. Linguine With Garlicky Kale And White Beans

Serving: Serves 4 (serving size: about 1 3/4 cups) | Prep: | Cook: | Ready in:

Ingredients

- 8 ounces uncooked linguine
- 3 tablespoons extra-virgin olive oil
- 1/4 cup chopped fresh garlic
- 1/2 cup water
- 1 (8-ounce) package prechopped kale
- 1 (15-ounce) can unsalted cannellini beans, rinsed and drained
- 3/4 teaspoon black pepper, divided
- 1/2 teaspoon salt

Direction

- Cook pasta according to package directions, omitting salt and fat. Drain in a colander over a bowl, reserving 1/4 cup cooking liquid.
- Heat oil and garlic in a large skillet over medium heat. When garlic begins to sizzle, add 1/2 cup water and kale; cover and cook 5 minutes or until kale is tender, stirring occa-sionally. Add beans, 1/2 teaspoon pepper, and salt; cook 1 minute or until

thoroughly heated, stirring occasionally. Add pasta and reserved 1/4 cup cooking liquid to pan; toss to coat. Sprinkle remaining 1/4 teaspoon pepper over pasta. Serve immediately.

Nutrition Information

- Calories: 381
- Protein: 13 g
- Total Carbohydrate: 58 g
- Sodium: 341 mg
- Cholesterol: 0.0 mg
- Fiber: 5 g
- Saturated Fat: 1.7 g
- Total Fat: 11.8 g

141. Linguine With Ricotta Meatballs

Serving: Serves 4 (serving size: about 1 cup pasta mixture, 4 meatballs, and 1 1/2 teaspoons cheese) | Prep: | Cook: | Ready in: 25mins

Ingredients

- 1 (9-ounce) package refrigerated fresh linguine
- 1 ounce pecorino Romano cheese, grated and divided (about 1/4 cup)
- 1/2 cup panko
- 1/3 cup part-skim ricotta cheese
- 8 ounces ground sirloin (90% lean)
- 1 large egg, lightly beaten
- 1 garlic clove, grated
- Cooking spray
- 2 cups lower-sodium marinara sauce (such as Dell'Amore)
- Small basil leaves (optional)

Direction

- Cook pasta according to package directions, omitting salt and fat; drain and keep pasta warm.
- While water for pasta comes to a boil, combine 2 tablespoons pecorino Romano, panko, and next 4 ingredients (through garlic) in a medium bowl. Shape mixture into 16 (1-inch) meatballs. Heat a large skillet over medium-high heat. Coat pan with cooking spray. Add meatballs to pan; cook 6 minutes, turning to brown on all sides. Add marinara; bring to a boil. Cover, reduce heat to medium, and cook 5 minutes or until meatballs are done. Remove pan from heat; remove meatballs from pan with a slotted spoon. Add pasta to pan; toss to coat. Top with meatballs and remaining 2 tablespoons pecorino Romano. Garnish with basil, if desired.

Nutrition Information

- Calories: 459
- Cholesterol: 129 mg
- Total Fat: 15 g
- Saturated Fat: 5.3 g
- Fiber: 5 g
- Protein: 26 g
- Sodium: 623 mg
- Total Carbohydrate: 50 g

142. Linguine With Seafood Sauce

Serving: 12 servings | Prep: | Cook: | Ready in:

Ingredients

- Two 28-ounce cans peeled Italian plum tomatoes
- 2 tablespoons extra-virgin olive oil
- 2 large garlic cloves, smashed
- 2 cups bottled clam juice (16 ounces)
- 2 large thyme sprigs
- 4 large basil leaves

- Pinch of sugar
- Salt and freshly ground pepper
- 2 pounds cleaned baby squid, bodies sliced crosswise into
- 1/2 - inch rings, large tentacles halved
- 1 1/2 pounds thin linguine
- 2 pounds mussels, scrubbed and debearded
- 3 dozen cockles--scrubbed, soaked in cold water for 2 hours and drained
- 1 pound medium shrimp, shelled and deveined
- Crushed red pepper

Direction

- Puree the Italian plum tomatoes in a food processor or blender. Strain them through a fine sieve set over a large bowl; discard the tomato seeds.
- In a large enameled cast-iron casserole, heat the extra-virgin olive oil until shimmering. Add the smashed garlic and cook over moderately high heat until fragrant, about 30 seconds. Add the pureed tomatoes, the clam juice, thyme, basil and sugar. Season with salt and pepper and bring to a boil. Cook over moderately low heat until it is reduced by one-third, about 45 minutes. Add the squid and cook over low heat until very tender, about 45 minutes longer.
- In a large pot of boiling salted water, cook the linguine until al dente. Drain the pasta well and return it to the pot.
- Add the mussels and cockles to the tomato sauce, cover and cook the sauce over moderately high heat until most of the shells have opened, 3 to 5 minutes. Add the shrimp and cook until they are pink and firm, about 2 minutes longer. Discard any unopened mussels and cockles. Pour the tomato-seafood sauce over the cooked pasta and toss over high heat for 2 minutes. Transfer the pasta and sauce to a large warmed bowl, sprinkle with crushed red pepper and serve.
- Make Ahead: The tomato-seafood sauce can be prepared through Step 2 and refrigerated overnight. Bring to a simmer before proceeding.
- Wine Recommendation: A light, bright white with sharp acidity will point up the shellfish and hint of red pepper in this dish. Try a Gavi such as the 1999 Coppo La Rocca or the superb 1999 La Scolca White Label.

143. Linguine With Spinach Herb Pesto

Serving: Serves 4 | Prep: | Cook: | Ready in: 28mins

Ingredients

- 4 ounces fresh baby spinach
- 1/4 cup slivered blanched almonds
- 1/4 cup fresh basil leaves
- 2 teaspoons chopped fresh oregano
- 1 teaspoon chopped fresh thyme
- 1/4 teaspoon black pepper
- 1 large garlic clove, chopped
- 2 tablespoons organic vegetable broth
- 2 teaspoons fresh lemon juice
- 1/4 teaspoon salt
- 2 tablespoons extra-virgin olive oil
- 1 ounce Parmigiano-Reggiano cheese, grated and divided (about 1/4 cup)
- 8 ounces uncooked linguine

Direction

- Place spinach in a microwave-safe bowl; cover bowl with plastic wrap. Microwave at HIGH 2 minutes or until spinach wilts. Remove plastic wrap; cool slightly.
- Place spinach, almonds, and next 5 ingredients (through garlic) in a food processor. Process until chopped. Add broth, juice, and salt; pulse 5 times. With processor on, slowly pour oil through food chute; process until well blended. Scrape into a bowl; stir in half of cheese. Cover with plastic wrap.
- Cook pasta according to package directions, omitting salt and fat. Drain. Toss pasta with

1/2 cup pesto. Arrange about 1 1/2 cups pasta mixture in each of 4 bowls; top each serving with 2 tablespoons remaining pesto and 1 1/2 teaspoons remaining cheese.

Nutrition Information

- Calories: 353
- Sodium: 327 mg
- Cholesterol: 5 mg
- Total Fat: 13.2 g
- Fiber: 4.3 g
- Protein: 12.9 g
- Total Carbohydrate: 48.2 g
- Saturated Fat: 2.6 g

144. Linguine With Sweet Pepper Sauce

Serving: Serves 4 | Prep: | Cook: | Ready in: 33mins

Ingredients

- 8 ounces uncooked linguine
- 1 pound red bell peppers, halved and seeded
- 1 pound yellow bell peppers, halved and seeded
- 3 tablespoons extra-virgin olive oil
- 6 garlic cloves, thinly sliced
- 3/4 teaspoon kosher salt
- 1/4 teaspoon freshly ground black pepper
- 1/4 cup small basil leaves
- 1 (4-ounce) ball Burrata cheese

Direction

- Preheat broiler to high.
- Cook pasta according to package directions until al dente, omitting salt and fat. Drain pasta, reserving 1/4 cup cooking liquid.
- While pasta cooks, place bell peppers, skin sides up, on a foil-lined baking sheet; flatten with hand. Broil 8 minutes or until blackened. Wrap peppers in foil. Let stand 10 minutes; peel. Set aside half of 1 of each color bell pepper. Puree remaining peppers in a food processor.
- Heat a large skillet over medium-low heat. Add oil to pan; swirl. Add garlic; cook 2 minutes or until fragrant and soft, stirring occasionally. Add reserved 1/4 cup cooking liquid, pureed bell pepper, salt, and black pepper; stir with a whisk. Simmer 5 minutes or until thickened. Add pasta; cook 1 minute, tossing to combine.
- Thinly slice reserved bell pepper. Place about 1 cup pasta mixture in each of 4 bowls; top each serving with sliced bell peppers, 1 tablespoon basil, and 1 ounce cheese. Serve immediately.

Nutrition Information

- Calories: 412
- Fiber: 6 g
- Protein: 14 g
- Total Carbohydrate: 55 g
- Total Fat: 14.2 g
- Saturated Fat: 5.3 g
- Cholesterol: 20 mg
- Sodium: 442 mg

145. Linguine With Turkey, Basil, And Crème Fraîche

Serving: Makes 4 servings | Prep: | Cook: | Ready in: 25mins

Ingredients

- 1 (9-ounce) package refrigerated fresh linguine pasta
- 1 (8-ounce) container crème fraîche
- 1 teaspoon lemon zest
- 1/2 teaspoon salt
- 1/4 teaspoon pepper
- 3 cups shredded cooked turkey
- 2 teaspoons fresh lemon juice
- 1/4 cup thinly sliced fresh basil

Direction

- Cook pasta in boiling salted water according to package directions.
- Meanwhile, whisk together crème fraîche and next 3 ingredients in a large bowl. Drain pasta, reserving 1/4 cup cooking water. Toss pasta and turkey in sauce mixture, adding enough cooking water to evenly coat pasta. Stir in lemon juice and basil. Serve immediately.
- *Crème fraîche is a cultured cream product similar to sour cream, but with a less tangy taste and a softer texture. You can substitute Mexican crema or a mixture of equal parts sour cream and whipping cream.

146. Lobster Mac And Cheese

Serving: 8 servings | Prep: 15mins | Cook: 50mins | Ready in:

Ingredients

- 16 ounces corkscrew pasta
- 6 tablespoons melted butter, divided
- 2 large garlic cloves, minced
- 1/2 cup finely chopped red onion
- 1/4 cup all-purpose flour
- 3 cups whole milk, at room temperature
- 1 1/2 cups (6 ounces) grated sharp Cheddar cheese
- 1 1/2 cups (6 ounces) grated Gruyère cheese
- 1 tablespoon Dijon mustard
- 1/2 cup minced fresh chives
- 1/8 teaspoon cayenne pepper
- 1/2 teaspoon salt, divided
- 1/2 teaspoon freshly ground black pepper, divided
- 1 pound coarsely chopped cooked lobster meat
- 2 cups oyster crackers, crushed

Direction

- Cook pasta until al dente according to package directions. Drain, rinse with cold water, and drain again.
- Place 4 tablespoons melted butter in a saucepot over medium-low heat. Add garlic and onion; cook 5 minutes or until onion is softened. Whisk in flour; cook 1 minute. Pour in milk; bring mixture to a boil over medium-high heat, whisking frequently. Reduce heat to medium-low, and simmer 3 minutes or until sauce is smooth and thickened.
- Remove from heat, and whisk in cheeses and next 3 ingredients. Stir in 1⁄4 teaspoon salt and 1⁄4 teaspoon pepper. Fold in pasta and lobster. Pour into a greased 3-quart baking dish.
- Combine crushed crackers and remaining 2 tablespoons melted butter. Stir in remaining 1⁄4 teaspoon salt and 1⁄4 teaspoon pepper. Sprinkle over casserole. Bake at 375° for 30 minutes or until crust is crisp and sauce bubbles. Let stand 5 minutes before serving.

147. Macaroni Salad

Serving: Serves 10 to 12 | Prep: | Cook: | Ready in: 30mins

Ingredients

- 1 pound ditalini or elbow pasta
- Olive oil or vegetable oil
- 1 teaspoon salt
- 1 teaspoon pepper
- 3/4 cup mayonnaise
- 2 tablespoons French's mustard
- 3/4 cup sweet pickle relish
- 2/3 cup finely chopped jarred red peppers or roasted red peppers
- 2/3 cup sliced canned black olives

Direction

- Boil pasta in a large pot of salted water, with a dash of oil, until very tender, 12 to 15 minutes. Drain, then rinse with cold water until cool.

- Mix remaining ingredients in a large bowl. Stir in cooled pasta. Taste and add more of any of the seasonings if you like. Chill until very cold.
- Make ahead: Up to 2 days, covered and chilled.

Nutrition Information

- Calories: 228
- Protein: 5.6 g
- Saturated Fat: 1 g
- Sodium: 605 mg
- Cholesterol: 3.8 mg
- Total Fat: 6.6 g
- Total Carbohydrate: 38 g
- Fiber: 1.8 g

148. Macaroni Salad With Bacon, Peas, And Creamy Dijon Dressing

Serving: 8 servings (serving size: 1 cup salad and about 1 teaspoon bacon) | Prep: | Cook: | Ready in:

Ingredients

- Dressing:
- 1/2 cup (4 ounces) 1/3-less-fat cream cheese
- 1/4 cup chopped shallots
- 1/4 cup reduced-fat mayonnaise
- 2 tablespoons fat-free sour cream
- 2 tablespoons Dijon mustard
- 2 tablespoons lemon juice
- 1 tablespoon white wine vinegar
- 3/4 teaspoon black pepper
- 1/2 teaspoon kosher salt
- Salad:
- 8 ounces uncooked large elbow macaroni
- 2/3 cup fresh green peas
- 2/3 cup finely diced red bell pepper
- 2/3 cup finely diced red onion
- 1/2 cup thinly sliced green onions
- 1/4 cup chopped fresh flat-leaf parsley
- 1/2 teaspoon grated lemon rind
- 3 lower-sodium bacon slices, cooked and crumbled

Direction

- To prepare dressing, combine first 9 ingredients in a food processor, and process until smooth. Cover and chill.
- To prepare salad, cook pasta according to package directions, omitting salt and fat; add peas during the last 3 minutes of cooking time. Drain; rinse with cold water. Drain. Combine pasta mixture, bell pepper, and next 4 ingredients (through rind) in a large bowl. Toss pasta mixture with half of dressing. Cover and chill until ready to serve. Toss salad with remaining dressing, and sprinkle with crumbled bacon; serve immediately.

Nutrition Information

- Calories: 208
- Total Carbohydrate: 29.1 g
- Saturated Fat: 3.2 g
- Cholesterol: 16 mg
- Fiber: 2.3 g
- Protein: 8.6 g
- Sodium: 454 mg
- Total Fat: 7 g

149. Macaroni And Cheese

Serving: Makes 6 to 8 servings | Prep: | Cook: | Ready in:

Ingredients

- 1 pound elbow macaroni
- 5 tablespoons unsalted butter, plus more for the dish
- 1/2 cup all-purpose flour
- 6 cups whole or low-fat milk
- 1 1/2 cups (6 ounces) grated Cheddar
- 2 cups (8 ounces) grated Gruyère

- 1 1/2 teaspoons kosher salt
- 1/4 teaspoon cayenne (optional)

Direction

- Heat oven to 350° F. Cook the macaroni according to the package directions. Melt the butter in a saucepan over medium heat. Sprinkle the flour over the top. Cook, stirring constantly, for 2 minutes. Still stirring, slowly add the milk. Cook, stirring occasionally, until the sauce has thickened, about 7 minutes. Add the Cheddar, Gruyère, salt, and cayenne (if using) and heat until the cheeses melt. Drain and rinse the macaroni. Add it to the sauce and toss. Transfer to a buttered casserole. Bake for 25 to 30 minutes.In Advance: Assemble the macaroni and cheese but do not bake it. Cover and refrigerate for up to 24 hours. Bake as directed, adding 15 to 20 minutes to the cooking time.

Nutrition Information

- Calories: 581
- Protein: 27 g
- Saturated Fat: 17 g
- Sodium: 651 mg
- Total Fat: 27 g
- Fiber: 2 g
- Total Carbohydrate: 57 g
- Sugar: 11 g
- Cholesterol: 86 mg

150. Macaroni And Cheese With Cauliflower

Serving: Makes 6 servings | Prep: 15mins | Cook: | Ready in:

Ingredients

- 12 ounces multigrain elbow macaroni
- 1 head cauliflower, roughly chopped
- 4 slices multigrain bread, torn
- 1/2 cup fresh flat-leaf parsley, chopped
- 3 tablespoons olive oil
- Kosher salt and pepper
- 1 onion, finely chopped
- 1 1/2 cups grated extra-sharp Cheddar (6 ounces)
- 1 1/2 cups reduced-fat sour cream
- 1/2 cup 1 percent milk
- 1 tablespoon Dijon mustard

Direction

- Heat oven to 400° F. Cook the pasta according to the package directions, adding the cauliflower during the last 3 minutes of cooking time; drain. Meanwhile, pulse the bread in a food processor until coarse crumbs form. Add the parsley, 2 tablespoons of the oil, and 1/4 teaspoon each salt and pepper and pulse to combine; set aside. Return the pasta pot to medium heat and add the remaining tablespoon of oil. Add the onion, 3/4 teaspoon salt, and 1/2 teaspoon pepper and cook, stirring occasionally, just until soft, 5 to 7 minutes. Mix in the pasta, cauliflower, cheese, sour cream, milk, and mustard. Transfer to a shallow 3-quart baking dish, sprinkle with the bread crumbs, and bake until golden brown, 12 to 15 minutes.

Nutrition Information

- Calories: 537
- Saturated Fat: 9 g
- Protein: 24 g
- Cholesterol: 51 mg
- Sugar: 8 g
- Total Carbohydrate: 63 g
- Fiber: 8 g
- Sodium: 692 mg
- Total Fat: 23 g

151. Manicotti Florentine

Serving: 7 servings (serving size: 2 stuffed pasta shells and about 1/3 cup pasta sauce) | Prep: | Cook: | Ready in:

Ingredients

- 1 (8-ounce) package uncooked manicotti shells
- 1 cup (4 ounces) shredded part-skim mozzarella cheese, divided
- 1/2 cup grated fresh Parmesan cheese, divided
- 2 (10-ounce) packages frozen chopped spinach, thawed, drained, and squeezed dry
- 1 1/2 cups 2% low-fat cottage cheese
- 3/4 cup chopped green onions (about 6 onions)
- 1 teaspoon lemon pepper
- 1/2 teaspoon dried oregano
- 1/4 teaspoon garlic powder
- 1 (15-ounce) container part-skim ricotta cheese
- 3 large egg whites
- 1 (26-ounce) jar garlic-and-herb pasta sauce (such as Healthy Choice)
- Cooking spray
- 2 tablespoons chopped fresh parsley

Direction

- Preheat over to 350°.
- Cook pasta according to package directions, omitting salt and fat.
- While pasta cooks, combine 1/2 cup mozzarella, 1/4 cup Parmesan, spinach, and next 7 ingredients in a large bowl; stir well. Drain pasta, and rinse with cold water to prevent sticking; drain. Spoon spinach mixture evenly into pasta shells (about 1/3 cup filling in each).
- Spoon 1/2 cup pasta sauce in bottom of a 13 x 9-inch baking dish coated with cooking spray. Arrange stuffed pasta shells over sauce in dish; top with remaining sauce. Sprinkle evenly with remaining 1/2 cup mozzarella, remaining 1/4 cup Parmesan, and parsley. Cover and bake at 350° for 45 minutes or until thoroughly heated. Uncover and bake an additional 5 minutes.

Nutrition Information

- Calories: 367
- Total Fat: 10.3 g
- Saturated Fat: 6.3 g
- Sodium: 868 mg
- Total Carbohydrate: 41.8 g
- Fiber: 5.2 g
- Protein: 28.5 g
- Cholesterol: 43 mg

152. Meatball And Ziti Bake

Serving: Serves 4 (serving size: about 1 3/4 cups) | Prep: | Cook: | Ready in:

Ingredients

- 6 ounces uncooked whole-wheat ziti
- 1/3 cup panko (Japanese breadcrumbs)
- 2 tablespoons minced garlic, divided
- 1/2 teaspoon kosher salt, divided
- 1/4 teaspoon freshly ground black pepper
- 12 ounces 90% lean ground sirloin
- 1 large egg
- 1 tablespoon olive oil
- 1/4 cup chopped fresh basil, divided
- 1/2 teaspoon crushed red pepper
- 1 (28-ounce) can unsalted crushed tomatoes
- 2 ounces part-skim mozzarella cheese, shredded (about 1/2 cup)

Direction

- Preheat broiler to high.
- Cook pasta according to package directions, omitting salt and fat. Drain in a colander over a bowl; reserve 1/2 cup cooking liquid.
- Place panko, 1 tablespoon garlic, 1/4 teaspoon salt, black pepper, beef, and egg in a bowl, stirring just until combined. Shape beef

mixture into 12 (1-inch) meatballs. Heat a large ovenproof skillet over medium-high heat. Add oil; swirl to coat. Add meatballs to pan; cook 5 minutes, turning to brown on all sides. Add remaining 1 tablespoon garlic; cook 30 seconds. Add reserved 1/2 cup cooking liquid, remaining 1/4 teaspoon salt, 3 tablespoons basil, crushed red pepper, and tomatoes to pan. Reduce heat to medium; cover and simmer 15 minutes.

- Stir pasta into tomato mixture; spread evenly in skillet. Sprinkle cheese over top; broil 1 minute or until cheese melts. Sprinkle with remaining 1 tablespoon basil.

Nutrition Information

- Calories: 474
- Total Carbohydrate: 47 g
- Total Fat: 16.2 g
- Protein: 31 g
- Cholesterol: 106 mg
- Fiber: 7 g
- Saturated Fat: 5.7 g
- Sodium: 415 mg

153. Meatballs And Spaghetti

Serving: Serves 6 (serving size: 2/3 cup pasta, 3 meatballs, and 2/3 cup sauce) | Prep: | Cook: | Ready in: 100mins

Ingredients

- 1 tablespoon olive oil
- 2 cups minced onion
- 1/4 cup water
- 4 cups lower-sodium marinara sauce
- 1/2 cup chopped fresh basil
- 1/4 cup (1 ounce) grated fresh Parmesan cheese
- 1 teaspoon dried oregano
- 1/4 teaspoon salt
- 1/4 teaspoon crushed red pepper
- 1 garlic clove, minced
- 1 large egg, lightly beaten
- 3/4 pound ground sirloin
- 3/4 pound ground pork
- 1 (1.5-ounce) slice firm white bread, crumbled
- 8 ounces uncooked spaghetti
- Grated fresh Parmesan cheese (optional)

Direction

- Heat a large skillet over medium heat. Add oil to pan; swirl to coat. Stir in onion; cover and cook 10 minutes. Uncover; stir, and reduce heat to medium. Cook 15 minutes or until onion is tender, stirring frequently. Add 1/4 cup water, stirring to loosen browned bits; cook 10 minutes, stirring frequently. Remove from heat; cool 10 minutes.
- Place marinara sauce in a Dutch oven. Bring to a simmer over low heat.
- Combine onion mixture, basil, and next 6 ingredients (through egg) in a large bowl. Add ground sirloin, ground pork, and crumbled bread; stir gently to combine. Shape meat mixture into 18 (2-inch) balls. Place meatballs in sauce. Bring to a boil; cover, reduce heat, and simmer 30 minutes or until meatballs are done.
- While meatballs simmer, cook pasta according to package directions, omitting salt and fat; drain.
- Serve meatballs and sauce over pasta. Sprinkle with Parmesan cheese, if desired.

Nutrition Information

- Calories: 537
- Total Carbohydrate: 46.7 g
- Total Fat: 24.3 g
- Protein: 31.4 g
- Saturated Fat: 8.3 g
- Cholesterol: 113 mg
- Fiber: 3.8 g
- Sodium: 406 mg

154. Meaty Cheese Manicotti

Serving: Makes 6 servings | Prep: 15mins | Cook: 20mins | Ready in:

Ingredients

- 1 (8-ounce) package uncooked manicotti shells
- 1/2 pound hot Italian sausage
- 1/2 pound ground round
- 1 medium onion, chopped
- 1/2 cup dry white wine
- 2 cups whipping cream
- 1 teaspoon dried Italian seasoning
- 1/2 teaspoon salt
- 1/2 teaspoon pepper
- 1 (14 1/2-ounce) can diced tomatoes with basil, garlic, and oregano, drained
- 2 cups (8 ounces) shredded mozzarella cheese
- 3/4 cup shredded Parmesan cheese

Direction

- Cook pasta according to package directions; rinse in cold water. Drain. Place in a single layer on a wire rack; set aside.
- Remove casings from sausage, and discard. Cook sausage, ground round, and onion in a large skillet, stirring until meat crumbles and is no longer pink. Drain and set aside.
- Add wine to skillet, stirring to loosen browned bits; bring to a boil. Add whipping cream and next 3 ingredients; reduce heat, and simmer, stirring often, 15 minutes or until thickened. Remove from heat; cover and set aside.
- Combine meat mixture, tomatoes, and mozzarella cheese. Spoon mixture evenly into 12 manicotti shells; arrange shells in a lightly greased 13- x 9-inch baking dish.
- Bake, covered, at 350° for 20 minutes. Uncover and pour cream mixture evenly over shells; sprinkle with Parmesan cheese. Bake, uncovered, at 350° for 10 more minutes. Broil, 5 1/2 inches from heat, 2 to 3 minutes or until cheese is lightly browned.

155. Mexican Mac And Cheese

Serving: Makes 6 to 8 servings | Prep: | Cook: | Ready in: 20mins

Ingredients

- 1/4 cup plus 1 1/2 tsp. kosher salt, divided
- 1 qt. milk
- 6 tablespoons butter, cut into pieces
- 6 tablespoons all-purpose flour
- 1 pound pasta (such as penne, cavatappi, or rotini)
- 1 pound Mexican chorizo
- 1 tablespoon olive oil
- 1 (8-oz.) package shredded extra-sharp Cheddar cheese
- 1 (8-oz.) package shredded pepper Jack cheese
- 1 teaspoon hot sauce (such as Tabasco)
- 1/2 teaspoon freshly ground black pepper
- 1 1/2 cups crushed tortilla chips
- 2 teaspoons olive oil
- 2 cups cherry tomatoes, halved

Direction

- Preheat broiler with oven rack 8 to 9 inches from heat.
- Bring 1/4 cup salt and 4 qt. water to a boil in a large covered Dutch oven over high heat.
- Meanwhile, microwave milk in a microwave-safe 1-qt. glass measuring cup covered with plastic wrap at HIGH 3 minutes. While milk is heating, melt butter in a 12-inch cast-iron skillet over medium heat. Reduce heat to medium-low; add flour, and cook, whisking constantly, 2 minutes. Gradually whisk in hot milk. Increase heat to medium-high, and bring to a low boil, whisking often.
- Add pasta to boiling water, and cook 8 minutes.
- While pasta cooks, sauté chorizo in 1 Tbsp. hot olive oil in a large skillet over medium-high heat 4 to 5 minutes or until crumbled and cooked.

- Meanwhile, continue to cook sauce, whisking often, 6 minutes. Remove from heat; whisk in cheeses, hot sauce, 1 1/2 tsp. salt, and 1/2 tsp. pepper. Cover.
- Stir together crushed tortilla chips and 2 tsp. olive oil.
- Drain pasta, and fold into cheese sauce. Fold in cooked chorizo and cherry tomato halves. Sprinkle with tortilla chips mixture.
- Broil 1 to 2 minutes or until breadcrumbs are golden brown. Serve immediately.

156. Mini Bow Ties With Bacon And Peas

Serving: Serves 4 (serving size: 1 1/4 cups) | Prep: | Cook: | Ready in:

Ingredients

- 8 ounces uncooked mini farfalle (bow tie pasta)
- 3 center-cut bacon slices, chopped
- 1/2 cup prechopped onion
- 2 medium carrots, peeled and diced
- 1 cup unsalted chicken stock
- 1 cup frozen green peas
- 1 tablespoon chopped fresh thyme
- 5/8 teaspoon kosher salt
- 1/2 teaspoon black pepper
- 3 ounces 1/3-less-fat cream cheese

Direction

- Cook pasta according to package directions, omitting salt and fat. Drain pasta, reserving 1/4 cup cooking liquid; set aside.
- Heat a large nonstick skillet over medium-high heat. Add bacon; cook 4 minutes, stirring frequently. Remove bacon with a slotted spoon.
- Add onion and carrot to drippings in pan; cook 5 minutes. Add stock; bring to a boil. Add peas; cook 2 minutes.
- Remove pan from heat; stir in reserved 1/4 cup cooking liquid, bacon, thyme, salt, pepper, and cream cheese. Add pasta to pan; toss to coat. Serve immediately.

Nutrition Information

- Calories: 333
- Total Carbohydrate: 53 g
- Protein: 15 g
- Fiber: 5 g
- Sugar: 7 g
- Total Fat: 7.4 g
- Saturated Fat: 3.8 g
- Cholesterol: 21 mg
- Sodium: 566 mg

157. Miso Vegetable Noodle Bowl

Serving: 6 servings (serving size: 1 1/2 cups) | Prep: | Cook: | Ready in:

Ingredients

- 4 ounces uncooked udon noodles (thick, round fresh Japanese wheat noodles) or spaghetti
- 3 cups water
- 3 cups vegetable broth
- 1 1/2 cups frozen shelled edamame, thawed
- 1 cup thinly sliced napa (Chinese) cabbage
- 1 cup (1/8-inch) diagonally cut carrot
- 1 cup thinly sliced red bell pepper
- 1 cup diagonally cut snow peas
- 1 cup thinly sliced shiitake mushroom caps
- 1/2 cup finely chopped green onions
- 2 tablespoons fresh lime juice
- 1 tablespoon minced peeled fresh ginger
- 3 tablespoons yellow miso (soybean paste)
- 2 teaspoons chile paste with garlic
- 2 tablespoons minced fresh cilantro
- Lime wedges (optional)

Direction

- Cook noodles in a Dutch oven according to package directions, omitting salt and fat. Rinse with cold water; drain.
- Bring water and broth to a boil in pan. Add noodles, edamame, and next 6 ingredients (edamame through onions). Remove from heat.
- Combine juice, ginger, miso, and chile paste, stirring with a whisk; stir into soup. Sprinkle with cilantro; serve with lime wedges, if desired.

Nutrition Information

- Calories: 214
- Total Carbohydrate: 29.5 g
- Cholesterol: 0.0 mg
- Saturated Fat: 0.5 g
- Fiber: 5.8 g
- Sodium: 948 mg
- Total Fat: 5.9 g
- Protein: 14.2 g

158. Mushroom Gnocchi

Serving: Makes 4 servings | Prep: | Cook: | Ready in:

Ingredients

- 1 (16-oz.) package gnocchi (such as Gia Russa)
- 2 tablespoons butter
- 1 (16-oz.) package fresh button mushrooms, quartered
- 1 (4-oz.) package fresh gourmet mushroom blend
- 3 tablespoons sliced fresh shallots
- 4 garlic cloves, thinly sliced
- 2 tablespoons butter
- 1/2 cup loosely packed fresh flat-leaf parsley leaves
- 1/2 teaspoon kosher salt
- 1/2 teaspoon pepper

Direction

- Prepare gnocchi according to package directions. Melt 2 Tbsp. butter in a large skillet over medium-high heat. Add button mushrooms and mushroom blend; sauté 3 minutes or until lightly browned and liquid evaporates. Add shallots and garlic; sauté 2 minutes or until shallots are tender. Add 2 Tbsp. butter to skillet; cook 2 minutes or until lightly browned. Add gnocchi; gently toss. Stir in parsley, salt, and pepper.

159. Mushroom Lasagna

Serving: Serves 6 | Prep: | Cook: | Ready in: 85mins

Ingredients

- 1 cup boiling water
- 1 ounce dried porcini mushrooms
- 1 tablespoon butter
- 2 tablespoons olive oil, divided
- 1 1/4 cups chopped shallots (about 4)
- 1 (8-ounce) package presliced cremini mushrooms
- 1 (4-ounce) package presliced exotic mushroom blend
- 1 teaspoon salt, divided
- 1/2 teaspoon freshly ground black pepper, divided
- 1 1/2 tablespoons chopped fresh thyme
- 6 garlic cloves, minced and divided
- 1/2 cup white wine
- 1/3 cup (3 ounces) 1/3-less-fat cream cheese
- 2 tablespoons chopped fresh chives, divided
- 3 cups 2% reduced-fat milk, divided
- 1.1 ounces all-purpose flour (about 1/4 cup)
- Cooking spray
- 9 no-boil lasagna noodles
- 1/2 cup (2 ounces) grated Parmigiano-Reggiano cheese

Direction

- Preheat oven to 350°.

- Combine 1 cup boiling water and porcini. Cover and let stand 30 minutes; strain mixture through a cheesecloth-lined sieve over a bowl, reserving liquid and mushrooms.
- Melt butter in a large skillet over medium-high heat. Add 1 tablespoon oil to pan; swirl to coat. Add shallots to pan; sauté 3 minutes. Add cremini and exotic mushrooms, 1/2 teaspoon salt, and 1/4 teaspoon pepper; sauté 6 minutes or until mushrooms are browned. Add thyme and 3 garlic cloves; sauté 1 minute. Stir in wine; bring to a boil. Cook 1 minute or until liquid almost evaporates, scraping pan to loosen browned bits. Remove from heat; stir in cream cheese and 1 tablespoon chives. Add reserved porcini mushrooms.
- Heat a saucepan over medium-high heat. Add remaining 1 tablespoon oil to pan; swirl to coat. Add remaining 3 garlic cloves to pan; sauté 30 seconds. Add the reserved porcini liquid, 2 3/4 cups milk, remaining 1/2 teaspoon salt, and remaining 1/4 teaspoon pepper; bring to a boil. Combine remaining 1/4 cup milk and flour in a small bowl; stir with a whisk. Add flour mixture to milk mixture, and simmer 2 minutes or until slightly thick, stirring constantly with a whisk.
- Spoon 1/2 cup sauce into an 11 x 7-inch glass or ceramic baking dish coated with cooking spray, and top with 3 noodles. Spread half of mushroom mixture over noodles. Repeat layers, ending with remaining sauce. Sprinkle cheese over top. Bake at 350° for 45 minutes or until golden. Top with remaining 1 tablespoon chopped chives.

Nutrition Information

- Calories: 396
- Saturated Fat: 7.1 g
- Total Carbohydrate: 43.5 g
- Fiber: 3.2 g
- Sodium: 668 mg
- Cholesterol: 33 mg
- Total Fat: 15.4 g
- Protein: 17.1 g

160. Mustard Dill Tortellini Salad Skewers

Serving: Makes 12 servings | Prep: 25mins | Cook: 5mins | Ready in:

Ingredients

- 1 (9-oz.) package refrigerated cheese tortellini
- 1 (8-oz.) package frozen sugar snap peas
- 68 (4-inch) wooden skewers
- 1 pt. grape tomatoes, cut in half
- Mustard-Dill Vinaigrette*

Direction

- Cook tortellini according to package directions. Rinse under cold running water.
- Place sugar snap peas in a small bowl; cover with plastic wrap. Microwave at HIGH 2 minutes. Let stand, covered, 2 minutes. Rinse under cold running water.
- Thread each skewer with 1 sugar snap pea, 1 tortellini, and 1 tomato half. Place skewers in a 13- x 9-inch baking dish. Pour Mustard-Dill Vinaigrette over skewers, turning to coat. Cover and chill 4 hours. Transfer skewers to a serving platter; discard any remaining vinaigrette.
- *1 (12-oz.) bottle light Champagne vinaigrette may be substituted. For testing purposes only, we used Girard's Light Champagne Dressing.

161. One Pan Broccoli Bacon Mac 'n' Cheese

Serving: Serves 6 (serving size: about 1 1/3 cups) | Prep: | Cook: | Ready in: 25mins

Ingredients

- 2 center-cut bacon slices, chopped

- 3 garlic cloves, minced
- 2 cups unsalted chicken stock (such as Swanson)
- 1 cup 1% low-fat milk
- 1 (10-ounce) package frozen butternut squash puree, thawed
- 10 ounce uncooked large elbow macaroni
- 3 cups chopped broccoli florets
- 1/2 teaspoon salt
- 1/2 teaspoon freshly ground black pepper
- 5 ounces sharp cheddar cheese, shredded and divided (about 1 1/4 cups)

Direction

- 1 Heat a large skillet over medium-high heat. Add bacon; cook 4 minutes or until crisp, stirring occasionally. Remove bacon from pan.
- Remove all but 2 teaspoons bacon drippings from pan. Add garlic to -drippings in pan; sauté 30 seconds.
- Add stock, milk, and squash to pan; bring to a boil, stirring occasionally.
- Add pasta; cover, -reduce heat, and -simmer 5 minutes, -stirring occasionally. Stir in broccoli; cover and cook 3 minutes or until pasta is done and sauce is thickened.
- 5 Stir in salt, pepper, and 4 ounces cheese. Sprinkle bacon and remaining cheese on top. Cover; let stand 1 minute.

Nutrition Information

- Calories: 339
- Protein: 18 g
- Sodium: 566 mg
- Total Carbohydrate: 45 g
- Cholesterol: 29 mg
- Total Fat: 10 g
- Fiber: 4 g
- Saturated Fat: 5.7 g

162. One Pan Mac 'n' Cheese

Serving: Serves 4 (makes 6 1/2 cups) | Prep: | Cook: | Ready in: 50mins

Ingredients

- BREAD CRUMBS AND SAUCE
- 1 1/2 cups fresh ciabatta bread crumbs*
- 1 1/2 tablespoons olive oil
- 1 1/8 teaspoons kosher salt, divided
- About 3/4 tsp. pepper, divided
- 3/4 teaspoon smoked sweet paprika
- 1/4 cup salted butter
- 1/4 cup flour
- 2 cups milk
- 2 cups shredded sharp cheddar cheese
- PASTA
- 12 ounces Barilla Pronto elbow macaroni (a one-pan, no-drain pasta)* or regular macaroni

Direction

- AT HOME
- Toast bread crumbs: In a large frying pan over medium heat, cook crumbs with oil and 1/8 tsp. each salt and pepper, stirring often, until crumbs begin to crisp, 4 to 5 minutes. Add paprika and cook, stirring, until crunchy, 2 to 4 more minutes. Pour from pan to a bowl and let cool; then seal in a lidded container or resealable plastic bag.
- Make sauce: Melt butter in a medium saucepan over medium-high heat. Add flour and remaining 1 tsp. salt and 1/2 tsp. pepper; whisk until bubbling and light tan, 1 1/2 to 2 minutes. Add milk and cook, whisk-ing, until sauce bubbles and thickens, 3 to 5 minutes. Remove from heat, add cheese, and whisk until melted. Let cool, then transfer to a lidded container and chill in refrigerator or cooler.
- IN CAMP
- Pour no-drain pasta into a 12-in. cast-iron skillet or other large, deep frying pan on a camp stove; add 3 cups cold water. Cook over high heat, stirring often, until all but about 1/2 cup water is absorbed, 10 to 15 minutes. (For regular pasta, cook in a large pot of boiling

water until just tender. Set aside 1/2 cup cooking water; drain pasta and return to pot with reserved water.)

- Add cheese sauce to pasta and bring to a simmer, stirring often. Spoon into bowls and scatter bread crumbs over each serving.
- *Whirl a few slices of bread in a food processor to make crumbs. Find Pronto pasta at well-stocked grocery stores.
- Make ahead: Through step 2, up to 3 days.

Nutrition Information

- Calories: 834
- Protein: 32 g
- Total Carbohydrate: 88 g
- Fiber: 3.4 g
- Saturated Fat: 21 g
- Cholesterol: 104 mg
- Total Fat: 40 g
- Sodium: 990 mg

163. Orange And Fennel Couscous

Serving: Serves 4 (serving size: about 1 cup) | Prep: | Cook: | Ready in:

Ingredients

- 3/4 cup unsalted chicken stock
- 3/4 cup uncooked couscous
- 1/2 teaspoon kosher salt, divided
- 2 tablespoons extra-virgin olive oil
- 1 tablespoon fresh lemon juice
- 1/4 teaspoon crushed red pepper
- 3/4 cup rinsed and drained unsalted canned chickpeas
- 3/4 cup thinly sliced fennel bulb
- 3/4 cup orange sections
- 1/3 cup chopped fresh flat-leaf parsley

Direction

- Bring stock to a boil in a small saucepan over high heat. Place couscous and 1/4 teaspoon salt in a small baking dish. Pour stock over couscous; stir to combine. Cover tightly with plastic wrap; let stand 8 minutes. Fluff with a fork.
- Combine olive oil, lemon juice, remaining 1/4 teaspoon kosher salt, and crushed red pepper in a bowl, stirring with a whisk. Add chickpeas, fennel, orange sections, and parsley; toss. Stir in couscous.

Nutrition Information

- Calories: 251
- Total Fat: 8.1 g
- Sodium: 340 mg
- Total Carbohydrate: 38 g
- Protein: 8 g
- Saturated Fat: 1.1 g
- Cholesterol: 0.0 mg
- Fiber: 3 g

164. Orange And Tomato Simmered Chicken With Couscous

Serving: Serves 4 (serving size: about 1/2 cup couscous, 2 chicken thighs, and about 1/2 cup sauce) | Prep: | Cook: | Ready in: 30mins

Ingredients

- 1 medium fennel bulb with stalks
- 2 teaspoons olive oil
- 8 skinless, bone-in chicken thighs (about 1 1/2 pounds)
- 1/4 teaspoon kosher salt
- 1/4 teaspoon freshly ground black pepper
- 3/4 cup prechopped onion
- 1 carrot, cut into 1/4-inch-thick slices
- 1/4 teaspoon ground cinnamon
- 1/4 teaspoon ground red pepper (optional)
- 1/3 cup orange juice

- 10 pitted kalamata olives, quartered
- 1 (14.5-ounce) can unsalted diced tomatoes, drained
- 1 1/4 cups water
- 1 cup whole-wheat couscous

Direction

- Trim tough outer leaves from fennel; mince feathery fronds to measure 2 tablespoons. Remove and discard stalks. Cut fennel bulb in half lengthwise; discard core. Vertically slice fennel bulb.
- Heat a large skillet over medium-high heat. Add oil to pan; swirl to coat. Sprinkle chicken with salt and black pepper. Add chicken to pan; cook 3 minutes on each side or until well browned. Transfer chicken to a plate.
- Add sliced fennel, onion, and carrot to pan; cook 3 minutes. Add cinnamon and red pepper, if desired; cook 1 minute. Add orange juice, olives, and tomatoes. Increase heat to high, and bring to a boil. Add chicken and accumulated juices to pan. Reduce heat to medium, and cook 20 minutes or until chicken is done.
- Bring 1 1/4 cups water to a boil in a medium saucepan. Stir in couscous; cover. Remove from heat; let stand 5 minutes. Fluff with a fork.
- Serve chicken and vegetables over couscous. Top with fennel fronds.

Nutrition Information

- Calories: 466
- Sodium: 374 mg
- Protein: 35 g
- Saturated Fat: 3.3 g
- Cholesterol: 99 mg
- Total Fat: 15.3 g
- Total Carbohydrate: 47 g
- Fiber: 6 g

165. Oysters Over Angel Hair

Serving: 6 servings (serving size: 1 1/3 cups) | Prep: | Cook: | Ready in:

Ingredients

- 3 tablespoons olive oil
- 1 cup sliced green onions
- 1/2 cup chopped fresh parsley
- 3 garlic cloves, minced
- 4 cups standard oysters (about 3 [12-ounce] containers), drained
- 2 tablespoons fresh lemon juice
- 1/4 teaspoon salt
- 1/8 teaspoon ground red pepper
- 1/8 teaspoon black pepper
- 6 cups hot cooked angel hair (about 14 ounces uncooked pasta)
- 1/2 cup (2 ounces) grated fresh Parmesan cheese

Direction

- Heat oil in a large nonstick skillet over medium heat. Add onions, parsley, and garlic; cook 8 minutes or until tender, stirring frequently. Add oysters; reduce heat, and cook 5 minutes or until edges of oysters curl. Stir in lemon juice, salt, and peppers. Add pasta and cheese; tossing well to coat.

Nutrition Information

- Calories: 470
- Total Fat: 14.5 g
- Total Carbohydrate: 58.9 g
- Cholesterol: 100 mg
- Sodium: 450 mg
- Fiber: 2.3 g
- Protein: 24.4 g
- Saturated Fat: 3.7 g

166. Pasta Primavera

Serving: 4 servings (serving size: 2 cups) | Prep: | Cook: | Ready in:

Ingredients

- 1 1/2 cups baby carrots, trimmed (about 6 ounces)
- 3 cups uncooked cavatappi or penne pasta (about 8 ounces)
- 1 teaspoon olive oil
- 2 cups pattypan squash, halved (about 8 ounces)
- 3/4 cup shelled green peas
- 1 teaspoon salt
- 1/4 teaspoon freshly ground black pepper
- 2 garlic cloves, minced
- 1/4 cup dry white wine
- 1/3 cup whipping cream
- 1 tablespoon fresh lemon juice
- 1/4 cup (1 ounce) grated fresh Parmesan cheese
- 1/4 cup thinly sliced fresh basil
- 1/4 cup chopped fresh parsley

Direction

- Bring 2 quarts of water to a boil in a stockpot. Add carrots; cook 3 minutes. Remove with a slotted spoon. Add pasta to boiling water; cook according to package directions, omitting salt and fat. Drain.
- Heat oil in a large nonstick skillet over medium-high heat. Add squash; sauté 3 minutes. Add carrots, peas, salt, pepper, and garlic; sauté 2 minutes. Stir in wine, scraping pan to loosen browned bits. Stir in cream and juice; cook 1 minute. Add pasta and cheese; stir well to coat. Remove from heat; stir in basil and parsley.
- Wine Note: Squash, peas, carrots, and an ample amount of herbs give this pasta a satisfying freshness that's made luxurious by cream and Parmesan. A crisp Sauvignon Blanc would be perfect, especially one that's refined and effortless to drink. Try Robert Mondavi Funé Blanc from the Napa Valley (about $18). (Note: Fumé Blanc is just another name for Sauvignon Blanc. See my wine column, page)
- Pasta Primavera with Shrimp and Sugar Snap Peas: Substitute 2 cups sugar snap peas for the green peas; cook sugar snap peas in boiling water with carrots. Substitute 1 pound peeled and deveined medium shrimp for pattypan squash; sauté 2 minutes. Stir in 2 cups trimmed arugula and 2 tablespoons chopped green onions with the basil and parsley. Yield: 4 servings (serving size: 2 1/4 cups.
- CALORIES 501 (24% from fat); FAT 5 (sat 4g, mono 9g, poly 7g); PROTEIN 4g; CARB 3g; CHOL 204mg; IRON 5mg; SODIUM 972mg; CALC 252mg.
- Pasta Primavera with Chicken and Asparagus: Substitute 2 cups (1-inch) sliced asparagus for carrot. Substitute 12 ounces skinless, boneless chicken breast for pattypan squash. Cut the chicken crosswise into 1/4-inch-wide strips; sauté 5 minutes. Increase green peas to 1 cup. Stir in 2 tablespoons green onions with basil ana parsley. Yeild: 4 servings (serving size:2 cups.)
- CALORIES 463 (24% from fat); FAT 6g (sat 4g, mono 9g, poly 2g); Protein 6g; CARB 1g; FIBER 1g; CHOL 81mg; IRON 4mg; SODIUM 773mg; CALC 154mg.

Nutrition Information

- Calories: 373
- Protein: 13.9 g
- Total Carbohydrate: 53.8 g
- Cholesterol: 32 mg
- Fiber: 4.5 g
- Saturated Fat: 6.1 g
- Sodium: 731 mg
- Total Fat: 11.8 g

167. Pasta Primavera With Arugula Pesto

Serving: Serves 6 (serving size: 1 1/2 cups pasta) | Prep: | Cook: | Ready in:

Ingredients

- 2 zucchini, thinly sliced
- 2 red onions, thinly sliced
- 1 tablespoon olive oil
- 1/4 teaspoon salt
- 1/4 teaspoon pepper
- 2 cups arugula
- 1 garlic clove, minced
- 3 walnut halves, toasted and chopped
- 1 tablespoon lemon juice
- 1 teaspoon lemon zest
- 1/4 cup grated Parmesan
- 1/4 teaspoon salt
- 1/4 teaspoon pepper
- 3 tablespoons olive oil
- 1 pound cooked penne
- 1/2 cup halved grape tomatoes
- 2 tablespoons lemon juice

Direction

- Preheat oven to 425°. In a bowl, toss zucchini and onions with 1 tablespoon olive oil and 1/4 tsp each salt and pepper. Spread on 2 baking sheets. Roast until tender (about 15 minutes), stirring once. In a food processor or blender, process arugula, garlic, walnuts, 1 tablespoon lemon juice, lemon zest, Parmesan, and 1/4 tsp each salt and pepper, pouring in 3 tablespoons olive oil in a slow stream. In a large bowl, toss arugula pesto with penne, roasted vegetables, grape tomatoes, and 2 tablespoons lemon juice.

Nutrition Information

- Calories: 414
- Protein: 12 g
- Fiber: 3 g
- Sodium: 254 mg
- Total Carbohydrate: 62 g
- Total Fat: 12.3 g
- Saturated Fat: 2 g
- Cholesterol: 3 mg

168. Pasta With Shrimp And Tomato Caper Sauce

Serving: Serves 4 (serving size: 1 1/2 cups) | Prep: | Cook: | Ready in: 28mins

Ingredients

- 8 ounces uncooked linguine
- 2 1/2 teaspoons olive oil, divided
- 12 ounces medium shrimp, peeled and deveined
- 1 cup chopped zucchini
- 1/2 cup chopped onion
- 3 garlic cloves, minced
- 1/4 teaspoon kosher salt
- 1/4 teaspoon crushed red pepper
- 1 (28-ounce) can whole plum tomatoes, rinsed and drained
- 1/4 cup fat-free, lower-sodium chicken broth
- 1 tablespoon capers, drained and chopped
- 1/4 cup small fresh basil leaves

Direction

- Cook pasta according to package directions, omitting salt and fat; drain.
- Heat a large nonstick skillet over medium-high heat. Add 1 1/2 teaspoons oil; swirl. Add shrimp; cook 3 minutes or until done. Remove shrimp from pan.
- Wipe out pan with a paper towel. Return pan to medium-high heat. Add remaining 1 teaspoon oil; swirl to coat. Add zucchini and onion; sauté 3 minutes. Add garlic; sauté 30 seconds. Add salt, red pepper, and tomatoes; lightly mash tomatoes with a potato masher. Reduce heat to medium, and simmer 8 minutes. Stir in broth; return to a simmer. Stir in pasta, shrimp, and capers; toss to coat.

Remove pan from heat; top with basil. Serve immediately.

Nutrition Information

- Calories: 340
- Total Carbohydrate: 53 g
- Sodium: 654 mg
- Saturated Fat: 0.8 g
- Fiber: 4 g
- Protein: 22 g
- Total Fat: 4.7 g
- Cholesterol: 107 mg

169. Penne All'Amatriciana

Serving: Serves 4 | Prep: | Cook: | Ready in: 30mins

Ingredients

- 8 ounces penne pasta
- 4 ounces pancetta or good-quality bacon, cubed
- 1 cup chopped onion
- 1 tablespoon minced garlic
- 1 large can (28 oz.) diced tomatoes
- 1 teaspoon kosher salt
- 1 teaspoon freshly ground black pepper
- 1 teaspoon red chile flakes
- 1/4 cup grated parmesan cheese

Direction

- Cook pasta according to package directions; drain and set aside.
- Cook pancetta in a large frying pan over medium-high heat until partly translucent. Spoon off most of drippings. Add onion and garlic; cook, stirring often, until browned, 5 minutes. Add remaining ingredients except parmesan and cook over high heat until juices have reduced by half, about 10 minutes. Add pasta, stir to coat, and transfer to a bowl. Sprinkle with parmesan.
- Note: Nutritional analysis is per serving.

Nutrition Information

- Calories: 362
- Saturated Fat: 3.3 g
- Fiber: 3.7 g
- Protein: 14 g
- Total Fat: 9.4 g
- Cholesterol: 13 mg
- Sodium: 856 mg
- Total Carbohydrate: 56 g

170. Penne And Chicken Tenderloins With Spiced Tomato Sauce

Serving: 4 servings (serving size: about 1 1/2 cups) | Prep: | Cook: | Ready in: 36 minutesmins

Ingredients

- 1 teaspoon ground fennel seed
- 1 teaspoon dried basil
- 1/2 teaspoon salt
- 1/2 teaspoon ground coriander
- 1/4 teaspoon freshly ground black pepper
- 1 pound chicken breast tenders, cut into (1-inch) pieces
- 1 tablespoon olive oil
- 4 garlic cloves, minced
- 4 cups canned diced tomatoes, undrained
- 1 cup white wine
- 8 ounces uncooked penne
- 1/4 cup (1 ounce) freshly grated Parmigiano-Reggiano cheese
- 1/4 cup chopped fresh basil

Direction

- Combine first 5 ingredients in a small bowl; rub over chicken.
- Heat oil in a large nonstick skillet over medium-high heat. Add chicken; cook 4

minutes, turning once. Remove from heat; set aside.

- Reduce heat to medium. Add garlic; sauté 30 seconds or until garlic is soft. Add tomatoes and wine, scraping pan to loosen browned bits. Bring to a boil. Reduce heat, and simmer 15 minutes. Add chicken, and simmer 5 minutes.
- Cook pasta according to package directions, omitting salt and fat. Drain. Toss pasta with sauce in a large bowl. Sprinkle with cheese and basil.

Nutrition Information

- Calories: 446
- Saturated Fat: 1.9 g
- Fiber: 6.5 g
- Cholesterol: 70 mg
- Total Fat: 7.2 g
- Sodium: 774 mg
- Total Carbohydrate: 57.1 g
- Protein: 38.5 g

171. Penne With Asparagus, Pistachios, And Mint

Serving: Serves 4 (serving size: about 2 cups pasta mixture, 1 tablespoon pistachios, and 1 1/2 teaspoons mint) | Prep: | Cook: | Ready in:

Ingredients

- 8 ounces uncooked whole-grain penne pasta
- 5 teaspoons extra-virgin olive oil, divided
- 1 pound asparagus, trimmed and cut diagonally into 1 1/2-inch pieces
- 3 green onions, chopped, white and green parts divided
- 2 large garlic cloves, minced
- 1/4 cup dry white wine
- 1/2 teaspoon kosher salt
- 1/4 teaspoon freshly ground black pepper
- 2 teaspoons butter
- 1.5 ounces pecorino Romano cheese, grated (about 1/3 cup)
- 1/4 cup chopped pistachios
- 2 tablespoons chopped fresh mint

Direction

- Cook pasta according to package directions, omitting salt and fat. Drain in a colander over a bowl, reserving 1/4 cup cooking liquid. Return pasta and 1/4 cup reserved cooking liquid to pan. Cover and keep warm over low heat.
- Heat a nonstick skillet over medium-high heat. Add 1 tablespoon oil to pan; swirl to coat. Add asparagus; sauté 3 minutes or until crisp-tender. Stir in white parts of green onions and garlic; cook 30 seconds. Add wine; cook 1 minute. Add asparagus mixture, salt, and pepper to pasta mixture. Stir in remaining 2 teaspoons oil, remaining green onions, butter, and cheese. Divide pasta evenly among 4 bowls. Sprinkle evenly with pistachios and mint.

Nutrition Information

- Calories: 400
- Total Fat: 15.4 g
- Fiber: 5 g
- Protein: 15 g
- Cholesterol: 16 mg
- Saturated Fat: 5.4 g
- Sodium: 474 mg
- Total Carbohydrate: 51 g

172. Penne With Asparagus, Spinach, And Bacon

Serving: 4 servings (serving size: about 1 1/2 cups pasta mixture and 1 tablespoon cheese) | Prep: | Cook: | Ready in:

Ingredients

- 8 ounces uncooked penne pasta
- 2 bacon slices
- 1/2 cup chopped sweet onion
- 2 1/2 cups (1-inch) slices asparagus (about 1 pound)
- 1 1/2 cups fat-free, less-sodium chicken broth
- 4 cups bagged baby spinach leaves
- 1/2 cup (2 ounces) preshredded Parmesan cheese, divided
- 1/4 teaspoon black pepper

Direction

- Cook pasta according to the package directions, omitting salt and fat. Drain; keep warm.
- Cook bacon in a large nonstick skillet over medium heat until crisp. Remove bacon from pan; crumble. Add onion to drippings in pan; sauté 1 minute. Add asparagus and broth to pan; bring to a boil. Reduce heat, and simmer 5 minutes or until asparagus is crisp-tender. Add pasta, spinach, 1/4 cup cheese, and pepper to pan; toss well. Sprinkle with remaining 1/4 cup cheese and bacon.

Nutrition Information

- Calories: 363
- Sodium: 501 mg
- Protein: 17.8 g
- Cholesterol: 18 mg
- Total Fat: 10.2 g
- Total Carbohydrate: 49.1 g
- Fiber: 4.6 g
- Saturated Fat: 4.2 g

173. Penne With Ricotta And Greens

Serving: Serves 4 (serving size: about 2 cups) | Prep: | Cook: | Ready in:

Ingredients

- 12 ounces uncooked whole-wheat penne rigate
- 2 teaspoons extra-virgin olive oil
- 1/2 cup finely chopped onion
- 1/4 teaspoon crushed red pepper
- 1 garlic clove, minced
- 1/2 cup part-skim ricotta cheese
- 2 teaspoons fresh lemon juice
- 1/2 teaspoon kosher salt
- 1/4 teaspoon black pepper
- 1 (5-ounce) package fresh baby spinach, coarsely chopped
- 2 ounces baby arugula
- 1 bunch watercress, trimmed
- 3 tablespoons shaved pecorino Romano cheese

Direction

- Cook pasta according to package directions, omitting salt and fat. Drain in a colander over a bowl, reserving 1/4 cup pasta water.
- Heat a large skillet over medium-high heat. Add oil, onion, red pepper, and garlic; sauté 2 minutes. Add pasta, reserved 1/4 cup pasta water, ricotta, lemon juice, salt, and black pepper; cook 1 to 2 minutes. Remove from heat.
- Combine spinach, arugula, and pasta mixture in a large bowl, stirring until spinach begins to wilt. Stir in watercress. Top with pecorino cheese.

Nutrition Information

- Calories: 388
- Protein: 18 g
- Fiber: 11 g
- Sodium: 421 mg
- Cholesterol: 14 mg
- Total Fat: 9.4 g
- Saturated Fat: 2.8 g
- Total Carbohydrate: 71 g

174. Penne With Sausage And Peppers

Serving: Serves 6 | Prep: | Cook: | Ready in: 40mins

Ingredients

- Salt and pepper
- 1 pound penne
- 1 tablespoon olive oil
- 1 pound sweet or hot Italian sausage, removed from casings
- 1 large red bell pepper, seeded, thinly sliced
- 1 large green bell pepper, seeded, thinly sliced
- 1 small onion, halved, thinly sliced
- 2 teaspoons garlic-herb seasoning
- 1 teaspoon Italian seasoning
- Grated Parmesan for serving, optional

Direction

- Bring a large pot of salted water to a boil. Cook penne until al dente, approximately 9 minutes or as package label directs. Drain, reserving 1/2 cup cooking liquid. Return pasta to pot.
- Warm oil in a large skillet over medium heat. Add sausage and cook, stirring to break up chunks, until no longer pink, 5 to 6 minutes. Remove sausage to a plate, and pour off all but 1 Tbsp. fat.
- In same skillet, cook peppers, onion and seasonings over medium heat, stirring occasionally, until vegetables are tender, about 12 minutes. Add sausage to pepper mixture; cook, stirring, until warmed through, about 30 seconds. Taste and season with salt and pepper, if desired.
- Add sausage mixture to pasta. Toss to combine, adding cooking liquid as necessary to moisten. Serve hot, topped with Parmesan if desired.

Nutrition Information

- Calories: 412
- Total Carbohydrate: 61 g
- Fiber: 3 g
- Cholesterol: 23 mg
- Total Fat: 8 g
- Protein: 22 g
- Saturated Fat: 3 g
- Sodium: 531 mg

175. Penne With Spicy Vodka Cream Sauce

Serving: Makes 4 entrée servings or 8 side dish servings | Prep: 10mins | Cook: 25mins | Ready in:

Ingredients

- 16 ounces uncooked penne or other short pasta
- 4 pancetta slices or thick bacon slices
- 1 tablespoon butter
- 1 tablespoon olive oil
- 2 shallots, chopped
- 1 garlic clove, minced
- 1/4 teaspoon dried crushed red pepper
- 1/2 cup vodka
- 1/2 cup chicken stock or broth
- 2 (14.5-ounce) cans fire-roasted diced tomatoes, undrained
- 1 (8-ounce) can tomato sauce
- 3/4 teaspoon salt
- 1/4 teaspoon freshly ground black pepper
- 1/2 cup heavy whipping cream
- 2 tablespoons chopped fresh basil
- Garnishes: Parmesan cheese shavings, fresh basil leaves

Direction

- Prepare pasta according to package directions.
- Meanwhile, cook pancetta in a large nonstick skillet over medium-high heat until crisp. Remove pancetta, and drain on paper towels. Wipe skillet clean.
- Melt butter in a large skillet over medium-high heat. Stir in oil, shallots, garlic, and red

pepper; sauté 3 to 4 minutes or until shallots are tender.

- Stir in vodka; bring to a boil, reduce heat, and simmer 3 minutes or until reduced by half. Stir in stock and next 4 ingredients, and simmer 15 more minutes.
- Reduce heat to low; stir in cream, basil, and pancetta. Cook 2 minutes or until heated through. (Do not boil.) Spoon pasta into serving bowls; top with sauce. Garnish, if desired.

176. Pesto Lasagna With Spinach And Mushrooms

Serving: 8 servings | Prep: | Cook: | Ready in:

Ingredients

- 4 cups torn spinach
- 2 cups sliced cremini mushrooms
- 1/2 cup commercial pesto
- 3/4 cup (3 ounces) shredded part-skim mozzarella cheese
- 3/4 cup (3 ounces) shredded provolone cheese
- 1 (15-ounce) carton fat-free ricotta cheese
- 1 large egg, lightly beaten
- 3/4 cup (3 ounces) grated fresh Parmesan cheese, divided
- 1 (25.5-ounce) bottle fat-free tomato-basil pasta sauce
- 1 (8-ounce) can tomato sauce
- Cooking spray
- 1 (8-ounce) package precooked lasagna noodles (12 noodles)

Direction

- Arrange the spinach in a vegetable steamer; steam, covered, 3 minutes or until spinach wilts. Drain, squeeze dry, and coarsely chop. Combine spinach, mushrooms, and pesto in a medium bowl, stirring to combine; set aside.
- Combine mozzarella, provolone, ricotta, and beaten egg in a medium bowl, stirring well to combine. Stir in 1/4 cup Parmesan, and set aside. Combine the pasta sauce and the tomato sauce in a medium bowl.
- Spread 1 cup pasta sauce mixture in the bottom of a 6-quart oval electric slow cooker coated with cooking spray. Arrange 3 noodles over pasta sauce mixture; top with 1 cup cheese mixture and 1 cup spinach mixture. Repeat the layers, ending with spinach mixture. Arrange 3 noodles over spinach mixture; top with remaining 1 cup cheese mixture and 1 cup pasta sauce mixture. Place remaining 3 noodles over sauce mixture; spread remaining sauce mixture over noodles. Sprinkle with the remaining 1/2 cup Parmesan. Cover with lid; cook on LOW 5 hours or until done.

Nutrition Information

- Calories: 398
- Total Fat: 18.2 g
- Total Carbohydrate: 38.5 g
- Cholesterol: 56 mg
- Protein: 22.2 g
- Sodium: 1036 mg
- Fiber: 2 g
- Saturated Fat: 7.8 g

177. Pesto Shrimp Pasta

Serving: 4 servings (serving size: 1 cup shrimp pasta and 1 tablespoon cheese) | Prep: 8mins | Cook: 15mins | Ready in:

Ingredients

- 4 ounces uncooked angel hair pasta
- 6 cups water
- 1 1/4 pounds peeled and deveined large shrimp
- 1/4 cup commercial pesto, divided
- 1 cup halved grape tomatoes

- 1/4 cup (1 ounce) shaved fresh Parmesan cheese
- Basil sprigs (optional)

Direction

- Cook pasta according to package directions, omitting salt and fat; drain.
- While pasta cooks, bring 6 cups water to a boil in a large saucepan. Add shrimp; cook 2 to 3 minutes or until done. Drain shrimp; toss with 2 tablespoons pesto and tomatoes. Stir in pasta and 2 tablespoons pesto. Top with cheese. Garnish with basil, if desired.

Nutrition Information

- Calories: 320
- Sodium: 505 mg
- Cholesterol: 220 mg
- Fiber: 1.9 g
- Total Carbohydrate: 23.6 g
- Total Fat: 11 g
- Protein: 31.4 g
- Saturated Fat: 2.7 g

178. Pizza Spaghetti Casserole

Serving: Makes 6 servings | Prep: 15mins | Cook: 15mins | Ready in:

Ingredients

- 12 ounces uncooked spaghetti
- 1/2 teaspoon salt
- 1 (1-lb.) package mild ground pork sausage
- 2 ounces turkey pepperoni slices (about 30), cut in half
- 1 (26-oz.) jar tomato-and-basil pasta sauce
- 1/4 cup grated Parmesan cheese
- 1 (8-oz.) package shredded Italian three-cheese blend

Direction

- Cook spaghetti with 1/2 tsp. salt according to package directions. Drain well, and place in a lightly greased 13- x 9-inch baking dish.
- Brown sausage in a large skillet over medium-high heat, stirring occasionally, 5 minutes or until meat crumbles and is no longer pink. Drain and set aside. Wipe skillet clean. Add pepperoni, and cook over medium-high heat, stirring occasionally, 4 minutes or until slightly crisp.
- Top spaghetti in baking dish with sausage; pour pasta sauce over sausage. Arrange half of pepperoni slices evenly over pasta sauce. Sprinkle evenly with cheeses. Arrange remaining half of pepperoni slices evenly over cheese. Cover with nonstick or lightly greased aluminum foil.
- Bake at 350° for 30 minutes; remove foil, and bake 10 more minutes or until cheese is melted and just begins to brown.

179. Pronto Stuffed Pasta Shells

Serving: Makes 4 to 6 servings | Prep: 30mins | Cook: | Ready in:

Ingredients

- 18 jumbo pasta shells
- 2 (10-oz.) packages frozen chopped spinach, thawed
- 2 cups chopped cooked Herb-Roasted Chickens
- 1 tablespoon chopped fresh basil
- 1 (16-oz.) container low-fat cottage cheese
- 1 large egg, lightly beaten
- 1/4 cup grated Parmesan cheese
- 1/4 teaspoon ground nutmeg
- 1 (16-oz.) jar Alfredo sauce

Direction

- Prepare pasta shells according to package directions.

- Meanwhile, drain chopped spinach well, pressing between paper towels.
- Stir together spinach, chicken, basil, and next 4 ingredients. Spoon mixture evenly into shells.
- Spread half of jarred Alfredo sauce in a lightly greased 13- x 9-inch baking dish. Arrange stuffed pasta shells over sauce, and pour remaining sauce over shells.
- Bake, covered, at 350° for 40 to 45 minutes or until filling is hot and sauce is bubbly. Remove from oven, and let stand 10 minutes.
- Note: To make ahead, prepare recipe as directed through Step Cover and freeze up to 1 month. Thaw in refrigerator 24 hours. Let stand at room temperature 30 minutes. Bake, covered, for 1 hour and 20 minutes.

180. Pumpkin Ravioli

Serving: 6 servings (serving size: 4 ravioli) | Prep: | Cook: | Ready in:

Ingredients

- 1 cup canned pumpkin
- 1/3 cup grated Parmesan cheese
- 1/4 teaspoon salt
- 1/8 teaspoon black pepper
- 24 wonton wrappers
- 1 teaspoon salt
- 1/2 cup chicken broth
- 1 1/2 tablespoons unsalted butter
- Chopped parsley

Direction

- Combine 1 cup pumpkin, 1/3 cup Parmesan, 1/4 teaspoon salt, and 1/8 teaspoon black pepper. Spoon about 2 teaspoons pumpkin mixture into center of each wonton wrapper. Moisten edges of dough with water; bring 2 opposite sides together to form a triangle, pinching edges to seal. Place ravioli into a large saucepan of boiling water with 1 teaspoon salt; cook 7 minutes, and drain in a colander. Place 1/2 cup broth and 1 1/2 tablespoons butter in pan; bring to a boil. Add ravioli, tossing to coat. Sprinkle with parsley.

Nutrition Information

- Calories: 162
- Total Fat: 5 g
- Fiber: 2 g
- Protein: 6 g
- Saturated Fat: 4 g
- Cholesterol: 17 mg
- Total Carbohydrate: 22 g
- Sodium: 505 mg

181. Pumpkin Ravioli With Gorgonzola Sauce

Serving: 6 servings | Prep: | Cook: | Ready in:

Ingredients

- 1 1/4 cups canned pumpkin
- 2 tablespoons dry breadcrumbs
- 2 tablespoons fresh grated Parmesan cheese
- 1/2 teaspoon salt
- 1/2 teaspoon minced fresh sage
- 1/4 teaspoon freshly ground black pepper
- 1/8 teaspoon ground nutmeg
- 30 round wonton wrappers
- 1 tablespoon cornstarch
- Cooking spray
- 1 cup fat-free milk
- 1 tablespoon all-purpose flour
- 1 1/2 tablespoons butter
- 1/2 cup (2 ounces) crumbled Gorgonzola cheese
- 3 tablespoons chopped hazelnuts, toasted

Direction

- Spoon pumpkin onto several layers of heavy-duty paper towels, and spread to 1/2-inch thickness. Cover with additional paper towels;

let stand 5 minutes. Scrape into a medium bowl using a rubber spatula. Stir in breadcrumbs, Parmesan, salt, minced sage, pepper, and nutmeg.

- Working with 1 wonton wrapper at a time (cover remaining wrappers with a damp towel to keep from drying), spoon 2 teaspoons pumpkin mixture into the center of wrapper. Brush edges of wrapper with water and fold in half, pressing edges firmly with fingers to form a half-moon. Place on a large baking sheet sprinkled with cornstarch. Repeat procedure with remaining wonton wrappers and pumpkin mixture.
- Fill a large Dutch oven with water; bring to a simmer. Add half of ravioli to pan (cover remaining ravioli with a damp towel to keep from drying). Cook 4 minutes or until done (do not boil), stirring gently. Remove ravioli with a slotted spoon; lightly coat with cooking spray, and keep warm. Repeat procedure with remaining ravioli.
- Combine milk and flour in a saucepan, stirring with a whisk. Bring to a boil; cook for 1 minute or until thick, stirring constantly. Remove from heat. Add butter, stirring until butter melts. Gently stir in Gorgonzola.
- Place 5 ravioli in each of 6 shallow bowls, and drizzle each serving with 3 tablespoons Gorgonzola mixture. Sprinkle each serving with 1 1/2 teaspoons hazelnuts. Serve immediately.

Nutrition Information

- Calories: 250
- Total Fat: 9.1 g
- Total Carbohydrate: 33 g
- Saturated Fat: 4.5 g
- Fiber: 3.1 g
- Sodium: 636 mg
- Cholesterol: 22 mg
- Protein: 9.5 g

182. Pumpkin Pecan Lasagna

Serving: Makes 8 servings | Prep: 47mins | Cook: 13mins | Ready in:

Ingredients

- 1 cup pecan halves
- 5 tablespoons butter, divided
- 5 cups peeled, cubed pumpkin or butternut squash (about 1 1/2 pounds)
- 1 onion, chopped
- 2 garlic cloves, minced
- 1 1/2 teaspoons salt, divided
- 9 (9 3/4- x 2-inch) uncooked lasagna noodles
- 1/4 cup all-purpose flour
- 2 cups whole milk
- 2 tablespoons minced fresh sage
- 1/2 teaspoon pepper
- 1 1/2 cups (6 ounces) freshly grated Parmesan cheese, divided
- 1 1/2 cups (6 ounces) shredded mozzarella cheese

Direction

- Preheat oven to 350°. Place pecans in a single layer on a baking sheet, and bake, stirring once, 7 minutes or until toasted. Transfer to a plate to cool; chop.
- Melt 2 tablespoons butter in a large nonstick skillet over medium heat. Add pumpkin, onion, garlic, and 3/4 teaspoon salt; cook, stirring often, 15 minutes or until pumpkin is just tender. Stir in pecans; set aside.
- Cook lasagna noodles according to package directions. Rinse with cool water, and cover with plastic wrap until ready to assemble.
- Melt remaining 3 tablespoons butter in a medium saucepan over medium heat. Add flour and cook, whisking constantly, 1 minute. Gradually whisk in milk. Add sage, pepper, and remaining 3/4 teaspoon salt; cook, whisking constantly, about 9 minutes or until thickened. Remove from heat, and whisk in 1 cup Parmesan cheese.
- Spread 1/3 cup sauce in a greased 13- x 9-inch baking dish. Top with 3 lasagna noodles.

Spread with about 2/3 cup sauce, half pumpkin mixture (about 2 1/4 cups), and 3/4 cup mozzarella. Top with 3 more lasagna noodles. Spread 2/3 cup sauce over noodles, top with remaining pumpkin mixture, and sprinkle with mozzarella. Top with remaining 3 lasagna noodles. Spread remaining sauce over noodles. Sprinkle with 1/4 cup Parmesan cheese. Cover tightly with aluminum foil, and bake 30 minutes.

- Remove foil; sprinkle with remaining 1/4 cup Parmesan, and bake 10 minutes or until golden brown. Let stand 10 minutes before serving.

183. Pumpkin And Turnip Green Lasagna

Serving: Makes 6-8 servings | Prep: | Cook: | Ready in: 115mins

Ingredients

- 1 pound mild Italian sausage, casings removed
- 2 tablespoons olive oil, divided
- 2 garlic cloves, finely chopped
- 2 1/2 teaspoons kosher salt, divided
- 1 (1-lb.) package fresh turnip greens, chopped
- 1 1/2 qt. milk
- 6 tablespoons butter
- 6 tablespoons all-purpose flour
- 1/2 teaspoon dry mustard
- 2 cups (8 oz.) shredded Parmesan cheese, divided
- 3/4 teaspoon freshly ground black pepper, divided
- 1/2 teaspoon ground nutmeg, divided
- 1 (29-oz.) can pumpkin
- 1 pound no-boil lasagna noodles
- Vegetable cooking spray

Direction

- Preheat oven to 375°. Cook sausage in 1 Tbsp. olive oil in a large skillet over medium-high heat, stirring often, 4 to 5 minutes or until meat crumbles and is no longer pink. Remove sausage to a plate, using a slotted spoon; reserve drippings in skillet. Reduce heat to medium.
- Stir garlic, 1/2 tsp. salt, half of turnip greens, 1/2 cup water, and remaining 1 Tbsp. oil into hot drippings. Cook 1 minute, stirring and scraping bottom of skillet to loosen browned bits. Stir in remaining turnip greens. Reduce heat to medium-low, and cook 5 to 6 minutes or until greens are tender and water has evaporated. Remove from heat.
- Microwave milk, in batches, in a microwave-safe measuring cup covered with plastic wrap at HIGH for 2 to 3 minutes or until very warm. Melt butter in a large saucepan over medium heat. Whisk in flour, and cook, whisking constantly, 1 minute. Gradually whisk in warm milk; cook, whisking often, 12 to 14 minutes or until mixture thickens and comes to a low boil. Remove from heat, and whisk in dry mustard, 1 cup Parmesan cheese, 1/4 tsp. pepper, 1/4 tsp. nutmeg, and 1 tsp. salt.
- Whisk together pumpkin, 3/4 cup Parmesan cheese, 1/4 tsp. ground nutmeg, 1 tsp. salt, and 1/2 tsp. pepper in a large bowl.
- Place 1 layer of lasagna noodles in a lightly greased (with cooking spray) 13- x 9-inch baking dish, covering bottom completely. (Use pieces of noodles to fill in any gaps.) Spread 1 cup sauce over noodles; top with cooked sausage. Add another layer of noodles and 1 cup sauce; top with half of pumpkin mixture. Add another layer of noodles and 1 cup sauce; top with turnip green mixture. Add another layer of noodles and 1 cup sauce; top with remaining pumpkin mixture. Add another layer of noodles and 1 cup sauce; top with remaining 1/4 cup Parmesan cheese.
- Bake at 375° for 40 minutes or until top is golden brown. Let stand 15 minutes before serving. Sprinkle with freshly grated Parmesan cheese. Serve with remaining sauce.

184. Pumpkin Filled Pasta

Serving: Makes 10 to 12 servings | Prep: | Cook: | Ready in:

Ingredients

- Filling:
- 1 cup canned pumpkin (about half of a 15-oz. can)
- 2 tablespoons finely chopped Cremona fruit in mustard syrup (see notes; optional)
- 1/4 cup fresh-grated parmesan cheese
- 2 tablespoons finely crushed amaretti or other almond macaroon cookies
- 1 tablespoon fine dried bread crumbs
- 1/8 teaspoon fresh-grated nutmeg
- 1/4 teaspoon salt
- 1 tablespoon brandy
- Pasta:
- About 2 cups unbleached or regular all-purpose flour
- 1/4 teaspoon salt
- 3 large eggs
- 2 large egg yolks
- Sauce:
- 1/2 cup (1/4 lb.) butter or margarine
- 1/3 cup lightly packed fresh sage leaves, rinsed and dried
- 1/2 cup fresh-grated parmesan cheese
- Salt and pepper

Direction

- To make filling: In a bowl, mix pumpkin, Cremona fruit in mustard syrup, parmesan cheese, crushed amaretti cookies, bread crumbs, nutmeg, salt, and brandy.
- To make pasta: In a food processor, whirl 2 cups flour and salt to blend; add eggs and egg yolks, and whirl until dough holds together (or in a bowl, mix ingredients with a fork). Scrape pasta dough onto a lightly floured board and roll to coat with flour. Knead until dough feels smooth, adding flour as required to prevent sticking, about 1 minute if mixed in a food processor, 15 minutes if stirred. Cover dough with plastic wrap and let rest 10 to 15 minutes.
- Divide dough in half and shape each portion into a smooth ball. Roll each ball through a pasta machine to 1/16 inch thick, or roll on a floured board. With a floured 2 3/4-inch round cutter, cut out 48 to 50 pasta rounds. Reroll dough as needed; discard excess.
- Spoon an equal portion of filling onto center of each pasta round (about 1 teaspoon). Moisten pasta rims with water, fold over to enclose filling, and press edges with fork tines to seal. Arrange filled pasta on a floured surface (or 10- by 15-in. baking pans, if making ahead); let dry 10 minutes, turn over, and dry 20 minutes longer (or cover airtight and chill).
- Bring 4 quarts water to a boil in a 7- to 8-quart pan over high heat; add half the pasta and cook, stirring occasionally, until tender to bite, 8 to 10 minutes. As they are cooked, transfer with a slotted spoon to a rimmed ovenproof platter; cover with foil and keep warm on an electric warming tray or in a 250° oven. Repeat to cook remaining pasta.
- To make sauce: In an 8- to 10-inch nonstick frying pan over high heat, melt butter. Add sage leaves and stir often until darker green, about 30 seconds. Immediately, pour over the filled pasta, sprinkle with 1/2 cup parmesan cheese, and add salt and pepper to taste.

Nutrition Information

- Calories: 221
- Sodium: 311 mg
- Saturated Fat: 6.6 g
- Protein: 7.3 g
- Cholesterol: 114 mg
- Fiber: 1 g
- Total Fat: 12 g
- Total Carbohydrate: 20 g

185. Quick Chicken Pho

Serving: Serves 4 | Prep: | Cook: | Ready in: 45mins

Ingredients

- 2 bone-in, skin-on chicken breast halves, plus 4 thighs
- 9 cups reduced-sodium chicken broth
- 1 stalk lemongrass
- 2 ounces fresh ginger, peeled and cut into 1/2-in.-thick slices
- 1 large yellow onion, peeled and halved
- 8 ounces rice noodles
- 1 tablespoon Thai or Vietnamese fish sauce
- 1/8 teaspoon ground white pepper
- 1/2 bunch cilantro, washed, dried, and torn into 3-in. sprigs
- 1 lime, cut into wedges
- 4 ounces bean sprouts
- 1 jalapeño, cut into 1/4-in.-thick slices

Direction

- Put chicken in a medium pot. Add broth, cover, and bring to a boil over high heat. Bruise lemongrass by chopping it a few times with the back side of a knife (blade up). Bend the stalk in half and add to pot along with ginger and onion. As soon as broth boils, reduce heat to medium and simmer, partially covered, until chicken is cooked through, about 20 minutes more.
- Bring a small pot of water to a boil over high heat. Add rice noodles and cook, stirring to keep them from sticking, until just cooked through, about 4 minutes. Drain in a colander and rinse with cold water. Set aside.
- Transfer chicken pieces from broth to a large plate to let cool. Add fish sauce and white pepper to broth, cover, and keep warm over lowest heat. Remove and discard lemongrass, ginger, and onion.
- When chicken is cool enough to handle, remove skin and bones. Thinly slice meat. Arrange cilantro, lime wedges, bean sprouts, and sliced jalapeño on a platter.
- Divide noodles among four large soup bowls. Put some chicken into each bowl, then pour 2 cups hot broth into each bowl. Serve with platter of toppings.

Nutrition Information

- Calories: 422
- Sodium: 590 mg
- Total Carbohydrate: 67 g
- Cholesterol: 76 mg
- Protein: 28 g
- Fiber: 3.4 g
- Total Fat: 4 g
- Saturated Fat: 1.1 g

186. Quick Rotini With Sausage And Tomato Sauce

Serving: Serves 4 (serving size: 1 1/2 cups pasta and 1 teaspoon cheese) | Prep: | Cook: | Ready in:

Ingredients

- 8 ounces uncooked rotini
- Cooking spray
- 3 (4-ounce) sweet turkey Italian sausage links, casings removed
- 1 1/2 cups finely chopped arugula, divided
- 1 cup minced onion
- 1 tablespoon chopped fresh oregano
- 1/2 teaspoon crushed red pepper
- 4 garlic cloves, thinly sliced
- 2 cups unsalted canned crushed tomatoes
- 1/2 teaspoon sugar
- 1/2 teaspoon freshly ground black pepper
- 1/4 teaspoon kosher salt
- 4 teaspoons grated Parmesan cheese

Direction

- Bring a large saucepan of water to a boil. Add pasta; cook 7 minutes or until al dente. Drain pasta in a colander over a bowl, reserving 1 cup cooking liquid.

- Heat a large skillet over medium-high heat. Coat pan with cooking spray. Add sausage to pan; cook 5 minutes or until browned, stirring to crumble. Add 1 cup arugula, onion, oregano, crushed red pepper, and garlic; cook 2 minutes, stirring frequently.
- Add reserved 1 cup cooking liquid, tomatoes, sugar, black pepper, and salt to pan; bring to a boil. Add pasta; cook 2 minutes. Stir in remaining 1/2 cup arugula. Divide pasta mixture among 4 shallow bowls; top with Parmesan cheese.

Nutrition Information

- Calories: 387
- Sodium: 558 mg
- Total Fat: 8.3 g
- Saturated Fat: 2.8 g
- Protein: 22 g
- Cholesterol: 39 mg
- Fiber: 5 g
- Total Carbohydrate: 55 g

187. Ravioli And Edamame In Parmesan Sauce

Serving: Makes 4 servings (serving size: about 2 ounces pasta and 3 tablespoons edamame) | Prep: 3mins | Cook: 7mins | Ready in:

Ingredients

- 1 (9-ounce) package whole-wheat cheese ravioli (such as Buitoni brand)
- 3/4 pound frozen shelled edamame
- 1 teaspoon chopped fresh thyme
- 1/2 cup reduced-fat sour cream
- 1/2 cup preshredded fresh Parmesan cheese
- 1/2 teaspoon freshly ground black pepper

Direction

- Bring a large pot of water to a boil. While the water is heating, measure remaining ingredients.
- Add the ravioli to the boiling water and cook for 5 minutes. Add the soybeans and cook an additional 1-2 minutes or until tender. Drain the ravioli and soybeans, reserving 1/4 cup of the cooking liquid.
- Return ravioli to the pot and stir in thyme. Whisk together sour cream, Parmesan, salt, pepper, and reserved cooking liquid. Toss the pasta mixture with the sour cream mixture, divide among 4 bowls, and serve immediately.

Nutrition Information

- Calories: 394
- Cholesterol: 62 mg
- Total Fat: 16 g
- Total Carbohydrate: 37 g
- Protein: 23 g
- Saturated Fat: 7 g
- Fiber: 8 g
- Sodium: 634 mg

188. Ravioli With Herbed Ricotta Filling

Serving: 4 servings | Prep: | Cook: | Ready in:

Ingredients

- Ravioli:
- 3/4 cup (6 ounces) whole-milk ricotta cheese
- 1/4 cup (1 ounce) grated fresh Parmigiano-Reggiano cheese
- 2 tablespoons finely chopped fresh basil
- 1/2 teaspoon grated lemon rind
- 1/4 teaspoon freshly ground black pepper
- 1 large egg
- Classic Pasta Dough
- 6 quarts water
- 2 tablespoons fine sea salt
- Sauce:

- 2 tablespoons extra-virgin olive oil
- 2 garlic cloves, minced
- 1/4 cup chopped fresh basil
- 1/4 cup (1 ounce) shaved fresh Parmigiano-Reggiano cheese

Direction

- To prepare ravioli, place ricotta in a cheesecloth-lined colander; drain 30 minutes. Combine ricotta, 1/4 cup Parmigiano-Reggiano, and next 4 ingredients (through egg), stirring until well combined.
- Place 1 (15 x 3-inch) Classic Pasta Dough sheet on a lightly floured surface. Spoon 1 1/2 teaspoons filling mixture 1 1/2 inches from left edge in the center of sheet. Spoon 1 1/2 teaspoons filling mixture at 3-inch intervals along the length of sheet. Moisten edges and in between each filling portion with water; place 1 (15 x 3-inch) pasta sheet on top, pressing to seal. Cut pasta sheet crosswise into 5 (3 x 3-inch) ravioli, trimming edges with a sharp knife or pastry wheel. Place ravioli on a lightly floured baking sheet (cover with a damp towel to prevent drying). Repeat procedure with remaining pasta sheets and filling mixture to form 20 ravioli.
- Bring 6 quarts water and salt to a boil in an 8-quart pot. Add half of ravioli to pot; cook 1 1/2 minutes or until no longer translucent. Remove ravioli from water with a slotted spoon. Repeat procedure with remaining ravioli.
- To prepare sauce, heat oil in a large skillet over low heat. Add garlic to pan; cook 6 minutes or until garlic is tender. Remove from heat. Place 5 ravioli in each of 4 shallow bowls; drizzle each serving with 1 1/2 teaspoons garlic oil. Top each serving with 1 tablespoon basil and 1 tablespoon shaved Parmigiano-Reggiano. Serve immediately.

Nutrition Information

- Calories: 394
- Total Fat: 20.5 g
- Fiber: 0.4 g
- Total Carbohydrate: 33 g
- Protein: 19 g
- Saturated Fat: 8.1 g
- Cholesterol: 193 mg
- Sodium: 731 mg

189. Rigatoni With Kale And Butternut Squash

Serving: Serves 4 | Prep: | Cook: | Ready in: 60mins

Ingredients

- 4 slices bacon, chopped
- 1 medium onion, chopped
- 2 cloves garlic, finely chopped
- 1/2 teaspoon allspice
- 1/2 teaspoon pumpkin pie spice
- 4 cups packed stemmed and chopped kale leaves
- 1 cup low-sodium chicken broth
- Salt and pepper
- 1 1/2 pounds butternut squash, peeled, cubed
- 8 ounces rigatoni
- 1/2 cup grated Parmesan
- 1/2 cup half-and-half
- 1/4 cup ricotta

Direction

- In a large skillet over medium heat, cook bacon, stirring, until crispy, about 5 minutes. Transfer bacon to paper towels to drain. Discard all but 1 Tbsp. bacon fat from skillet.
- In same skillet over medium heat, sauté onion until translucent, about 4 minutes. Add garlic, spices, kale and 1/4 cup broth. Cook until kale is wilted, 2 to 3 minutes. Season with salt and pepper. Remove from heat.
- Bring a large pot of salted water to a boil. In a medium pot, bring squash and remaining broth to a boil. Cover, reduce heat to low and simmer until squash is tender, 12 to 14 minutes. Transfer 1/2 of squash to skillet.

Using an immersion blender, puree remaining squash until chunky; add to skillet.

- Add rigatoni to boiling water; cook until al dente, about 12 minutes or as package label directs. Drain, reserving 1/2 cup cooking water. Add pasta, Parmesan and half-and-half to skillet. Toss quickly over low heat until warmed through, adding pasta water to thin if needed. Season with salt and pepper. Divide into 4 bowls; top with ricotta and bacon.

Nutrition Information

- Calories: 442
- Fiber: 6 g
- Total Carbohydrate: 70 g
- Cholesterol: 28 mg
- Total Fat: 11 g
- Protein: 21 g
- Sodium: 535 mg
- Saturated Fat: 5 g

190. Roast Turkey Pho

Serving: Serves 6 | Prep: | Cook: | Ready in: 120mins

Ingredients

- Stock:
- 1 leftover Rosemary-Orange Roast Turkey carcass, picked over, plus reserved turkey neck
- 1 large yellow onion, quartered
- 1 garlic head, halved crosswise
- 1 lemon, quartered
- 3 tablespoons canola oil
- 6 cups water, divided
- 3 cups unsalted chicken stock
- 1 tablespoon whole black peppercorns
- 2 teaspoons brown sugar
- 3 star anise
- 1 (3-inch) piece peeled fresh ginger, sliced
- Remaining ingredients:
- 1 1/2 tablespoons fish sauce
- 3/8 teaspoon kosher salt
- 5 ounces shredded skinless, boneless turkey breast
- 5 ounces shredded skinless, boneless turkey thigh or drumstick
- 4 ounces uncooked wide brown rice noodles (banh pho or pad Thai)
- 1 tablespoon chili oil
- 2 cups mung bean sprouts
- 1 cup basil leaves
- 1/2 cup cilantro leaves
- 1/2 cup thinly vertically sliced red onion
- 6 lime wedges
- 1 jalapeño pepper, thinly sliced

Direction

- Preheat oven to 425°.
- To prepare stock, place first 4 ingredients on a jelly-roll pan. Drizzle with canola oil; toss. Roast at 425° for 40 minutes or until deep golden brown, turning once.
- Transfer roast turkey parts and vegetables to a large stockpot. Discard fat from jelly-roll pan. Pour 1 cup water into jelly-roll pan; carefully scrape up browned bits, and add to pot. Stir in remaining 5 cups water, chicken stock, peppercorns, sugar, star anise, and ginger. Bring to a boil. Reduce heat to low; simmer stock mixture 1 hour. Strain through a fine sieve into a large bowl. Discard solids.
- Wipe out pot; return strained stock to pot. Stir in fish sauce, salt, and leftover turkey; cook over medium heat 5 minutes or until thoroughly heated.
- Prepare noodles according to package directions, omitting salt and fat; drain and divide evenly among 6 bowls. Ladle about 1 1/3 cups stock over each serving; drizzle each serving with 1/2 teaspoon chili oil. Top evenly with bean sprouts and remaining ingredients.

Nutrition Information

- Calories: 268
- Sodium: 639 mg
- Total Fat: 9.3 g

- Fiber: 2 g
- Saturated Fat: 1.8 g
- Cholesterol: 53 mg
- Protein: 24 g
- Total Carbohydrate: 22 g

191. Roasted Red Pepper And Herb Pasta With Shrimp

Serving: 4 servings (serving size: 1 1/2 cups shrimp and pasta mixture and 1 1/2 teaspoons cheese) | Prep: | Cook: | Ready in: 55mins

Ingredients

- 2 red bell peppers
- 8 ounces uncooked fettuccine
- 2 tablespoons extra-virgin olive oil
- 1 tablespoon unsalted butter
- 1 cup finely chopped onion
- 1 tablespoon minced garlic
- 1/2 pound peeled and deveined large shrimp
- 1/4 cup fresh lemon juice (about 2 lemons)
- 2 tablespoons chopped fresh flat-leaf parsley
- 1 teaspoon chopped fresh thyme
- 1/2 teaspoon chopped fresh sage
- 3/4 teaspoon salt
- 1/2 teaspoon freshly ground black pepper
- 1/2 teaspoon crushed red pepper
- 1 teaspoon extra-virgin olive oil
- 2 tablespoons shaved fresh Parmesan cheese

Direction

- Preheat broiler.
- Cut bell peppers in half lengthwise; discard seeds and membranes. Place pepper halves, skin sides up, on a foil-lined baking sheet; flatten with hand. Broil 15 minutes or until blackened. Place in a paper bag; fold to close tightly. Let stand 20 minutes. Peel and chop; set aside.
- Cook fettuccine according to the package directions, omitting salt and fat; drain well. Set aside; keep warm.
- Heat 2 tablespoons olive oil and butter in a large skillet over medium-high heat. Add chopped onion and garlic to pan, and cook for 4 minutes or until the onion is tender, stirring frequently. Add shrimp to the pan, and cook for 2 minutes. Add bell peppers and 1/4 cup lemon juice to the pan, and cook for 4 minutes or until the shrimp are done and half of the liquid has evaporated. Add chopped parsley and the next 5 ingredients (through 1/2 teaspoon crushed red pepper) to the shrimp mixture. Remove pan from heat.
- Combine cooked fettuccine and 1 teaspoon olive oil in a large bowl; toss well. Add shrimp mixture, tossing gently to coat. Top each serving with cheese.

Nutrition Information

- Calories: 378
- Total Carbohydrate: 51 g
- Total Fat: 10.5 g
- Sodium: 573 mg
- Cholesterol: 96 mg
- Fiber: 4.9 g
- Saturated Fat: 3.3 g
- Protein: 20.7 g

192. Roasted Tomato Mac And Cheese

Serving: Serves 12 (serving size: 1 cup) | Prep: | Cook: | Ready in: 42mins

Ingredients

- Cooking spray
- 5 plum tomatoes, cut into 1/2-inch-thick slices (about 16 slices)
- 2 tablespoons brown rice flour or all-purpose flour
- 2 tablespoons butter, softened
- 4 cups unsalted chicken stock
- 3 cups 1% low-fat milk, divided

- 3/4 teaspoon salt
- 3/4 teaspoon Dijon mustard
- 18 ounces brown rice elbows (such as Tinkyáda) or whole-grain pasta shells
- 4 1/2 ounces (1/2 package) frozen artichoke hearts, thawed and halved
- 6 ounces reduced-fat sharp cheddar cheese, shredded (about 1 1/2 cups)
- 3 ounces fontina cheese, shredded (about 3/4 cup)
- 2.5 ounces Parmesan cheese, grated and divided (about 10 tablespoons)
- 1/2 teaspoon freshly ground black pepper

Direction

- Remove top oven rack, and cover with foil; lightly coat with cooking spray. Preheat broiler to high.
- Arrange tomato slices on prepared rack; lightly coat with cooking spray. Broil 8 to 10 minutes or until tomatoes are lightly browned. Transfer tomatoes to a plate; set aside.
- Combine flour and butter in a bowl until a paste forms.
- Place a large high-sided sauté pan over medium-high heat. Add stock, 2 cups milk, salt, and mustard, stirring with a whisk. Add pasta to pan; bring to a boil. Cook 12 minutes or until pasta is done, stirring frequently. Stir in remaining 1 cup milk and artichokes; cook 2 minutes. Add butter-flour paste, in pieces, stirring constantly to blend and thicken. Remove from heat; stir in cheddar, fontina, 6 tablespoons Parmesan, and pepper.
- Arrange broiled tomato slices on top of pasta. Sprinkle with remaining 4 tablespoons Parmesan. Broil 2 minutes or until cheese begins to brown.

Nutrition Information

- Calories: 299
- Sugar: 5 g
- Cholesterol: 29 mg
- Sodium: 489 mg
- Fiber: 4 g
- Total Fat: 11.3 g
- Saturated Fat: 6 g
- Protein: 15 g
- Total Carbohydrate: 37 g

193. Roasted Vegetable Lasagna

Serving: 9 servings | Prep: | Cook: | Ready in:

Ingredients

- Vegetables:
- 4 red bell peppers
- 1 teaspoon olive oil
- 1/2 teaspoon salt
- 1/2 teaspoon black pepper
- 6 yellow squash, halved lengthwise and cut into 1-inch pieces (about 1 1/2 pounds)
- 1 large onion, cut into 16 wedges
- 4 garlic cloves, minced
- Cheese mixture:
- 2 cups 2% low-fat cottage cheese
- 1 1/2 cups (6 ounces) grated sharp provolone cheese
- 1/4 cup chopped fresh basil
- 1 teaspoon dried oregano
- White sauce:
- 3 tablespoons all-purpose flour
- 1 1/2 cups 2% reduced-fat milk
- 2 tablespoons chopped fresh basil
- 1/4 teaspoon black pepper
- Cooking spray
- 9 cooked lasagna noodles
- 2 cups spinach leaves, divided
- 1/2 cup (2 ounces) shredded part-skim mozzarella cheese
- Fresh basil sprigs (optional)

Direction

- Preheat broiler.
- To prepare vegetables, cut bell peppers in half lengthwise; discard seeds and membranes.

Place pepper halves, skin sides up, on a foil-lined baking sheet; flatten with hand. Broil 15 minutes or until blackened. Place in a zip-top plastic bag; seal. Let stand 15 minutes. Peel; set aside.

- Preheat oven to 450°.
- Combine oil, salt, 1/2 teaspoon black pepper, squash, and onion on a baking sheet; toss well. Bake at 450° for 20 minutes. Remove from oven; combine squash mixture and garlic in a bowl.
- Decrease oven temperature to 375°.
- To prepare cheese mixture, combine cottage cheese and next 3 ingredients (cottage cheese through oregano) in a bowl.
- To prepare white sauce, place flour in a medium saucepan. Gradually add milk; stir with a whisk. Place over medium heat. Cook until thick; stir constantly. Remove from heat; stir in 2 tablespoons chopped basil and 1/4 teaspoon black pepper.
- Spread 1/4 cup white sauce in bottom of a 13 x 9-inch baking dish coated with cooking spray. Arrange 3 noodles over sauce; top with 1 1/4 cups cheese mixture, 1 cup spinach, 4 bell pepper halves, 2 cups vegetable mixture, and 1/4 cup white sauce. Repeat layers, ending with noodles. Spread remaining white sauce over noodles. Cover and bake at 375° for 15 minutes. Uncover; sprinkle with mozzarella cheese. Bake an additional 20 minutes. Garnish with basil sprigs, if desired.

Nutrition Information

- Calories: 275
- Sodium: 564 mg
- Total Fat: 9.1 g
- Saturated Fat: 5.2 g
- Total Carbohydrate: 29.3 g
- Cholesterol: 24 mg
- Protein: 19.3 g
- Fiber: 2.9 g

194. Rotini And Cheese

Serving: 4 servings (serving size: about 1 1/2 cups) | Prep: | Cook: | Ready in:

Ingredients

- 2 bacon slices
- 1 tablespoon butter
- 1 tablespoon olive oil
- 1 cup finely chopped onion
- 2 garlic cloves, minced
- 1 1/2 teaspoons all-purpose flour
- 2 teaspoons Dijon mustard
- 1 cup 1% low-fat milk
- 3/4 cup (3 ounces) shredded sharp cheddar cheese
- 1/2 teaspoon kosher salt
- 1/4 teaspoon freshly ground black pepper
- 5 cups hot cooked rotini (about 8 ounces uncooked pasta)
- 3/4 cup frozen green peas, thawed

Direction

- Cook bacon in a large nonstick skillet over medium heat until crisp. Remove bacon from pan; crumble. Increase heat to medium-high. Add butter and oil to drippings in pan; swirl to coat. Add onion; sauté for 5 minutes, stirring occasionally. Add garlic; sauté for 30 seconds, stirring constantly. Add flour, and sauté 1 minute, stirring frequently. Stir in mustard. Gradually add 1 cup milk, stirring constantly with a whisk, and bring to a boil. Cook for 3 minutes or until slightly thickened. Remove from heat. Let stand 5 minutes. Add cheese, salt, and pepper, stirring with a whisk until smooth.
- Place pan over low heat. Stir in bacon, pasta, and peas; cook for 1 minute or until thoroughly heated, tossing to coat.

Nutrition Information

- Calories: 470
- Total Fat: 19.9 g

- Fiber: 3.7 g
- Saturated Fat: 9.1 g
- Total Carbohydrate: 54.8 g
- Cholesterol: 40 mg
- Sodium: 667 mg
- Protein: 18.4 g

195. Rotini And Cheese With Broccoli And Ham

Serving: 6 servings (serving size: 1 3/4 cups) | Prep: | Cook: | Ready in:

Ingredients

- 4 quarts water
- 2 cups uncooked rotini (about 8 ounces corkscrew pasta)
- 1 (10-ounce) package frozen chopped broccoli
- 1/4 cup all-purpose flour
- 2 cups fat-free milk
- 1 1/2 cups (6 ounces) cubed light processed cheese (such as Velveeta Light)
- 2 teaspoons Dijon mustard
- 1/2 teaspoon salt
- 1/4 teaspoon garlic powder
- 1/4 teaspoon black pepper
- 1 cup chopped reduced-fat ham

Direction

- Bring water to a boil in a large stockpot. Add pasta; cook 5 minutes. Add broccoli; cook an additional 5 minutes or until pasta is done; drain.
- While pasta cooks, lightly spoon flour into a dry measuring cup; level with a knife. Place flour in a medium saucepan; gradually add milk, stirring with a whisk until blended. Cook over medium heat 8 minutes or until mixture is thick, stirring frequently.
- Remove from heat; stir in cheese and next 4 ingredients (cheese through pepper). Combine pasta mixture, cheese sauce, and ham.

Nutrition Information

- Calories: 288
- Sodium: 937 mg
- Total Carbohydrate: 42.6 g
- Cholesterol: 23 mg
- Fiber: 2.6 g
- Protein: 19.1 g
- Total Fat: 4.7 g
- Saturated Fat: 2.5 g

196. Rotini, Summer Squash, And Prosciutto Salad With Rosemary Dressing

Serving: 4 servings (serving size: 2 1/4 cups salad) | Prep: | Cook: | Ready in:

Ingredients

- 3 cups uncooked rotini (corkscrew pasta; about 8 ounces)
- 1 1/2 cups coarsely chopped yellow squash
- 1 1/2 cups coarsely chopped zucchini
- 4 ounces thinly sliced prosciutto, chopped
- 3 tablespoons chopped red onion
- 2 ounces fresh mozzarella cheese, chopped
- 1/4 teaspoon salt
- 1/4 teaspoon freshly ground black pepper
- 2 tablespoons white balsamic vinegar
- 1 tablespoon extravirgin olive oil
- 1 1/2 teaspoons Dijon mustard
- 1/2 teaspoon finely chopped fresh rosemary

Direction

- Cook pasta according to package directions, omitting salt and fat. Add squash and zucchini during the last minute of cooking. Drain pasta mixture; rinse under cold water.
- Heat a large nonstick skillet over medium-high heat until hot. Add prosciutto; cook 5 minutes or until crisp, stirring frequently.
- Combine the pasta mixture, prosciutto, onion, and cheese in a large bowl; sprinkle with salt

and pepper. Combine white balsamic vinegar, olive oil, Dijon mustard, and rosemary in a small bowl, stirring with a whisk. Add vinegar mixture to pasta mixture, tossing gently to coat.

Nutrition Information

- Calories: 359
- Saturated Fat: 4 g
- Total Carbohydrate: 46.3 g
- Cholesterol: 36 mg
- Protein: 18.7 g
- Fiber: 2.4 g
- Sodium: 771 mg
- Total Fat: 11.1 g

197. Sausage And Bean Ragù On Quinoa Macaroni

Serving: 8 servings (serving size: 1 1/2 cups pasta and 1 tablespoon cheese) | Prep: | Cook: | Ready in:

Ingredients

- 1 (16-ounce) package quinoa macaroni
- 1 tablespoon olive oil
- 1 cup finely chopped onion (about 1 medium)
- 2 garlic cloves, minced
- 1 pound bulk turkey Italian sausage
- 1/2 cup dry white wine
- 1/2 cup fat-free, less-sodium chicken broth
- 1/2 teaspoon fennel seeds
- 1/4 teaspoon freshly ground black pepper
- 2 (16-ounce) cans cannellini beans or other white beans, rinsed and drained
- 2 (14.5-ounce) cans diced tomatoes, undrained
- 1/2 cup (2 ounces) shaved Romano cheese

Direction

- Cook pasta according to package directions, omitting salt and fat.
- Heat oil in a large nonstick skillet over medium-high heat. Add onion and garlic; sauté 3 minutes. Add sausage; cook until browned, stirring to crumble. Stir in wine, scraping pan to loosen browned bits. Add broth and next 4 ingredients (through tomatoes); bring to a boil. Reduce heat, and simmer 15 minutes.
- Add pasta, stirring well. Top evenly with cheese. Serve immediately.

Nutrition Information

- Calories: 410
- Sodium: 729 mg
- Total Carbohydrate: 58.9 g
- Cholesterol: 41 mg
- Total Fat: 10.7 g
- Saturated Fat: 3.6 g
- Fiber: 8.9 g
- Protein: 23.4 g

198. Sausage Stuffed Manicotti

Serving: 10 servings (serving size: 1 stuffed manicotti) | Prep: | Cook: | Ready in:

Ingredients

- 10 uncooked manicotti
- Cooking spray
- 1 pound sweet turkey Italian sausage
- 1 1/2 cups chopped onion
- 1 cup chopped green bell pepper
- 2 tablespoons butter
- 2 tablespoons all-purpose flour
- 2 cups fat-free milk
- 1/8 teaspoon black pepper
- 1 1/2 cups (6 ounces) shredded part-skim mozzarella cheese
- 2 cups tomato-basil pasta sauce (such as Newman's Own)
- 1/4 cup (1 ounce) grated fresh Parmesan cheese

Direction

- Cook pasta according to package directions, omitting salt and fat.
- Heat a large nonstick skillet over medium-high heat. Coat pan with cooking spray. Remove casings from sausage. Add sausage to pan; cook 5 minutes or until browned, stirring to crumble. Add onion and bell pepper to pan; sauté 5 minutes or until tender.
- Melt butter in a medium saucepan over medium heat. Stir in flour; cook 2 minutes, stirring constantly with a whisk. Remove from heat; gradually add milk, stirring with a whisk. Return pan to heat; bring to a boil. Cook 6 minutes or until thickened, stirring constantly with a whisk. Remove from heat; stir in black pepper. Add 1/2 cup milk mixture to sausage mixture; stir well.
- Preheat oven to 350°.
- Spoon about 1/3 cup sausage mixture into each manicotti; arrange manicotti in a single layer in a 13 x 9-inch baking dish coated with cooking spray. Sprinkle mozzarella over manicotti; spread remaining milk mixture evenly over mozzarella. Top milk mixture with pasta sauce, spreading to cover. Sprinkle with Parmesan. Bake at 350° for 35 minutes or until bubbly.

Nutrition Information

- Calories: 292
- Cholesterol: 57 mg
- Sodium: 719 mg
- Saturated Fat: 4.9 g
- Total Fat: 11.5 g
- Fiber: 1.4 g
- Protein: 19.6 g
- Total Carbohydrate: 25.8 g

199. Seafood Ragù With Cavatappi

Serving: 6 servings (serving size: 1 1/2 cups) | Prep: | Cook: | Ready in:

Ingredients

- 2 tablespoons olive oil, divided
- 1 1/2 cups finely chopped red onion
- 2 teaspoons minced garlic cloves
- 1/2 teaspoon crushed red pepper
- 1 cup dry red wine
- 1 1/2 cups canned crushed plum tomatoes
- 3 tablespoons minced fresh flat-leaf parsley, divided
- 1/2 teaspoon salt
- 24 littleneck clams
- 16 medium shrimp, peeled and deveined (about 1/2 pound)
- 1 pound skinless halibut fillets, cut into 1/2-inch pieces
- 1/2 cup water
- 4 cups hot cooked cavatappi (about 10 ounces uncooked pasta)

Direction

- Heat 1 tablespoon oil in a large Dutch oven over medium heat. Add onion, garlic, and pepper; cover and cook 10 minutes or until tender, stirring occasionally.
- Add wine; bring to a boil. Reduce heat; simmer, uncovered, 10 minutes or until liquid almost evaporates. Stir in tomatoes, 2 tablespoons parsley, and salt; bring to a boil. Cover, reduce heat, and simmer 10 minutes.
- Add clams. Cover and cook 2 minutes. Stir in shrimp and fish. Increase heat to medium-high; cook 2 minutes. Add water. Cover, reduce heat, and simmer 5 minutes or until clams open. Discard any unopened shells. Add 1 tablespoon oil and pasta; toss to coat. Sprinkle with 1 tablespoon parsley.

Nutrition Information

- Calories: 361
- Total Fat: 8.7 g
- Protein: 37.8 g
- Total Carbohydrate: 31.3 g
- Fiber: 3 g
- Saturated Fat: 1.2 g
- Sodium: 390 mg
- Cholesterol: 154 mg

200. Sesame Noodles

Serving: | Prep: | Cook: | Ready in: 31mins

Ingredients

- Peanut Sauce:
- 1/2 cup creamy peanut butter (not natural or old-fashioned)
- 1/2 cup low-sodium chicken or vegetable broth
- 3 tablespoons low-sodium soy sauce
- 2 tablespoons rice vinegar
- 2 tablespoons sugar
- 1 tablespoon toasted sesame oil
- 1 teaspoon freshly grated ginger
- 1/2 teaspoon sriracha
- Noodle Salad:
- Salt
- 3/4 cup whole-wheat penne
- 1/4 cup frozen edamame
- 1/4 cup small broccoli florets
- 1/4 cup snow peas
- 1/4 cup diced cucumber
- 1/4 cup diced red bell pepper
- 1/4 cup chopped radish
- 1/4 cup shredded carrots
- 2 scallions, sliced

Direction

- Make peanut sauce: Combine all ingredients in a medium pan. Bring to a boil over medium heat, stirring constantly. Continue cooking and stirring until sauce is thick, about 2 minutes. Let cool.
- Make noodle salad: Bring a pot of salted water to a boil. Cook pasta until al dente, about 10 minutes, adding edamame for last 3 minutes and broccoli and snow peas for last minute. Drain; run under cold water. Transfer to a large bowl, shaking off excess water. Add remaining vegetables. Toss with 1/4 cup sauce.

Nutrition Information

- Calories: 522
- Sodium: 731 mg
- Protein: 22 g
- Total Carbohydrate: 69 g
- Saturated Fat: 4 g
- Cholesterol: 0.0 mg
- Total Fat: 20 g
- Fiber: 10 g

201. Sesame Oil Noodles

Serving: Serves 8 | Prep: | Cook: | Ready in: 30mins

Ingredients

- About 2 lbs. fresh Chinese egg or wheat noodles* (or about 1 3/4 lbs. dried)
- 3 tablespoons toasted sesame oil
- 2 tablespoons vegetable oil
- 2 tablespoons soy sauce
- 2 tablespoons sliced green onions

Direction

- Bring 4 qts. water to a boil in a pot. Gently pull fresh noodles apart and add to pot, stirring to keep from sticking. Cook, stirring often, until noodles are tender, 3 minutes for fresh and 6 minutes for dried.
- Drain noodles well, rinse with hot water, and drain again. Transfer to a serving bowl.
- Toss noodles with oils and soy sauce and sprinkle with green onions.

- *Buy noodles in Asian markets and some supermarkets.

Nutrition Information

- Calories: 459
- Sodium: 247 mg
- Total Carbohydrate: 71 g
- Saturated Fat: 2.3 g
- Total Fat: 13 g
- Fiber: 3.4 g
- Cholesterol: 83 mg
- Protein: 14 g

202. Shrimp Couscous With Seafood Broth

Serving: 6 servings (serving size: 1 cup) | Prep: | Cook: | Ready in:

Ingredients

- 1 1/2 pounds unpeeled rock shrimp or medium shrimp
- 1 teaspoon unsalted butter
- 1 1/3 cups chopped onion
- 1/2 cup chopped celery
- 1/3 cup chopped carrot
- 1 teaspoon chopped fresh or 1/4 teaspoon dried thyme
- 4 garlic cloves, chopped
- 6 cups coarsely chopped tomato
- 4 cups water
- 1 cup dry white wine
- 1 tablespoon tomato paste
- 1 teaspoon unsalted butter
- 1/2 teaspoon salt
- 1/8 teaspoon pepper
- 1 cup uncooked couscous
- 1 tablespoon olive oil
- 1 cup diced red bell pepper
- 1 cup diced yellow bell pepper
- 1/2 cup diced yellow squash
- 1/2 cup diced zucchini

Direction

- Peel shrimp, reserving shells, and set shrimp aside.
- Melt 1 teaspoon butter in a large Dutch oven over medium heat. Add reserved shrimp shells, onion, celery, carrot, thyme, and garlic; sauté 3 minutes. Add tomato, water, wine, and tomato paste; bring to a boil. Reduce heat, and simmer, uncovered, 35 minutes. Place half of seafood broth in a blender, and process until smooth. Strain pureed seafood broth through a sieve into a bowl; discard solids. Repeat process with remaining seafood broth.
- Combine 1 cup seafood broth, 1 teaspoon butter, salt, and pepper in a medium saucepan, and bring to a boil; gradually stir in couscous. Remove from heat; cover and let stand 5 minutes. Fluff with a fork before serving.
- Heat oil in a large nonstick skillet over medium-high heat. Add shrimp, and sauté 1 minute. Add bell peppers, squash, and zucchini; sauté 3 minutes. Stir in couscous and an additional 1 1/2 cups seafood broth; cook 1 minute.
- Note: Store remaining seafood broth in an airtight container in refrigerator for up to 1 week, or freeze for up to three months.

Nutrition Information

- Calories: 276
- Total Fat: 6.3 g
- Cholesterol: 176 mg
- Fiber: 3.2 g
- Saturated Fat: 1.6 g
- Protein: 27.8 g
- Sodium: 381 mg
- Total Carbohydrate: 27.7 g

203. Shrimp Destin Linguine

Serving: Makes 2 to 3 servings | Prep: | Cook: | Ready in: 30mins

Ingredients

- 1 1/2 pounds unpeeled, large raw shrimp (2 1/25 count)
- 1 (9-oz.) package refrigerated linguine
- 1/4 cup butter
- 1/4 cup olive oil
- 1/4 cup chopped green onions
- 2 garlic cloves, minced
- 1 tablespoon dry white wine
- 2 teaspoons fresh lemon juice
- 1/2 teaspoon salt
- 1/4 teaspoon coarsely ground pepper
- 1 tablespoon chopped fresh dill
- 1 tablespoon chopped fresh parsley

Direction

- Peel shrimp, leaving tails on, if desired. Devein, if desired.
- Prepare pasta according to package directions.
- Meanwhile, melt butter with oil in a large skillet over medium-high heat; add green onions and garlic, and sauté 4 to 5 minutes or until onions are tender. Add shrimp, wine, and next 3 ingredients. Cook over medium heat, stirring occasionally, 3 to 5 minutes or just until shrimp turn pink. Stir in dill and parsley. Remove shrimp with a slotted spoon, reserving sauce in skillet.
- Add hot cooked pasta to sauce in skillet, tossing to coat. Transfer pasta to a serving bowl, and top with shrimp.

Nutrition Information

- Calories: 728
- Saturated Fat: 0.0 g
- Total Fat: 49.9 g
- Sodium: 1064 mg
- Protein: 0.0 g
- Cholesterol: 384 mg
- Total Carbohydrate: 0.0 g
- Fiber: 0.0 g

204. Shrimp Fettuccine Alfredo

Serving: Serves 4 (serving size: about 1 cup) | Prep: | Cook: | Ready in:

Ingredients

- 1 (9-ounce) package refrigerated fettuccine
- 1 pound peeled and deveined medium shrimp
- 2 green onions, chopped
- 2 garlic cloves, minced
- 2 teaspoons olive oil
- 1/2 cup (2 ounces) grated Parmigiano-Reggiano cheese
- 1/3 cup half-and-half
- 3 tablespoons (1 1/2 ounces) 1/3-less-fat cream cheese
- 1/4 teaspoon freshly ground black pepper
- 2 tablespoons chopped fresh parsley

Direction

- Cook the pasta according to package directions, omitting salt and fat. Drain pasta in a colander over a bowl, reserving 1/4 cup cooking liquid. Combine shrimp, onions, and garlic in a small bowl. Heat a large skillet over medium-high heat. Add olive oil; swirl to coat. Add shrimp mixture, and sauté for 4 minutes or until shrimp are done. Remove from pan; keep warm.
- Reduce heat to medium. Add reserved cooking liquid, Parmigiano-Reggiano, half-and-half, cream cheese, and pepper to pan. Cook 2 minutes or until cheeses melt. Combine pasta, cheese mixture, and shrimp mixture. Sprinkle with parsley.

Nutrition Information

- Calories: 442
- Saturated Fat: 6.1 g
- Sodium: 565 mg
- Total Fat: 14.3 g
- Protein: 37.4 g
- Total Carbohydrate: 40 g
- Cholesterol: 200 mg
- Fiber: 2.1 g

205. Shrimp Linguine With Ricotta, Fennel, And Spinach

Serving: Serves 4 (serving size: 1 cup) | Prep: | Cook: | Ready in:

Ingredients

- 9 ounces fresh linguine
- 1 tablespoon olive oil
- 8 ounces medium shrimp, peeled and deveined
- 1 cup vertically sliced fennel bulb
- 1/2 cup thinly sliced shallots
- 2 garlic cloves, thinly sliced
- 1 (6-ounce) package fresh baby spinach
- 1 tablespoon grated lemon rind
- 2 tablespoons fresh lemon juice
- 1/2 teaspoon freshly ground black pepper
- 1/4 teaspoon salt
- 2 ounces grated fresh Parmesan cheese (about 1/2 cup)
- 1/4 cup part-skim ricotta cheese

Direction

- Cook pasta according to package directions, omitting salt and fat. Drain in a colander over a bowl, reserving 1/2 cup cooking liquid.
- Heat a large skillet over medium-high heat. Add oil; swirl to coat. Add shrimp, fennel, and shallots; sauté 3 minutes. Add garlic; sauté 30 seconds. Add spinach; cook 2 minutes or until spinach wilts.
- Stir in rind and next 3 ingredients (through salt). Stir in reserved cooking liquid; cook 1 minute or until slightly thickened. Add pasta and Parmesan cheese; toss to coat. Top each serving with 1 tablespoon ricotta.

Nutrition Information

- Calories: 377
- Protein: 23.9 g
- Cholesterol: 122 mg
- Fiber: 4.8 g
- Total Fat: 10.6 g
- Saturated Fat: 4.1 g
- Total Carbohydrate: 43.6 g
- Sodium: 650 mg

206. Shrimp Lo Mein

Serving: Serves 4 (serving size: 1 1/4 cups) | Prep: | Cook: | Ready in: 35mins

Ingredients

- 1/2 pound multigrain spaghetti
- 1 1/2 cups unsalted chicken stock
- 2 tablespoons plus 2 teaspoons lower-sodium soy sauce
- 1 teaspoon cornstarch
- 1 teaspoon dark sesame oil
- 1/2 teaspoon sugar
- 1/2 teaspoon black pepper
- 2 teaspoons canola oil
- 2 cups small broccoli florets
- 3/4 cup thinly sliced carrot
- 3/4 cup thinly sliced red bell pepper
- 1 pound peeled and deveined extra-large shrimp
- 1 tablespoon minced garlic
- 1 teaspoon grated peeled fresh ginger
- 1 tablespoon rice vinegar

Direction

- Cook pasta according to package directions, omitting salt and fat, and removing from heat

2 minutes earlier than recommended for al dente texture. Drain.
- Combine chicken stock, soy sauce, cornstarch, sesame oil, sugar, and black pepper, stirring well.
- Heat a large skillet or wok over high heat. Add canola oil to pan; swirl to coat. Add broccoli, carrot, and red bell pepper; sauté 5 minutes or until vegetables soften. Add 1/4 cup stock mixture; sauté 2 minutes. Add shrimp, garlic, ginger, and 1/4 cup stock mixture; sauté 3 minutes or until shrimp are almost done. Add pasta and remaining stock mixture. Cook over medium heat 1 minute, stirring constantly. Remove from heat; stir in vinegar.

Nutrition Information

- Calories: 373
- Total Fat: 6.9 g
- Protein: 30 g
- Fiber: 6 g
- Total Carbohydrate: 48 g
- Sodium: 625 mg
- Sugar: 5 g
- Saturated Fat: 0.5 g
- Cholesterol: 143 mg

207. Shrimp Scampi Linguine

Serving: Makes 4 servings | Prep: 8mins | Cook: 15mins | Ready in:

Ingredients

- 8 ounces linguine
- 3 tablespoons extra virgin olive oil, divided
- 1 pound large shrimp, peeled and deveined
- 6 tablespoons unsalted butter
- 6 garlic cloves, minced
- 1/4 teaspoon dried crushed red pepper
- 1/4 cup coarsely chopped fresh parsley
- 2 teaspoons lemon zest
- 1 tablespoon fresh lemon juice
- 3/4 teaspoon salt

Direction

- Cook pasta in boiling salted water according to package directions; drain.
- Heat 1 tablespoon oil in a large nonstick skillet over medium-high heat. Add half of shrimp, and cook 1 minute on each side or until opaque. Transfer shrimp to a plate, cover, and keep warm. Repeat with 1 tablespoon oil and remaining shrimp.
- Melt butter over medium heat in same skillet. Add remaining 1 tablespoon oil, garlic, and red pepper; sauté 3 minutes or until garlic starts to brown. Stir in cooked shrimp, parsley, lemon zest and juice, and salt; cook 1 minute. Add pasta, and cook 1 minute or until hot, tossing constantly. Serve immediately.

208. Shrimp Vodka Pasta

Serving: Serves 4 (serving size: 1 1/4 cups) | Prep: | Cook: | Ready in: 18mins

Ingredients

- 9 ounces refrigerated fettuccine
- 1 tablespoon olive oil, divided
- 12 ounces large shrimp, peeled and deveined
- 3 garlic cloves, thinly sliced
- 1/3 cup vodka
- 1 1/3 cups lower-sodium marinara sauce
- 1/3 cup chopped fresh basil, divided
- 1/4 cup heavy whipping cream
- 1/2 teaspoon kosher salt
- 1/4 teaspoon black pepper
- Creamed Spinach and Mushrooms

Direction

- Cook pasta per directions. Drain.
- Heat 1 1/2 teaspoons oil in a large skillet over medium-high heat. Add shrimp; sauté for 4 minutes or until done. Remove shrimp from pan.

- Add 1 1/2 teaspoons oil and garlic to pan; sauté 1 minute. Carefully add vodka; cook 1 minute. Add marinara, 1/4 cup basil, cream, salt, and pepper; bring to a simmer. Stir in pasta and shrimp. Sprinkle with remaining basil.

Nutrition Information

- Calories: 427
- Total Carbohydrate: 60.1 g
- Fiber: 2.4 g
- Protein: 24.6 g
- Sodium: 632 mg
- Cholesterol: 184 mg
- Total Fat: 12.6 g
- Saturated Fat: 4.9 g

209. Shrimp And Broccoli Rotini

Serving: Serves 4 (serving size: about 1 1/2 cups) | Prep: | Cook: | Ready in:

Ingredients

- 6 cups water
- 8 ounces uncooked rotini
- 3 cups packaged fresh broccoli florets
- 2 tablespoons olive oil
- 1 pound peeled and deveined large shrimp
- 2 teaspoons grated lemon rind
- 2 1/2 tablespoons unsalted butter
- 2 tablespoons fresh lemon juice
- 5/8 teaspoon kosher salt
- 1/2 teaspoon freshly ground black pepper

Direction

- Bring 6 cups water to a boil in a large saucepan. Add pasta, and cook according to package directions, omitting salt and fat. Add broccoli during last 3 minutes of cooking; drain.
- Heat a large skillet over high heat. Add oil; swirl to coat. Add shrimp to pan; sauté 2 minutes. Stir in lemon rind; sauté 1 minute. Add pasta mixture, butter, lemon juice, and salt to pan. Sauté 1 minute, stirring occasionally; toss to coat. Sprinkle with black pepper; serve immediately.

Nutrition Information

- Calories: 428
- Cholesterol: 162 mg
- Protein: 25 g
- Saturated Fat: 5.9 g
- Total Carbohydrate: 47 g
- Fiber: 4 g
- Total Fat: 16.1 g
- Sodium: 486 mg

210. Shrimp And Noodle Salad With Asian Vinaigrette Dressing

Serving: 4 servings (serving size: 2 cups) | Prep: 9mins | Cook: 5mins | Ready in:

Ingredients

- 2 ounces dried rice noodles (such as Hokan)
- Asian Vinaigrette Dressing
- 4 cups thinly sliced napa (Chinese) cabbage
- 3/4 pound cooked peeled and deveined large shrimp
- 1 cup snow peas, trimmed and cut diagonally in half
- 3 cups fresh bean sprouts
- 3 tablespoons thinly sliced green onions (optional)
- 1/4 cup chopped fresh cilantro (optional)

Direction

- Cook noodles in boiling water 5 minutes, omitting salt and fat; drain and rinse with cold water. Drain.

- While noodles cook, prepare Asian Vinaigrette Dressing; set aside.
- Combine noodles, cabbage, and next 3 ingredients. Add dressing, and toss well. Sprinkle salad with green onions and cilantro, if desired.

Nutrition Information

- Calories: 243
- Sodium: 288 mg
- Total Fat: 6.2 g
- Fiber: 2 g
- Total Carbohydrate: 21.4 g
- Cholesterol: 166 mg
- Protein: 26.9 g
- Saturated Fat: 0.9 g

211. Shrimp, Broccoli, And Sun Dried Tomatoes With Pasta

Serving: 4 servings (serving size: 2 cups) | Prep: | Cook: | Ready in:

Ingredients

- 1/2 cup sun-dried tomatoes, packed without oil
- 1/2 cup boiling water
- 3 cups uncooked farfalle (bow tie pasta)
- 1 1/2 cups chopped broccoli
- Cooking spray
- 1 garlic clove, minced
- 1 pound large shrimp, peeled and deveined
- 1/2 cup fat-free, less-sodium chicken broth
- 1/2 cup (4 ounces) 1/3-less-fat cream cheese
- 1/2 teaspoon dried basil
- 1/4 cup (1 ounce) grated fresh Parmesan cheese
- 2 teaspoons fresh lemon juice

Direction

- Place tomatoes and boiling water in a bowl. Cover and let stand 30 minutes or until tender; drain and chop.
- While tomatoes steep, cook pasta according to package directions, omitting salt and fat. Drain.
- Steam broccoli, covered, 4 minutes or until crisp-tender. Set aside.
- Heat a large nonstick skillet over medium-high heat. Coat pan with cooking spray. Add garlic to pan; sauté 30 seconds. Add shrimp; cook 4 minutes. Add broth and cream cheese, stirring to combine; bring to a boil. Reduce heat, and simmer 2 minutes. Add tomatoes, broccoli, and basil; stir well. Cook 2 minutes or until thoroughly heated, stirring frequently. Remove from heat. Stir in pasta, Parmesan cheese, and juice. Serve immediately.

Nutrition Information

- Calories: 493
- Protein: 39.8 g
- Saturated Fat: 5.7 g
- Fiber: 5.6 g
- Cholesterol: 198 mg
- Sodium: 862 mg
- Total Fat: 12 g
- Total Carbohydrate: 58.7 g

212. Shrimp Stuffed Shells

Serving: Serves 5 (serving size: 4 stuffed shells) | Prep: | Cook: | Ready in: 70mins

Ingredients

- 20 uncooked jumbo pasta shells (about 8 ounces)
- 1 1/2 tablespoons olive oil
- 1/2 cup chopped shallots
- 2 tablespoons minced garlic (about 6 cloves)
- 1/2 cup (4 ounces) 1/3-less-fat cream cheese
- 1/4 cup 2% reduced-fat milk

- 1/4 teaspoon ground red pepper
- 1/3 cup chopped fresh basil
- 1 pound medium shrimp, peeled, deveined, and coarsely chopped
- 1 tablespoon potato starch
- Cooking spray
- 3 cups lower-sodium marinara sauce (such as McCutcheon's), divided
- 1/3 cup (1 1/2 ounces) grated fresh Parmigiano-Reggiano cheese

Direction

- Preheat oven to 400°.
- Cook pasta 7 minutes or until almost al dente, omitting salt and fat. Drain well.
- Heat a medium skillet over medium heat. Add oil to pan; swirl to coat. Add shallots; cook 4 minutes, stirring occasionally. Add garlic; cook 1 minute, stirring constantly. Add cream cheese, milk, and pepper; cook until cheese melts, stirring until smooth. Remove from heat. Stir in basil. Place shrimp in a bowl. Sprinkle with potato starch; toss well to coat. Add cream cheese mixture to shrimp; toss well.
- Divide shrimp mixture evenly among pasta shells. Coat a 13 x 9-inch glass or ceramic baking dish with cooking spray; spread 1 cup marinara over bottom of dish. Arrange shells in prepared dish; top with remaining 2 cups marinara. Sprinkle shells evenly with Parmigiano-Reggiano cheese. Bake at 400° for 30 minutes or until shrimp is done.

Nutrition Information

- Calories: 496
- Saturated Fat: 6.2 g
- Sodium: 575 mg
- Cholesterol: 163 mg
- Protein: 31.1 g
- Total Carbohydrate: 85.6 g
- Total Fat: 16 g
- Fiber: 1.6 g

213. Skillet Toasted Penne With Bacon And Spinach

Serving: Serves 4 (serving size: 1 cup) | Prep: | Cook: | Ready in: 55mins

Ingredients

- 6 cups unsalted chicken stock (such as Swanson)
- 2 tablespoons olive oil, divided
- 8 ounces uncooked penne pasta
- 1/2 cup sliced shallots
- 8 garlic cloves, sliced
- 4 center-cut bacon slices, chopped
- 1 tablespoon fresh lemon juice
- 1/2 teaspoon grated lemon rind
- 6 ounces baby spinach
- 1/4 teaspoon kosher salt
- 0.5 ounces grated Parmigiano-Reggiano cheese (about 2 tablespoons)
- Oregano leaves (optional)

Direction

- Bring stock to a simmer in a saucepan (do not boil). Keep warm over low heat.
- Heat a large skillet over medium heat. Add 1 tablespoon oil to pan; swirl to coat. Add pasta; cook 5 minutes or until toasted, stirring frequently. Remove pasta from pan.
- Add the remaining 1 tablespoon oil, shallots, garlic, and bacon to pan; cook 4 minutes or until browned. Remove bacon mixture from pan. Reduce heat to medium-low. Return pasta to pan. Add stock, 1 cup at a time, stirring constantly until each portion of stock is nearly absorbed before adding the next (about 35 minutes total), stirring frequently. Stir in bacon mixture, juice, rind, spinach, salt, and cheese. Garnish with oregano, if desired.

Nutrition Information

- Calories: 394

- Sodium: 601 mg
- Total Fat: 11.8 g
- Saturated Fat: 3.1 g

214. Skillet Toasted Penne With Chicken Sausage

Serving: Serves 4 (serving size: 1 cup) | Prep: | Cook: | Ready in: 55mins

Ingredients

- 6 cups unsalted chicken stock (such as Swanson)
- 2 tablespoons olive oil, divided
- 8 ounces uncooked penne pasta
- 1 cup sliced sweet onion
- 13 ounces Italian chicken sausage, casings removed
- 2 tablespoons fresh lemon juice
- 1 tablespoon minced Calabrian chiles or hot red chiles
- 1/4 teaspoon kosher salt
- 0.5 ounces grated Parmigiano-Reggiano cheese (about 2 tablespoons)
- Oregano leaves (optional)

Direction

- Bring stock to a simmer in a saucepan (do not boil). Keep warm over low heat.
- Heat a large skillet over medium heat. Add 1 tablespoon oil to pan; swirl to coat. Add pasta; cook 5 minutes or until toasted, stirring frequently. Remove pasta from pan.
- Add the remaining 1 tablespoon oil, onion, and sausage to pan; cook 4 minutes or until browned, stirring to crumble. Remove sausage mixture from pan. Reduce heat to medium-low. Return pasta to pan. Add stock, 1 cup at a time, stirring constantly until each portion of stock is nearly absorbed before adding the next (about 35 minutes total), stirring frequently. Stir in sausage mixture, juice, chiles, salt, and cheese. Garnish with oregano, if desired.
- Skillet-Toasted Penne with Bacon and Spinach: Follow steps 1 and Substitute 4 chopped center-cut bacon slices for the sausage, and 1/2 cup sliced shallots and 8 sliced garlic cloves for the onion. Substitute 1 tablespoon fresh lemon juice and 1/2 teaspoon grated lemon rind for the 2 tablespoons lemon juice. Substitute 6 ounces baby spinach for the chiles. Serves 4 (serving size: 1 cup) Calories 394; Fat 8g (sat 1g); Sodium 601mg

Nutrition Information

- Calories: 411
- Total Carbohydrate: 46.1 g
- Fiber: 2.4 g
- Protein: 22.3 g
- Sodium: 620 mg
- Cholesterol: 63 mg
- Total Fat: 14.6 g
- Saturated Fat: 3.1 g

215. Slow Cooker Ramen Bowls

Serving: Serves 8 (serving size: 2 1/2 ounces pork, 3/4 cup noodles, 1 egg, 1 cup broth, 1/2 teaspoon sesame seeds, and 1 tablespoon nori) | Prep: | Cook: | Ready in: 495mins

Ingredients

- 2 tablespoons canola oil
- 1 (2-pound) boneless pork shoulder roast
- 2 onions, peeled and halved horizontally
- 4 cups unsalted chicken stock
- 4 cups water
- 1/4 cup lower-sodium soy sauce, divided
- 12 ounces shiitake mushrooms
- 2 tablespoons dark sesame oil
- 1 (7 x 3-inch) piece kombu
- 1 (2-inch) piece peeled ginger, cut into 6 slices

- 12 ounces uncooked fresh Chinese noodles (or brown rice fresh ramen, such as Lotus Foods)
- 8 large eggs
- 3 green onions, cut into 1/3-inch pieces
- 2 Fresno chiles, thinly sliced
- 4 teaspoons toasted sesame seeds
- 1 sheet nori, cut into very thin strips

Direction

- Heat a large skillet over medium heat. Add oil to pan. Add pork; cook 12 minutes, turning to brown on all sides. Place pork in a 6-quart slow cooker. Increase heat to medium-high. Add onions, cut side down, to skillet. Cook 5 minutes or until charred; transfer to slow cooker. Add stock, 4 cups water, and 2 tablespoons soy sauce to slow cooker. Remove stems from mushrooms; add stems to cooker. Reserve caps. Cover; cook on LOW for 7 hours.
- Remove pork from cooker. Let stand 5 minutes; shred. Strain liquid through a fine sieve into a bowl. Discard solids. Return liquid to slow cooker; increase heat to HIGH. Thinly slice mushroom caps. Add remaining 2 tablespoons soy sauce, mushroom caps, sesame oil, kombu, and ginger to slow cooker. Cook on HIGH for 20 minutes. Discard kombu and ginger. Add noodles to slow cooker; cook 5 minutes.
- Bring a pot of water to a boil. Carefully lower eggs into water; cook 6 minutes. Place eggs in a bowl of ice water for 2 minutes; peel and halve lengthwise. For each serving, place 3/4 cup noodles in a wide bowl; pour 1 cup broth over noodles. Top with pork, mushrooms, green onions, and chiles. Place 2 egg halves toward one side of bowl. Sprinkle with sesame seeds and nori.

Nutrition Information

- Calories: 455
- Fiber: 2 g
- Sugar: 2 g
- Saturated Fat: 5.4 g
- Cholesterol: 262 mg
- Total Fat: 21.1 g
- Total Carbohydrate: 26 g
- Protein: 39 g
- Sodium: 632 mg

216. Slow Cooker Baked Ziti

Serving: Serves 6 | Prep: 10mins | Cook: 180mins | Ready in:

Ingredients

- 1 15-oz. container part-skim ricotta
- 1 cup shredded mozzarella
- 1 cup grated Parmesan
- 1 teaspoon salt
- 1 pound ziti
- 2 25-oz. jars marinara sauce
- 2 tablespoons finely chopped fresh basil leaves

Direction

- Combine all three cheeses and salt in a medium bowl. Rinse ziti under cold water in a colander, allowing some water to cling to pasta.
- Mist inside of slow cooker with cooking spray. Place half of pasta in an even layer over bottom of cooker. Spoon half of sauce over pasta. Dot with half of cheese mixture and half of basil. Repeat with remaining pasta, sauce, cheese and basil. Pour in 2/3 cup water.
- Cover and cook on high until pasta is tender, 2 to 3 hours.

Nutrition Information

- Calories: 671
- Sodium: 1984 mg
- Fiber: 4 g
- Protein: 33 g
- Total Carbohydrate: 88 g
- Cholesterol: 51 mg

- Total Fat: 22 g
- Saturated Fat: 10 g

217. Slow Cooker Chicken Cacciatore With Spaghetti

Serving: Makes 6 to 8 servings | Prep: | Cook: | Ready in: 550mins

Ingredients

- 6 garlic cloves, minced
- 2 green bell peppers, chopped
- 2 red bell peppers, chopped
- 1 yellow onion, chopped
- 1 (8-oz.) package sliced cremini mushrooms
- 1 tablespoon kosher salt
- 1 teaspoon dried crushed red pepper
- 1 teaspoon freshly ground black pepper
- 3 tablespoons tomato paste
- 1/2 cup white wine
- 1 (28-oz.) can fire-roasted diced tomatoes, drained
- 2 skinned, bone-in chicken breasts (about 1 1/2 lb.)
- 2 skinned, bone-in chicken leg quarters (about 1 1/2 lb.)
- 1 (16-oz.) box spaghetti
- 1 1/2 cups pitted kalamata olives, halved
- 1/4 cup freshly grated Parmesan cheese
- 2 tablespoons butter
- Garnishes: fresh basil, fresh parsley, shaved fresh Parmesan cheese

Direction

- Place first 5 ingredients in a 6-qt. slow cooker; stir in salt, crushed red pepper, and black pepper. Whisk together tomato paste and wine, and add to slow cooker. Add drained tomatoes and chicken. Cover and cook on LOW 8 hours.
- Uncover and carefully remove chicken from slow cooker, using tongs. Increase slow cooker temperature to HIGH. Cover and cook tomato mixture 30 more minutes or until sauce thickens to desired consistency.
- Meanwhile, cook pasta according to package directions. Remove chicken meat from bones; discard bones. Shred meat. Stir olives and next 2 ingredients into sauce. Serve immediately over spaghetti.

218. Slow Cooker Lasagna

Serving: Makes 6 servings | Prep: 25mins | Cook: | Ready in:

Ingredients

- 2 28-ounce cans diced tomatoes, drained
- 3 cloves garlic, finely chopped
- 1/4 cup fresh oregano, chopped
- Kosher salt and pepper
- 16 ounces fresh ricotta
- 1/2 cup fresh flat-leaf parsley, chopped
- 1/2 cup grated Parmesan
- 12 ounces dry lasagna noodles
- 1 bunch Swiss chard, tough stems removed and torn into large pieces
- 12 ounces mozzarella, grated

Direction

- In a medium bowl, combine the tomatoes, garlic, oregano, 1/2 teaspoon salt, and 1/2 teaspoon pepper. In another medium bowl, combine the ricotta, parsley, Parmesan, and 1/4 teaspoon pepper. Spoon 1/3 cup of the tomato mixture into the bowl of a slow cooker. Top with a single layer of noodles, breaking them to fit as necessary. Add half the Swiss chard. Dollop with a third of the ricotta mixture and a third of the remaining tomato mixture. Sprinkle with a third of the mozzarella. Add another layer of noodles and repeat with the other ingredients. Finish with a layer of noodles and the remaining ricotta mixture, tomato mixture, and mozzarella. Set the slow cooker to low and cook, covered, until the noodles are tender, 2 to 3 hours.If You Don't Have a Slow Cooker: Heat oven to 375° F. Follow the recipe above using no-boil lasagna noodles in place of the dried ones and layer the ingredients in a Dutch oven or large casserole. Cover and bake until the noodles are tender, 50 minutes to 1 hour.

Nutrition Information

- Calories: 790
- Sugar: 13 g
- Protein: 45 g
- Cholesterol: 99 mg
- Total Fat: 39 g
- Total Carbohydrate: 69 g
- Fiber: 7 g
- Saturated Fat: 11 g
- Sodium: 1003 mg

219. Smokin' Macaroni And Cheese

Serving: Makes 8 servings | Prep: 20mins | Cook: 37mins | Ready in:

Ingredients

- 1 pound uncooked cellentani pasta
- 2 tablespoons butter
- 3 tablespoons flour
- 1 cup milk
- 1 (12-oz.) can evaporated milk
- 2 cups (8 oz.) shredded smoked Gouda cheese
- 1 (3-oz.) package cream cheese, softened
- 3/4 teaspoon salt
- 1/2 teaspoon ground red pepper, divided
- 1 (8-oz.) package chopped cooked, smoked ham
- 2 cups cornflakes cereal, crushed
- 2 tablespoons butter, melted

Direction

- Preheat oven to 350°. Prepare cellentani pasta according to package directions. Transfer hot pasta to a large bowl.
- Melt 2 Tbsp. butter in a medium saucepan over medium heat. Gradually whisk in flour until smooth; cook, whisking constantly, 1 minute. Gradually whisk in milk and evaporated milk; cook, whisking constantly, 3 to 5 minutes or until thickened. Whisk in Gouda, cream cheese, salt, and 1/4 tsp. ground red pepper until smooth. Remove from heat, and stir in chopped ham.
- Combine pasta and Gouda cheese mixture, and pour into a lightly greased 13- x 9-inch baking dish. Stir together 2 cups crushed cereal, 2 Tbsp. melted butter, and remaining 1/4 tsp. ground red pepper; sprinkle over pasta mixture.
- Bake at 350° for 30 minutes or until golden and bubbly. Let stand 5 minutes before serving.
- Note: For testing purposes only, we used Barilla Cellentani Pasta.

220. Soba Edamame Noodle Bowl

Serving: Serves 4 (serving size: about 1 1/2 cups) | Prep: | Cook: | Ready in:

Ingredients

- 1 cup frozen shelled edamame
- 6 ounces uncooked soba noodles
- 1 cup thinly vertically sliced snow peas
- 2 tablespoons dark sesame oil
- 2 tablespoons rice vinegar
- 1 tablespoon lower-sodium soy sauce or tamari
- 1 tablespoon yellow miso
- 1 1/2 teaspoons brown sugar
- 1 1/2 teaspoons grated peeled fresh ginger
- 1/4 teaspoon kosher salt
- 2 cups very thinly sliced red cabbage
- 2/3 cup thinly sliced green onions

- 2 large carrots, peeled and shaved into ribbons
- 1/4 cup fresh cilantro leaves (optional)

Direction

- Bring a large saucepan of water to a boil. Add edamame and soba noodles; cook 2 minutes. Add snow peas; cook 1 minute or until noodles are tender. Drain; rinse noodle mixture well with cold water. Drain.
- Combine oil and next 6 ingredients (through salt) in a large bowl. Add noodle mixture, cabbage, onions, and carrots; toss gently to combine. Sprinkle with cilantro, if desired.

Nutrition Information

- Calories: 304
- Sodium: 577 mg
- Total Carbohydrate: 48 g
- Sugar: 7 g
- Protein: 13 g
- Saturated Fat: 1 g
- Total Fat: 8.8 g
- Cholesterol: 0.0 mg
- Fiber: 4 g

221. Southern Barbecue Bowl

Serving: Serves 1 | Prep: | Cook: | Ready in:

Ingredients

- 1/2 cup cooked bulgur
- 1/2 cup oil-based coleslaw
- 1/3 cup unsalted pinto beans
- 1/4 cup charred corn
- 4 bread-and-butter pickle slices
- 2 ounces roasted pork shoulder
- Tangy White Sauce:
- 1 tablespoon cider vinegar
- 2 teaspoons canola mayonnaise
- 1/8 teaspoon freshly ground black pepper
- Dash of kosher salt

Direction

- Top cooked bulgur with coleslaw, pinto beans, corn, pickle slices, and roasted pork.
- In a small bowl, combine vinegar, mayonnaise, pepper, and salt, stirring well with a whisk. Drizzle over bowl.

Nutrition Information

- Calories: 395
- Protein: 24 g
- Saturated Fat: 2.9 g
- Total Carbohydrate: 44 g
- Fiber: 10 g
- Sugar: 9 g
- Cholesterol: 54 mg
- Total Fat: 13.5 g
- Sodium: 403 mg

222. Southern Pimiento Mac And Cheese

Serving: Makes 6 to 8 servings | Prep: | Cook: | Ready in: 20mins

Ingredients

- 1/4 cup plus 1 1/2 tsp. kosher salt, divided
- 1 qt. milk
- 6 tablespoons butter, cut into pieces
- 6 tablespoons all-purpose flour
- 1 pound pasta (such as penne, cavatappi, or rotini)
- 2 (8-oz.) packages shredded extra-sharp Cheddar cheese
- 1/2 cup grated sweet onion
- 2 tablespoons fresh lemon juice
- 1 tablespoon Worcestershire sauce
- 1 teaspoon hot sauce (such as Tabasco)
- 1/2 teaspoon freshly ground black pepper
- 1 1/2 cups panko (Japanese breadcrumbs)

- 2 teaspoons olive oil
- 2 (7-oz.) jars diced pimiento, drained
- 2 (2.52-oz.) packages fully cooked bacon, diced
- 2 tablespoons chopped fresh chives

Direction

- Preheat broiler with oven rack 8 to 9 inches from heat.
- Bring 1/4 cup salt and 4 qt. water to a boil in a large covered Dutch oven over high heat.
- Meanwhile, microwave milk in a microwave-safe 1-qt. glass measuring cup covered with plastic wrap at HIGH 3 minutes. While milk is heating, melt butter in a 12-inch cast-iron skillet over medium heat. Reduce heat to medium-low; add flour, and cook, whisking constantly, 2 minutes. Gradually whisk in hot milk. Increase heat to medium-high, and bring to a low boil, whisking often.
- Add pasta to boiling water, and cook 8 minutes.
- Meanwhile, continue to cook sauce, whisking often, 6 minutes. Remove from heat; whisk in cheese, onion, lemon juice, Worcestershire sauce, hot sauce, 1 1/2 tsp. salt, and 1/2 tsp. pepper. Cover.
- Stir together panko and olive oil.
- Drain pasta, and fold into cheese sauce. Stir pimiento and bacon into pasta mixture. Sprinkle with panko mixture.
- Broil 1 to 2 minutes or until breadcrumbs are golden brown. Sprinkle with chives; serve immediately.

223. Spaghetti Aglio E Olio

Serving: Serves 4 (serving size: about 1 cup) | Prep: | Cook: | Ready in: 21mins

Ingredients

- 10 ounce refrigerated fresh spaghetti noodles
- 1/3 cup extra-virgin olive oil
- 5 garlic cloves, thinly sliced
- 2 dried red Chinese chiles or chiles de arbol, seeded and sliced into rings
- 2 tablespoons fresh lemon juice
- 1 tablespoon fish sauce
- 3/8 teaspoon kosher salt
- 2 tablespoons chopped fresh Thai basil
- 1 tablespoon chopped fresh parsley
- 1 tablespoon fried garlic (optional)

Direction

- Bring a large pot of water to a boil over high heat; add pasta to pan. Cook 1 to 3 minutes or until al dente. Drain, reserving 1/2 cup cooking liquid.
- Heat oil in a large skillet over medium heat; add sliced garlic to pan. Cook 30 seconds or until lightly browned. Add chiles to pan; cook 1 minute or until chiles are fragrant. Stir in juice, fish sauce, and reserved pasta water; bring to a boil. Cook 2 to 3 minutes or until reduced and saucy. Add pasta and salt to pan; toss well to coat. Sprinkle evenly with basil, parsley, and fried garlic, if desired.

Nutrition Information

- Calories: 381
- Cholesterol: 52 mg
- Fiber: 3 g
- Saturated Fat: 2.7 g
- Sodium: 554 mg
- Total Carbohydrate: 41 g
- Sugar: 1 g
- Total Fat: 20.1 g
- Protein: 9 g

224. Spaghetti Bolognese

Serving: 4 servings (serving size: 1 cup spaghetti, about 3/4 cup sauce, and 1 tablespoon cheese) | Prep: | Cook: | Ready in: 40mins

Ingredients

- 1 (3/4-ounce) slice French bread
- 1/4 cup 1% low-fat milk
- 2 teaspoons olive oil
- 1 cup finely chopped onion
- 1/2 cup finely chopped carrot
- 3 garlic cloves, minced
- 1 tablespoon tomato paste
- 2 tablespoons red wine vinegar
- 2 teaspoons dried oregano
- 1/2 teaspoon salt
- 1/4 teaspoon black pepper
- 1/8 teaspoon ground red pepper
- 12 ounces ground sirloin
- 1 (14.5-ounce) can diced tomatoes with basil, garlic, and oregano, undrained (such as Hunt's)
- 4 cups hot cooked spaghetti (about 8 ounces uncooked)
- 1/4 cup (1 ounce) shaved fresh Parmigiano-Reggiano cheese

Direction

- Pulse bread in a food processor until coarse crumbs measure 1/2 cup. Combine crumbs and milk in a bowl.
- Heat olive oil in a large skillet over medium-high heat. Add onion and carrot; sauté 8 minutes. Add garlic and tomato paste; sauté for 1 minute, stirring constantly. Add vinegar; cook for 30 seconds. Add oregano, salt, peppers, and beef; cook 7 minutes, stirring to crumble. Stir in breadcrumb mixture and tomatoes; bring to a boil. Reduce heat, and simmer for 6 minutes, stirring occasionally. Serve over spaghetti; top with cheese.

Nutrition Information

- Calories: 440
- Saturated Fat: 3.4 g
- Total Carbohydrate: 59.1 g
- Cholesterol: 51 mg
- Total Fat: 9.6 g
- Fiber: 6 g
- Sodium: 682 mg
- Protein: 29.8 g

225. Spaghetti Carbonara

Serving: Makes 4 to 6 servings | Prep: | Cook: | Ready in: 30mins

Ingredients

- 2 eggs
- 3 ounces parmesan cheese
- 1/2 cup loosely packed flat-leaf parsley leaves
- 1/4 teaspoon freshly ground black pepper, plus more for garnish
- 1/4 pound pancetta or thin-cut bacon
- 2 cloves garlic
- 3 tablespoons olive oil
- 1/2 cup dry white wine
- 1 tablespoon salt
- 1 pound spaghetti or spaghettini

Direction

- Put a large pot of water on to boil. Meanwhile, crack eggs into a large bowl and beat lightly. Finely shred or grate cheese, add 1/2 cup to eggs, and set the rest aside. Finely chop parsley and add to eggs. Add pepper and whisk to combine well. Set aside.
- Cut pancetta or bacon into 1/4-in.-thick slices, peel and chop garlic, and set both aside. Heat olive oil in a small frying pan over medium-high heat. Add pancetta and cook, stirring occasionally, until it starts to brown. Add garlic and cook, stirring, until fragrant, about 1 minute. Add wine and cook until liquid is reduced by about half. Remove from heat and set aside.
- When water boils, add salt and spaghetti. Boil pasta until it is tender to the bite. Drain well and immediately pour pasta into bowl with egg mixture. Toss to thoroughly coat pasta with egg mixture (the heat from the pasta will partly cook the egg and melt the cheese). Pour

pancetta mixture on top of pasta and toss to combine thoroughly. Sprinkle with remaining cheese and pepper to taste. Serve immediately.

- Variations:
- Peas, please: Add 3/4 cup frozen peas to the egg mixture.
- Add radicchio: Finely shred 1 small head radicchio and cook with the pancetta.
- Pick basil: Substitute 1/4 cup chopped fresh basil leaves for the parsley.
- Spice it up: Add 1/2 tsp. red chile flakes with the garlic.
- Change the cheese: Substitute other hard, aged cheese (such as asiago, pecorino, or aged gouda) for the parmesan.
- Go for whole grain: Try using whole-wheat spaghetti (the assertive, rich flavors of this dish will hold up to a heartier pasta beautifully).
- Note: Nutritional analysis is per serving.

Nutrition Information

- Calories: 625
- Protein: 25 g
- Saturated Fat: 10 g
- Sodium: 1999 mg
- Total Fat: 27 g
- Fiber: 2.6 g
- Cholesterol: 111 mg
- Total Carbohydrate: 71 g

226. Spaghetti Carbonara With Leeks And Pancetta

Serving: 4 servings (serving size: 1 1/4 cups) | Prep: | Cook: | Ready in:

Ingredients

- 8 ounces uncooked spaghetti
- 1/2 cup (2 ounces) finely grated Parmigiano-Reggiano cheese
- 1/4 teaspoon black pepper
- 1/8 teaspoon salt
- 1 large egg
- 1 large egg white
- 1/2 cup chopped pancetta (about 2 ounces)
- 2 cups thinly sliced leek (about 2 large)
- 2 garlic cloves, minced
- 2 tablespoons chopped fresh flat-leaf parsley

Direction

- Cook pasta according to the package directions, omitting salt and fat. Drain, reserving 1/4 cup cooking liquid.
- Combine cheese, pepper, salt, egg, and egg white in a small bowl, stirring with a whisk. Gradually add the reserved 1/4 cup cooking liquid to egg mixture, stirring constantly with a whisk.
- Cook pancetta in a large nonstick skillet over medium-high heat until crisp. Remove pancetta from pan, reserving drippings in pan; set pancetta aside. Add leek to drippings in pan, and sauté 4 minutes. Add garlic to pan; sauté for 1 minute. Add pasta, cheese mixture, and pancetta to pan; reduce heat, and cook 1 minute, tossing well to coat. Cook 1 minute. Sprinkle with parsley; serve immediately.

Nutrition Information

- Calories: 400
- Total Carbohydrate: 49.4 g
- Saturated Fat: 5.7 g
- Fiber: 2.7 g
- Cholesterol: 78 mg
- Total Fat: 12.8 g
- Protein: 22.1 g
- Sodium: 726 mg

227. Spaghetti Carbonara With Pancetta, Leeks, And Peas

Serving: Makes 4 to 6 servings | Prep: | Cook: | Ready in:

Ingredients

- 1 leek (about 8 oz.)
- 12 ounces dried spaghetti
- 8 ounces pancetta, diced (1/2 in.; see notes)
- 1 1/2 cups shelled fresh peas or thawed frozen petite peas
- About 1/2 cup whipping cream
- 3 large egg yolks (see notes)
- 3/4 cup fresh-grated parmesan cheese
- 1 teaspoon salt
- 1/4 teaspoon fresh-ground pepper
- 1 tablespoon chopped parsley

Direction

- Trim and discard root end and tough green top from leek; peel off and discard outer layer. Cut leek in half lengthwise and hold each half under cold running water, flipping layers to separate and remove grit. Thinly slice crosswise.
- In a 5- to 6-quart pan over high heat, bring 4 quarts water to a boil. Add pasta and cook, stirring occasionally, until tender to bite, 8 to 10 minutes. Drain.
- Meanwhile, in a 12-inch frying pan or 4- to 5-quart pan over medium-high heat, stir pancetta until fat is rendered and pancetta is crisp and brown, about 8 minutes. Transfer to a paper towel-lined plate. Discard all but 2 teaspoons fat from pan.
- Lower heat to medium and add leek to pan; stir often until limp and slightly golden, 2 to 3 minutes. Stir in peas and cook until warmed through, 2 minutes longer. Reduce heat to low.
- Whisk together 1/2 cup cream, egg yolks, cheese, salt, and pepper. Add hot pasta and cream mixture to pan with leek and peas; mix gently to coat. Stir in pancetta. If desired, add a little more cream to thin sauce. Pour into a large bowl and sprinkle with parsley.

Nutrition Information

- Calories: 551
- Protein: 19 g
- Cholesterol: 157 mg
- Total Fat: 30 g
- Saturated Fat: 13 g
- Sodium: 829 mg
- Fiber: 3 g
- Total Carbohydrate: 51 g

228. Spaghetti Minestrone

Serving: Serves: 6 | Prep: 15mins | Cook: 20mins | Ready in:

Ingredients

- 2 tablespoons olive oil
- 1 carrot, diced
- 1 onion, chopped
- 2 ribs celery, thinly sliced
- 1 clove garlic, minced
- 6 cups low-sodium chicken broth
- 1/2 cup canned white beans, rinsed and drained
- 12 green beans (about 2 1/2 oz.), cut into 1/4-inch pieces
- 1 cup small cauliflower florets
- 1 1/2 cups cooked spaghetti, chopped
- 1 zucchini, sliced lengthwise and cut into 1/4-inch-thick pieces
- 1 cup canned diced tomatoes, drained
- 2 tablespoons fresh parsley, chopped
- Salt and pepper
- Grated Parmesan, for garnish

Direction

- Warm oil in a large pot over medium-high heat. Add carrot, onion and celery; cook, stirring often, until softened, 3 to 5 minutes. Add garlic; sauté 1 minute. Pour in broth, increase heat to high and bring to boil. Add both types of beans. Cover, reduce heat to low and simmer 5 minutes.
- Add cauliflower, spaghetti, zucchini and tomatoes. Cook until vegetables are tender,

about 8 minutes. Add parsley; season with salt and pepper. Garnish with Parmesan.

Nutrition Information

- Calories: 184
- Saturated Fat: 2 g
- Protein: 10 g
- Cholesterol: 4 mg
- Fiber: 4 g
- Sodium: 896 mg
- Total Carbohydrate: 22 g
- Total Fat: 6 g

229. Spaghetti Pie

Serving: 6 Servings | Prep: 15mins | Cook: 30mins |Ready in:

Ingredients

- 8 ounces uncooked spaghetti
- 2 tablespoons unsalted butter
- 8 large eggs
- 1/2 cup milk
- 1/3 cup cooked bacon crumbles (such as Hormel brand)
- 3 scallions (green portions only), thinly sliced
- 1/4 teaspoon freshly ground pepper
- 1/4 cup finely shredded Parmesan cheese

Direction

- Bring a pot of salted water to a boil, add spaghetti and cook according to package directions, stirring often, until al dente. Drain pasta and rinse well with cold water.
- Preheat oven to 400°F. Grease an ovenproof 9- or 10-inch skillet with about 1/2 Tbsp. butter.
- In a bowl, whisk together eggs, milk, bacon, scallion, pepper and 3 Tbsp. Parmesan. Add spaghetti; mix well. Transfer mixture to skillet, spreading evenly. Dot with remaining butter and sprinkle remaining 1 Tbsp. Parmesan on top. Bake for 25 to 30 minutes, until center is set and top is golden. Let cool for 10 minutes before serving.

Nutrition Information

- Calories: 328
- Total Fat: 14 g
- Fiber: 1 g
- Protein: 18 g
- Saturated Fat: 6 g
- Cholesterol: 304 mg
- Total Carbohydrate: 31 g
- Sodium: 430 mg

230. Spaghetti Squash Lasagna With Spinach

Serving: Serves 4 (serving size: 1 squash half) | Prep: | Cook: |Ready in: 110mins

Ingredients

- 2 small spaghetti squash (about 1 1/2 pounds each)
- 2 teaspoons olive oil
- 4 garlic cloves, thinly sliced
- 1 (8-ounce) package fresh baby spinach
- 1/2 cup part-skim ricotta cheese
- 1/8 teaspoon kosher salt
- 2 ounces shredded part-skim mozzarella cheese (about 1/2 cup), divided
- 8 ounces 93% lean ground turkey
- 1 1/2 cups lower-sodium marinara sauce (such as Dell'Amore)
- 1 ounce Parmesan cheese, grated (about 1/4 cup)

Direction

- Preheat oven to 350°.
- Cut each squash in half lengthwise. Scoop out seeds; discard. Place squash halves, cut sides up, on a baking sheet. Bake at 350° for 50

minutes. Let stand 10 minutes. Scrape inside of squash with a fork to remove spaghetti-like strands. Place strands on a clean dish towel; squeeze until barely moist.

- Heat a large skillet over medium-high heat. Add oil to pan; swirl to coat. Add garlic; cook 30 seconds. Add spinach; cook 1 minute or until spinach wilts. Remove from heat. Combine spinach mixture, squash strands, ricotta cheese, salt, and half of mozzarella cheese in a medium bowl.
- Return skillet to medium-high heat. Add turkey to pan; cook 4 minutes or until browned, stirring to crumble. Add marinara sauce; cover, reduce heat to medium, and simmer 4 minutes. Remove from heat.
- Increase oven temperature to 425°.
- Spoon sauce evenly into the bottom of each squash half. Top evenly with squash mixture. Sprinkle evenly with remaining mozzarella cheese and Parmesan cheese. Bake at 425° for 20 minutes.
- Preheat broiler to high (keep squash in oven). Broil squash 1 to 2 minutes or until cheese is golden brown and bubbly. Remove from oven; let stand 10 minutes.

Nutrition Information

- Calories: 374
- Sodium: 613 mg
- Saturated Fat: 6.2 g
- Cholesterol: 65 mg
- Total Carbohydrate: 30 g
- Total Fat: 18.9 g
- Fiber: 6 g
- Protein: 25 g

231. Spaghetti And Easy Meatballs

Serving: 6 Servings | Prep: 10mins | Cook: 20mins | Ready in:

Ingredients

- 1 pound spaghetti
- 1 (25 oz.) jar tomato sauce
- 1 1/2 pounds ground beef
- 1/2 cup bread crumbs, soaked in 1/4 cup milk
- 1/2 cup grated
- Parmesan
- 1/2 cup chopped onion
- 1/4 cup chopped fresh parsley
- 1 egg, lightly beaten
- 2 cloves garlic, minced
- 1 1/2 teaspoons kosher salt

Direction

- Preheat oven to 375°F. In a large pot of boiling salted water, cook spaghetti, stirring often, until al dente, about 10 minutes. Drain well in a colander. In a large, wide saucepan or deep skillet, heat tomato sauce over low heat while you proceed.
- While pasta is cooking, combine beef, soaked bread crumbs, cheese, onion, parsley, egg, garlic and salt in a large bowl. Form mixture into balls slightly larger than golf balls. (They will shrink as they cook.) Lay meatballs out on two nonstick or oiled baking sheets and bake in oven until nicely browned, about 10 minutes.
- Transfer meatballs from oven with tongs and place into simmering sauce to combine. Serve meatballs and sauce on top of spaghetti.

Nutrition Information

- Calories: 754
- Total Fat: 35 g
- Saturated Fat: 14 g
- Sodium: 315 mg
- Protein: 36 g
- Cholesterol: 139 mg
- Fiber: 4 g
- Total Carbohydrate: 71 g

232. Spaghetti And Meatballs

Serving: 8 servings (serving size: 3/4 cup pasta and 1 cup plus 2 tablespoons sauce and meatballs) | Prep: | Cook: | Ready in:

Ingredients

- 1 (1.5-ounce) slice gluten-free baguette
- 1 garlic clove
- 1/2 small onion, cut into 3 wedges
- 1/2 cup fresh parsley leaves
- 1 pound ground round
- 2 (4-ounce) links sweet turkey Italian sausage, casings removed {Check for Gluten}
- 1/4 cup (1 ounce) grated fresh Parmesan cheese
- 1/4 cup fat-free, lower-sodium chicken broth {Check for Gluten}
- 1 large egg
- 1/2 teaspoon freshly ground black pepper
- 1/4 teaspoon crushed red pepper
- Cooking spray
- 12 ounces uncooked gluten-free spaghetti
- 2 (25.5-ounce) jars gluten-free Italian herb pasta sauce
- Chopped fresh parsley (optional)
- Grated fresh Parmesan cheese (optional)

Direction

- Preheat oven to 400°.
- Place bread in a food processor; pulse 10 times or until coarse crumbs measure 1/2 cup. Transfer to a bowl; set aside.
- Place garlic, onion, and parsley in processor; pulse 20 seconds or until chopped. Add breadcrumbs, ground round, and next 6 ingredients. Pulse 1 minute or until mixture is combined, stopping frequently to scrape down sides.
- Line a broiler pan with foil. Shape meat mixture into 48 (1 1/2-inch) balls. Place meatballs on broiler rack coated with cooking spray. Bake at 400° for 12 minutes or until meatballs are no longer pink in center.
- While meatballs cook, cook pasta according to package directions, omitting salt and fat.
- Bring pasta sauce to a simmer in a large saucepan. Add meatballs, and simmer 10 minutes or until sauce reaches desired consistency. Serve over spaghetti. Garnish with chopped parsley, and serve with additional Parmesan cheese, if desired.

Nutrition Information

- Calories: 452
- Saturated Fat: 4.8 g
- Fiber: 3.2 g
- Protein: 23.8 g
- Total Fat: 14.3 g
- Total Carbohydrate: 53.9 g
- Cholesterol: 96 mg
- Sodium: 850 mg

233. Spaghetti And Meatballs In Tomato Basil Sauce

Serving: Serves 8 (serving size: 5 meatballs, about 3/4 cup sauce, and about 3/4 cup pasta) | Prep: | Cook: | Ready in: 75mins

Ingredients

- SAUCE
- 1 tablespoon extra-virgin olive oil
- 1 cup chopped onion
- 5 garlic cloves, minced
- 1 1/2 teaspoons dried basil
- 1/4 cup tomato paste
- 1/3 cup dry red wine
- 2 (15-ounce) cans unsalted crushed tomatoes
- 2 (14.5-ounce) cans unsalted diced tomatoes, undrained
- 1 tablespoon sugar
- 1/2 teaspoon kosher salt
- 1/4 teaspoon black pepper
- MEATBALLS
- Cooking spray
- 2 (1-ounce) slices whole-grain bread
- 1/2 cup finely chopped onion

- 1/2 cup chopped fresh flat-leaf parsley, divided
- 1/2 teaspoon kosher salt
- 1/4 teaspoon black pepper
- 1 1/2 pounds 90% lean ground sirloin
- 6 ounces sweet Italian sausage, casings removed
- 3 garlic cloves, minced
- 2 eggs, lightly beaten
- 12 ounces uncooked whole-grain spaghetti

Direction

- To prepare sauce, heat a Dutch oven over medium-high heat. Add oil; swirl to coat. Add 1 cup chopped onion, 5 garlic cloves, and basil to pan; cook 4 minutes, stirring frequently. Add tomato paste; cook 1 minute, stirring constantly. Stir in wine; cook 2 minutes. Add tomatoes and sugar; bring to a boil. Reduce heat, and simmer 25 minutes or until thickened, stirring occasionally. Stir in 1/2 teaspoon salt and 1/4 teaspoon pepper.
- Preheat oven to 450°.
- To prepare meatballs, coat 2 baking sheets with cooking spray. Tear bread into pieces, and place in the bowl of a food processor; pulse until fine crumbs form. Place breadcrumbs, 1/2 cup chopped onion, 1/3 cup parsley, and next 6 ingredients (through eggs) in a large bowl; stir until combined. Shape into 40 meatballs (about 2 tablespoons each); arrange meatballs on prepared pans. Bake at 450° for 15 minutes. Add meatballs to tomato sauce; simmer 10 minutes, stirring occasionally. Follow freezing instructions, or continue recipe.
- Cook pasta according to package directions, omitting salt and fat. Drain. Top pasta with meatball mixture. Sprinkle with remaining 3 tablespoons parsley.

Nutrition Information

- Calories: 479
- Protein: 30 g
- Cholesterol: 105 mg
- Total Fat: 14.2 g
- Fiber: 6 g
- Saturated Fat: 4.7 g
- Sodium: 544 mg
- Total Carbohydrate: 53 g

234. Spaghetti And Turkey Meatballs In Tomato Sauce

Serving: Makes 5 servings (serving size: 1 cup pasta, 3 meatballs, and about 3/4 cup sauce) | Prep: | Cook: | Ready in:

Ingredients

- 1/2 pound whole-wheat spaghetti
- 1 pound ground lean turkey
- 1/2 cup finely grated Parmesan
- 1/4 cup chopped parsley
- 1/4 cup fresh whole-wheat bread crumbs
- 1 large egg, lightly beaten
- 1/2 teaspoon salt
- 1/4 teaspoon pepper
- 1 tablespoon olive oil
- 1 cup minced onion
- 2 garlic cloves, minced
- 1 (26-ounce) can low-sodium crushed tomatoes
- 1 cup canned pinto beans, rinsed and drained
- 1/4 teaspoon salt
- 1/4 teaspoon pepper
- Garnish: additional parsley, 1/4 cup Parmesan

Direction

- Cook spaghetti according to package directions; keep warm. Combine turkey, 1/2 cup Parmesan, 1/4 cup chopped parsley, bread crumbs, egg, 1/2 teaspoon salt, and 1/4 teaspoon pepper in a bowl. Form into 15 meatballs; set aside. Heat olive oil in a large saucepan over medium-high heat. Add onion; cook until soft (5 minutes). Add garlic; cook 2 minutes. Stir in tomatoes, pinto beans, 1/4 teaspoon each salt and pepper; bring to a boil.

Add meatballs; return to a boil. Reduce heat and simmer over low until meatballs are cooked through and sauce has thickened (15 minutes). Divide spaghetti, meatballs, and sauce among 5 bowls. Garnish with additional parsley and 1/4 cup Parmesan.

Nutrition Information

- Calories: 439
- Cholesterol: 98 mg
- Fiber: 9 g
- Sodium: 623 mg
- Saturated Fat: 3.4 g
- Total Fat: 12.2 g
- Protein: 33 g
- Total Carbohydrate: 55 g

235. Spaghetti With Anchovies And Bread Crumbs (Spaghetti Con Acciughe E Mollica)

Serving: Makes 8 servings | Prep: | Cook: | Ready in: 50mins

Ingredients

- 6 salt-packed anchovies or 12 best-quality anchovy fillets in olive oil (see Notes), divided
- 1 pound spaghetti
- 1/2 cup extra-virgin olive oil
- 6 large garlic cloves, minced
- 1 or 2 small fresh or dried hot red chiles such as peperoncini or Thai, thinly sliced
- 2 tablespoons minced flat-leaf parsley
- 3/4 cup Toasted Fresh Bread Crumbs, divided

Direction

- If using salt-packed anchovies, rinse them under cold water. With your fingers, pry them open along the back and lift out backbone to yield 2 fillets. Rinse fillets again to remove any fine bones; pat dry on paper towels. If using anchovy fillets in olive oil, lift out of jar or tin, leaving oil behind (no need to rinse oil-packed fillets). Finely chop 6 fillets; set aside. Cut remaining 6 fillets into 4 or 5 pieces each; set aside.
- In an 8-qt. pot, bring 5 qts. well-salted water to a boil over high heat. Add pasta and cook, stirring occasionally, until tender to the bite, about 10 minutes.
- Meanwhile, put olive oil, garlic, finely chopped anchovies, and chiles in a deep 12-in. frying pan (with at least 2-in. sides) or wide pot and cook over low heat, stirring, until anchovies dissolve. Stir in parsley and remaining anchovies; turn off heat.
- When pasta is almost done, set aside 1 cup of the cooking water, then drain pasta and transfer to pan of anchovy sauce. Toss quickly until all the strands are well coated. Add some reserved cooking water if pasta seems dry. Set aside 2 tbsp. bread crumbs, then add remainder to pasta and toss again.
- Divide pasta among 8 warm bowls and sprinkle each serving with some reserved bread crumbs. Serve immediately.
- Note: Nutritional analysis is per serving.

Nutrition Information

- Calories: 411
- Total Carbohydrate: 51 g
- Protein: 9.6 g
- Sodium: 440 mg
- Total Fat: 19 g
- Cholesterol: 1.7 mg
- Fiber: 1.9 g
- Saturated Fat: 2.8 g

236. Spaghetti With Anchovies, Garlic, And Red Pepper With Lemon Caper Broccoli

Serving: Serves 4 (serving size: about 1 cup pasta, 1 cup broccoli, and 1 tablespoon shallot mixture) | Prep: | Cook: | Ready in: 25mins

Ingredients

- 4 cups broccoli florets
- 16 ounces uncooked whole-grain spaghetti (such as Barilla)
- 5 tablespoons olive oil, divided
- 4 garlic cloves, sliced
- 4 anchovy fillets, drained
- 1/2 teaspoon crushed red pepper
- 1/4 cup chopped fresh flat-leaf parsley
- 1 1/2 tablespoons fresh lemon juice, divided
- 1 teaspoon kosher salt, divided
- 3 ounces Parmesan cheese, grated and divided (about 3/4 cup)
- 2 teaspoons chopped shallots
- 1 teaspoon chopped capers, drained
- 1/4 teaspoon freshly ground black pepper

Direction

- Bring a large saucepan of water to a boil. Add broccoli; cook 3 minutes or until crisp-tender. Remove broccoli from pan with a slotted spoon; set aside. Return water to a boil. Add pasta to pan; cook according to package directions, omitting salt and fat. Drain pasta in a colander over a bowl, reserving 1/2 cup cooking liquid.
- Place 1/4 cup oil, garlic, and anchovies in a large skillet. Heat over medium heat for 3 minutes or until garlic is golden brown and anchovies have melted into the oil, stirring occasionally. Add crushed red pepper to pan; cook 30 seconds, stirring constantly. Carefully add reserved 1/2 cup cooking liquid to pan. Add pasta to pan; toss to coat. Stir in parsley, 1 1/2 teaspoons juice, 3/4 teaspoon salt, and 2 ounces Parmesan cheese (about 1/2 cup). Reserve 4 cups pasta mixture. Divide remaining 4 cups pasta mixture among 4 plates; sprinkle evenly with remaining 1 ounce Parmesan cheese (about 1/4 cup).
- Combine remaining 1 tablespoon oil, remaining 1 tablespoon juice, remaining 1/4 teaspoon salt, shallots, capers, and black pepper in a small bowl, stirring with a whisk. Drizzle oil mixture over broccoli florets. Serve with pasta mixture.
- Italian Wedding Soup: Shape 12 ounces bulk hot Italian sausage into 42 meatballs. Heat 1 tablespoon oil in a large Dutch oven over medium-high heat. Add meatballs; cook 2 minutes on each side. Remove meatballs from pan. Add 3/4 cup chopped onion, 3/4 cup chopped carrot, and 2 minced garlic cloves to pan; sauté 4 minutes. Add 3 cups unsalted chicken stock and 2 cups water; bring to a simmer. Add meatballs; cook 2 minutes. Stir in 5 cups spinach, 1 1/2 cups chopped pasta mixture, 1/4 cup chopped fresh dill, 2 teaspoons lemon juice, 1/2 teaspoon kosher salt, and 1/2 teaspoon pepper; cook 2 minutes. Place 1 1/3 cups soup in each of 6 bowls; top each serving with 2 teaspoons grated Parmesan cheese.
- Serves 6
- Calories 234; Fat 15g (sat 8g, mono 1g, poly 7g); Protein 14g; Carb 11g; Fiber 2g; Chol 44mg; Iron 2mg; Sodium 634mg; Calc 81mg
- Tomato-Basil Spaghetti Frittata: Heat 1 1/2 teaspoons olive oil in a medium nonstick skillet over medium heat. Spread 2 1/2 cups pasta mixture in pan; cook 3 minutes. Combine 1/3 cup sliced green onions, 1/3 cup 2% reduced-fat milk, 2 tablespoons chopped fresh basil, 1/2 teaspoon kosher salt, 1/4 teaspoon pepper, 6 large eggs, and 1 1/3 ounces shredded whole-milk mozzarella cheese (about 1/3 cup) in a large bowl. Add egg mixture to pan. Reduce heat to medium-low; cover and cook 8 minutes or until set. Combine 3/4 cup quartered cherry tomatoes, 1 tablespoon sliced basil, 1 tablespoon olive oil, 1/2 teaspoon white wine vinegar, and 1/8

teaspoon kosher salt in a bowl. Cut frittata into 4 wedges; top with tomato mixture.

- Serves 4 (serving size: 1 wedge and about 3 tablespoons tomato mixture)
- Calories 302; FAT 2g (sat 4g, mono 4g, poly 5g); Protein 16g; Carb 18g; Fiber 1g; Chol 290mg; Iron 2mg; Sodium 594mg; Calc 157mg

Nutrition Information

- Calories: 238
- Total Carbohydrate: 26 g
- Cholesterol: 10 mg
- Protein: 11 g
- Saturated Fat: 2.9 g
- Sodium: 448 mg
- Total Fat: 10.7 g
- Fiber: 4 g

237. Spaghetti With Brussels Sprouts

Serving: Serves 4 | Prep: | Cook: | Ready in: 30mins

Ingredients

- Kosher salt for pasta water plus 1 1/4 tsp., divided
- 12 ounces whole-wheat spaghetti
- 1 pound brussels sprouts
- 4 tablespoons olive oil
- 1 garlic clove, minced
- 3 tablespoons butter, divided
- 1/2 teaspoon pepper, divided
- 4 eggs
- 1/2 lemon, zested and juiced
- 2 ounces grated pecorino cheese (1 scant cup), divided

Direction

- In a large pot of salted boiling water, cook pasta until just cooked through, 7 to 9 minutes.
- Meanwhile, trim brussels sprouts and slice very thin. Heat oil in a large nonstick pan over medium-high heat. Add sprouts and 1 tsp. salt and cook, stirring occasionally, until softened and beginning to brown, 8 to 10 minutes. Add garlic, 2 tbsp. butter, and 1/4 tsp. pepper and cook 30 seconds more. Transfer sprouts to a bowl. Wipe pan clean with a paper towel.
- Return pan to medium-high heat and add remaining 1 tbsp. butter. When it's melted, crack in eggs and cook, covered, until whites are just set and butter is starting to brown, about 2 minutes. Season eggs with remaining 1/4 tsp. each salt and pepper. Cover to keep warm.
- Reserve 1 cup pasta-cooking water. Drain pasta and return to pot. Add sprouts, three-fourths of reserved cooking water, and lemon zest and juice. Cook, stirring, until everything is heated through. Add more cooking water if necessary. Add half of cheese and stir to just combine.
- Divide pasta among 4 wide, shallow bowls and top each with some of the remaining cheese and an egg.

Nutrition Information

- Calories: 667
- Total Carbohydrate: 74 g
- Protein: 25 g
- Total Fat: 33 g
- Saturated Fat: 12 g
- Fiber: 14 g
- Cholesterol: 249 mg
- Sodium: 1195 mg

238. Spaghetti With Chorizo And Toasted Paprika Bread Crumbs

Serving: Serves 4 | Prep: | Cook: | Ready in: 35mins

Ingredients

- 8 ounces dried spaghetti
- 3 large slices crusty white bread, such as pain au levain
- 6 tablespoons extra-virgin olive oil, divided
- 6 1/2 ounces Spanish chorizo, sliced diagonally
- 3 garlic cloves, finely chopped
- 1 1/2 teaspoons smoked paprika
- 1/2 teaspoon kosher salt
- 1/2 cup roughly chopped flat-leaf parsley
- Pepper

Direction

- Cook pasta according to package instructions. Meanwhile, trim crusts from bread and toast bread. Whirl toast in a food processor just until rough crumbs form. You should have about 1 1/2 cups crumbs.
- Heat 2 tbsp. oil in a large frying pan over medium heat. Add chorizo slices and cook until browned on both sides, about 4 minutes. Add garlic and cook until fragrant, about 1 minute. Drain off any liquid and transfer chorizo and garlic to a plate. Wipe any blackened bits out of frying pan with a paper towel.
- Add 1 tbsp. oil to pan along with paprika and cook, stirring frequently, about 30 seconds. Add bread crumbs and salt and cook, stirring frequently, until bread crumbs are toasted and paprika is evenly distributed. Transfer crumbs to a plate. Keep pan hot over low heat.
- Drain cooked pasta, reserving cooking water, and add to hot frying pan along with 1/2 cup cooking water, remaining 3 tbsp. oil, the chorizo, 2/3 of the bread crumbs and parsley.
- Transfer pasta to a serving bowl and top with remaining crumbs, parsley, and pepper to taste.

Nutrition Information

- Calories: 729
- Fiber: 3.4 g
- Protein: 24 g
- Total Fat: 40 g
- Saturated Fat: 9.9 g
- Total Carbohydrate: 71 g
- Sodium: 1057 mg
- Cholesterol: 41 mg

239. Spaghetti With Creamy Broccoli Pesto

Serving: Serves: 6 | Prep: 5mins | Cook: 18mins | Ready in:

Ingredients

- Salt and pepper
- 1 pound broccoli, stems and florets chopped into 1-inch pieces
- 1 pound spaghetti
- 1/4 cup olive oil
- 1 clove garlic, chopped
- 1/2 cup heavy cream
- 1 cup grated Parmesan

Direction

- Bring a large pot of salted water to boil. Add broccoli and cook until soft, 7 to 9 minutes. Remove with a slotted spoon to a food processor. Add spaghetti to pot and cook until al dente, about 10 minutes or as package label directs.
- Add olive oil and garlic to broccoli and process until smooth. Transfer to a large bowl and stir in heavy cream and Parmesan. Season with salt and pepper.
- Drain pasta, reserving 1 cup of cooking water. Mix pasta with broccoli pesto, adding pasta water 1 Tbsp. at a time if pesto is too dry. Serve, passing additional Parmesan if desired.

Nutrition Information

- Calories: 530

- Cholesterol: 42 mg
- Fiber: 3 g
- Protein: 19 g
- Saturated Fat: 9 g
- Total Carbohydrate: 63 g
- Sodium: 482 mg
- Total Fat: 23 g

240. Spaghetti With Parmesan And Bacon

Serving: 8 servings (serving size: 1 1/4 cups) | Prep: | Cook: | Ready in:

Ingredients

- 1 pound uncooked spaghetti
- 12 bacon slices, chopped
- 3 garlic cloves, minced
- 1 cup 2% reduced-fat milk
- 1 teaspoon salt
- 1 teaspoon freshly ground black pepper
- 3 large eggs
- 1 cup frozen petite green peas, thawed
- 1 1/2 cups (6 ounces) grated fresh Parmesan cheese

Direction

- Cook pasta according to package directions. Drain in a colander over a bowl, reserving 1/2 cup hot cooking liquid.
- While pasta cooks, cook bacon in a large nonstick skillet over medium heat until crisp. Remove bacon from pan, reserving 1 tablespoon drippings in pan. Discard remaining drippings; set bacon aside. Add garlic to drippings in pan; cook 30 seconds, stirring constantly.
- Combine milk, salt, pepper, and eggs, stirring with a whisk. Gradually add reserved hot cooking liquid to milk mixture, stirring constantly with a whisk. Add pasta, milk mixture, and peas to skillet; cook over low heat 3 minutes or until sauce thickens. Add bacon and cheese; stir to combine.

Nutrition Information

- Calories: 359
- Sodium: 721 mg
- Fiber: 3.3 g
- Saturated Fat: 5.6 g
- Cholesterol: 99 mg
- Total Carbohydrate: 44.6 g
- Protein: 18.9 g
- Total Fat: 11.2 g

241. Spaghetti With Parsley Pesto And Sausage

Serving: Serves 4 (serving size: about 1 1/4 cups) | Prep: | Cook: | Ready in: 25mins

Ingredients

- 8 ounces uncooked spaghetti
- 3 ounces spicy pork Italian sausage, casings removed
- 4 garlic cloves, crushed and coarsely chopped
- 1/4 cup extra-virgin olive oil, divided
- 1 ounce fresh Parmigiano-Reggiano cheese, grated and divided (about 1/4 cup)
- 5 cups fresh flat-leaf parsley leaves, divided
- 1/2 teaspoon kosher salt

Direction

- Bring 4 quarts of water to a boil in a large saucepan or Dutch oven. Add pasta to pan, and cook 8 minutes or until almost al dente. Drain pasta in a colander over a bowl, reserving 3/4 cup cooking liquid. Discard the remaining cooking liquid.
- Heat a large heavy skillet over medium-high heat. Add Italian sausage to pan; sauté 6 minutes or until browned, stirring to crumble. Remove sausage from pan, reserving

drippings; drain on paper towels. Add garlic to drippings in pan; sauté 1 minute, stirring constantly. Add 1/2 cup reserved cooking liquid to pan; bring to a boil, scraping pan to loosen browned bits. Stir in 2 tablespoons olive oil; cook 30 seconds, stirring constantly with a whisk. Add pasta to pan; cook 1 minute, tossing to combine. Remove from heat.
- Combine about 2 tablespoons cheese and 4 3/4 cups parsley leaves in a food processor; process until finely ground. With motor running, add remaining 1/4 cup cooking liquid and remaining 2 tablespoons olive oil; process until smooth. Add parsley mixture and salt to pasta; toss well to coat. Divide pasta mixture evenly among 4 shallow bowls; top evenly with sausage, remaining 2 tablespoons cheese, and remaining 1/4 cup parsley leaves. Serve immediately.

Nutrition Information

- Calories: 342
- Total Carbohydrate: 21.6 g
- Total Fat: 24.5 g
- Fiber: 3.2 g
- Protein: 10.9 g
- Cholesterol: 22 mg
- Sodium: 607 mg
- Saturated Fat: 5.9 g

242. Spaghetti With Spinach Avocado Sauce

Serving: Serves 4 (serving size: about 1 cup) | Prep: | Cook: | Ready in:

Ingredients

- 8 ounces uncooked whole-grain spaghetti
- 1 cup baby spinach leaves
- 1/4 cup rinsed and drained unsalted cannellini beans
- 1/4 cup fresh basil leaves
- 2 tablespoons extra-virgin olive oil
- 2 teaspoons grated lemon rind
- 1 tablespoon fresh lemon juice
- 1 teaspoon kosher salt
- 2 garlic cloves
- 1 ripe peeled avocado
- 1/4 cup chopped tomato
- 2 tablespoons sliced almonds, toasted

Direction

- Prepare pasta according to package directions, omitting salt and fat. Reserve 1/2 cup cooking liquid. Drain pasta.
- Combine reserved 1/2 cup cooking liquid, spinach, and next 8 ingredients (through avocado) in a food processor; process until smooth. Combine pasta and spinach mixture; toss to coat. Sprinkle with tomato and almonds.

Nutrition Information

- Calories: 374
- Cholesterol: 0.0 mg
- Total Fat: 15.2 g
- Sodium: 502 mg
- Protein: 10 g
- Total Carbohydrate: 50 g
- Fiber: 6 g
- Sugar: 2 g
- Saturated Fat: 2 g

243. Spaghetti With Squash, Walnuts And Parmesan

Serving: Serves 6 | Prep: | Cook: | Ready in: 75mins

Ingredients

- 1 large butternut squash (2 1/2 to 3 lbs.), peeled, seeded, cut into 1-inch pieces
- 1/4 cup olive oil

- Salt and pepper
- 1 cup fresh bread crumbs
- 1 pound spaghetti
- 2 tablespoons unsalted butter
- 1 cup chopped walnuts
- 2 tablespoons chopped fresh parsley leaves
- 1/4 cup grated Parmesan

Direction

- Preheat oven to 400°F. In a bowl, toss squash with 2 Tbsp. oil; season with salt and pepper. Spread in a single layer on a baking sheet. Roast, turning often, until tender and lightly browned, 50 to 55 minutes. Add walnuts to sheet 12 minutes before squash is done, then toast.
- Warm 2 Tbsp. oil in a skillet over medium heat. Sauté bread crumbs until golden, 7 to 10 minutes. Transfer to a bowl and season with salt and pepper.
- Bring a pot of salted water to a boil. Cook spaghetti until al dente, about 10 minutes. Drain, reserving 1/2 cup water. Return pasta to pot over low heat; toss with butter. Stir in squash, nuts, parsley and Parmesan. Toss in 1/2 of the bread crumbs. Add some reserved pasta water if dish seems dry. Divide among 6 plates and sprinkle with remaining bread crumbs.

Nutrition Information

- Calories: 696
- Sodium: 592 mg
- Protein: 19 g
- Saturated Fat: 6 g
- Cholesterol: 13 mg
- Total Fat: 29 g
- Fiber: 8 g
- Total Carbohydrate: 95 g

244. Spaghetti With Turkey Meatballs

Serving: Serves 4 (serving size: about 1 1/4 cups) | Prep: | Cook: | Ready in:

Ingredients

- 1 (9-ounce) package refrigerated fettuccine
- 3 (4-ounce) links sweet Italian turkey sausage
- 1 tablespoon extra-virgin olive oil
- 2 cups sliced onions
- 1/4 teaspoon crushed red pepper
- 2 large garlic cloves, crushed
- 2 cups lower-sodium marinara sauce (such as McCutcheon's)
- 1/2 ounce pecorino cheese, grated (about 2 tablespoons packed)
- 8 basil leaves, torn

Direction

- Cook the pasta according to package directions, omitting salt and fat; drain.
- Remove casing from sausages. Shape sausages into 12 (1-inch) balls. Heat a large skillet over medium-high heat. Add oil to pan; swirl to coat. Add meatballs to pan; cook 7 minutes, browning on all sides. Remove the meatballs from pan. Add onions, red pepper, and garlic to pan; sauté for 2 minutes. Return meatballs and add marinara sauce to pan, and bring to a simmer over medium heat, scraping pan to loosen browned bits. Reduce heat to medium-low, and simmer 5 minutes or until meatballs are done. Add pasta to sauce mixture; toss well. Sprinkle with cheese and basil.

Nutrition Information

- Calories: 412
- Total Carbohydrate: 77.7 g
- Fiber: 2.6 g
- Total Fat: 14 g
- Cholesterol: 77 mg
- Saturated Fat: 4.2 g
- Protein: 19.2 g

- Sodium: 632 mg

245. Speedy Baked Ziti

Serving: 8 | Prep: | Cook: | Ready in: 45mins

Ingredients

- 1 pound ziti or penne
- 1 tablespoon extra-virgin olive oil
- 1 medium onion, finely chopped
- 3 garlic cloves, minced
- 1 pound lean ground sirloin
- 1/4 teaspoon crushed red pepper
- 1/2 teaspoon smoked paprika
- Salt
- 1 (3 cups) jar marinara sauce
- 1 1/2 cups (about 12 ounces) fresh ricotta
- 1/2 pound packaged mozzarella, shredded
- 1/4 cup freshly grated Parmigiano-Reggiano cheese

Direction

- Preheat the oven to 450° and bring a large pot of salted water to a boil. Add the ziti to the pot and boil until just al dente. Drain and return the ziti to the pot.
- Meanwhile, in a large, deep skillet, heat the olive oil. Add the onion and garlic, cover and cook until just softened, about 2 minutes. Add the ground sirloin, crushed red pepper and paprika and season with salt. Cook over high heat, stirring to break up the meat with a spoon, until the meat is no longer pink, about 3 minutes. Add the marinara sauce and bring to a boil. Cover partially and cook over moderate heat for 5 minutes.
- Add the sauce to the ziti in the pot and stir to coat it thoroughly. Add the ricotta in large dollops and stir gently, leaving it in large clumps. Pour half of the ziti into a 9-by-13-inch baking dish and top with half of the mozzarella and Parmigiano. Repeat with the remaining ziti and cheeses.
- Bake the ziti on the top rack of the oven for about 15 minutes, until it is bubbling and browned. Let the ziti rest for 10 minutes before serving.

246. Speedy Homemade Mac And Cheese

Serving: Makes 6 to 8 servings | Prep: | Cook: | Ready in: 20mins

Ingredients

- 1/4 cup plus 1 1/2 tsp. kosher salt, divided
- 1 qt. milk
- 6 tablespoons butter, cut into pieces
- 6 tablespoons all-purpose flour
- 1 pound pasta (such as penne, cavatappi, or rotini)
- 1 (8-oz.) package shredded extra-sharp Cheddar cheese
- 1 (8-oz.) package shredded Monterey Jack cheese
- 1 teaspoon hot sauce (such as Tabasco)
- 1/2 teaspoon freshly ground black pepper
- 1 1/2 cups panko (Japanese breadcrumbs)
- 2 teaspoons olive oil

Direction

- Preheat broiler with oven rack 8 to 9 inches from heat.
- Bring 1/4 cup salt and 4 qt. water to a boil in a large covered Dutch oven over high heat.
- Meanwhile, microwave milk in a microwave-safe 1-qt. glass measuring cup covered with plastic wrap at HIGH 3 minutes. While milk is heating, melt butter in a 12-inch cast-iron skillet over medium heat. Reduce heat to medium-low; add flour, and cook, whisking constantly, 2 minutes. Gradually whisk in hot milk. Increase heat to medium-high, and bring to a low boil, whisking often.
- Add pasta to boiling water, and cook 8 minutes.

- Meanwhile, continue to cook sauce, whisking often, 6 minutes. Remove from heat; whisk in cheeses, hot sauce, 1 1/2 tsp. salt, and 1/2 tsp. pepper. Cover.
- Stir together panko and olive oil.
- Drain pasta, and fold into cheese sauce. Sprinkle with panko mixture.
- Broil 1 to 2 minutes or until breadcrumbs are golden brown. Serve immediately.
- Southern Pimiento Mac and Cheese: Substitute extra-sharp Cheddar cheese for Monterey Jack cheese. Prepare recipe as directed through Step 5, whisking 2 Tbsp. fresh lemon juice, 1 Tbsp. Worcestershire sauce, and 1/2 cup grated sweet onion into sauce along with cheese. Proceed with recipe as directed, stirring 2 (7-oz.) jars diced pimiento, drained, and 2 (52-oz.) packages fully cooked bacon, diced, into pasta mixture just before topping with panko. Sprinkle with 2 Tbsp. chopped fresh chives before serving.
- Barbecue Mac and Cheese: Substitute Gouda cheese for Monterey Jack cheese and crumbled savory cornbread for panko. Prepare recipe as directed through Step 5, stirring 1 lb. pulled pork barbecue (without sauce) into pasta mixture after adding cheese. Sprinkle 1/2 cup chopped green onions over cornbread mixture before broiling, and drizzle with 1/2 cup bottled barbecue sauce after broiling.
- Mexican Mac and Cheese: Substitute pepper Jack cheese for Monterey Jack cheese and crushed tortilla chips for panko. Prepare recipe as directed through Step While pasta cooks, sauté 1 lb. Mexican chorizo in 1 Tbsp. hot olive oil in a large skillet over medium-high heat 4 to 5 minutes or until crumbled and cooked. Proceed with recipe, folding chorizo and 2 cups cherry tomatoes, halved, into cheese sauce along with pasta in Step

247. Speedy Lasagna

Serving: Makes 6 servings | Prep: 15mins | Cook: 40mins |Ready in:

Ingredients

- 1 pound Italian sausage, casings removed
- 1 (26-ounce) jar spaghetti sauce with onions and roasted garlic
- 1 tablespoon chopped fresh or 1 teaspoon dried basil
- 1/2 teaspoon pepper
- 6 no-cook lasagna noodles
- 2 cups ricotta cheese
- 2 cups shredded mozzarella cheese
- 3/4 cup grated Parmesan cheese

Direction

- Crumble sausage into a plastic colander; place over a large microwave-safe bowl. Microwave at HIGH 1 minute, and stir. Microwave at HIGH 3 to 3 1/2 minutes more, stirring every 30 seconds, or until sausage is done and no longer pink. Drain well on paper towels. Discard drippings. Rinse and wipe bowl clean.
- Stir together sausage, spaghetti sauce, basil, and pepper in large bowl.
- Spread one-third sausage mixture in bottom of a lightly greased 11- x 7-inch microwave-safe baking dish; top with 3 noodles, 1 cup ricotta cheese, and 1 cup mozzarella cheese. Repeat layers once.
- Top evenly with remaining sausage mixture and grated Parmesan cheese. Cover with double-thickness plastic wrap, and microwave at MEDIUM (50% power) 30 to 35 minutes. Using an oven mitt, carefully lift one corner of plastic wrap to allow steam to escape, and let stand in microwave 5 minutes before serving.

248. Spicy Seafood Fusilli

Serving: 4 servings (serving size: 2 cups) | Prep: | Cook: | Ready in:

Ingredients

- 4 quarts water
- 8 ounces uncooked long fusilli or 3 cups uncooked short fusilli (twisted spaghetti)
- 2 tablespoons olive oil
- 1/3 cup minced shallots
- 1/2 teaspoon fennel seeds, crushed
- Dash of powdered saffron (optional)
- 1/8 teaspoon salt
- 1 (14.5-ounce) can diced tomatoes, undrained
- 16 littleneck clams, scrubbed
- 3/4 pound large shrimp, peeled and deveined
- 2 teaspoons grated lemon rind
- 1 teaspoon minced seeded jalapeño pepper

Direction

- Bring water to a boil in a large stockpot. Add fusilli; return to a boil. Cook, uncovered, 10 minutes or until fusilli is al dente, stirring occasionally. Drain.
- Heat the olive oil in a large skillet over medium-low heat. Add the shallots, fennel seeds, and saffron (if desired). Cover and cook for 4 minutes or until shallots are tender, stirring occasionally. Stir in salt and tomatoes. Increase heat to medium; cover and cook for 5 minutes. Add the clams. Increase heat to high; cover and cook for 6 minutes or until clams open. Add shrimp, rind, and jalapeño. Stir gently. Cover and cook for 3 minutes or until the shrimp are done. Discard any unopened clamshells. Stir in fusilli.

Nutrition Information

- Calories: 396
- Total Carbohydrate: 50.8 g
- Fiber: 2.2 g
- Saturated Fat: 1.3 g
- Total Fat: 9.4 g
- Cholesterol: 109 mg
- Protein: 26.2 g
- Sodium: 358 mg

249. Spicy Shrimp And Fettuccine

Serving: 4 servings | Prep: | Cook: | Ready in:

Ingredients

- 8 ounces uncooked fettuccine
- 1 tablespoon olive oil
- 1/2 teaspoon crushed red pepper
- 4 garlic cloves, minced
- 1 pound large shrimp, peeled and deveined
- 2 cups chopped plum tomato (about 5)
- 2 tablespoons reduced-fat sour cream
- 1 tablespoon tomato paste
- 1 teaspoon dried basil
- 1/2 teaspoon kosher salt
- 1/4 cup freshly grated Parmesan cheese

Direction

- Cook pasta according to the package directions, omitting salt and fat. Drain.
- Heat oil in a Dutch oven over medium-high heat. Add red pepper and garlic to pan; sauté 1 minute. Add shrimp; sauté 1 minute. Stir in tomatoes and next 4 ingredients (through salt); bring to a boil. Reduce heat, and simmer 5 minutes. Stir in pasta; cook 1 minute or until thoroughly heated.
- Place 1 1/2 cups pasta mixture on each of 4 plates; top each serving with 1 tablespoon cheese. Serve immediately.

Nutrition Information

- Calories: 414
- Protein: 34.1 g
- Total Carbohydrate: 49.4 g
- Total Fat: 8.7 g

- Fiber: 3.3 g
- Cholesterol: 180 mg
- Saturated Fat: 2.5 g
- Sodium: 494 mg

250. Spicy Vegetables With Penne Pasta

Serving: Makes 6 servings | Prep: 30mins | Cook: 15mins | Ready in:

Ingredients

- 1/2 cup dried tomatoes
- 1/2 cup boiling water
- 12 ounces uncooked penne pasta
- 2 medium-size sweet onions, chopped
- 2 small zucchini, chopped
- 1 medium-size green bell pepper, chopped
- 1 medium-size red bell pepper, chopped
- 1 cup sliced fresh mushrooms
- 2 garlic cloves, minced
- 2 tablespoons olive oil
- 1 (26-ounce) jar hot-and-spicy pasta sauce
- 1/2 cup chopped fresh basil
- 1/2 teaspoon salt

Direction

- Stir together dried tomatoes and 1/2 cup boiling water in a bowl; let stand 30 minutes. Drain, chop, and set aside.
- Prepare pasta according to package directions; drain and set aside.
- Sauté onions and next 5 ingredients in hot olive oil in a large skillet over medium-high heat 6 to 8 minutes or until vegetables are tender. Stir in chopped tomatoes.
- Stir in pasta sauce, and bring to a boil. Reduce heat to medium; stir in basil and salt, and simmer, stirring occasionally, 5 minutes. Serve over hot cooked pasta.
- Note: For testing purposes only, we used Newman's Own Fra Diavolo Sauce for hot-and-spicy pasta sauce.

251. Spinach Lasagna

Serving: Makes 6 to 8 servings | Prep: | Cook: | Ready in: 155mins

Ingredients

- 1 (24-oz.) jar pasta sauce
- 1/4 teaspoon dried crushed red pepper
- 2 1/3 cups heavy cream, divided
- 32 ounces ricotta cheese
- 1 ounce fresh basil, chopped
- 1/2 teaspoon kosher salt
- 2 cups freshly shredded Parmesan cheese, divided
- 4 large shallots, thinly sliced
- 1/3 cup olive oil
- 8 garlic cloves, minced
- 2 (10-oz.) packages fresh baby spinach
- 2 tablespoons butter
- 1 tablespoon all-purpose flour
- 12 no-boil lasagna noodles
- 1 (12-oz.) jar roasted red bell pepper strips, drained

Direction

- Preheat oven to 350°. Combine first 2 ingredients and 1 cup cream. Separately combine ricotta, next 2 ingredients, and 1 cup Parmesan. Sauté shallots in hot oil in a Dutch oven over medium-high heat 3 minutes. Add garlic; sauté 1 minute. Remove shallot mixture.
- Add one-third of spinach to Dutch oven; cook over medium-high heat 1 minute or until wilted. Place spinach in a colander; drain. Repeat with remaining spinach.
- Cook butter and flour in Dutch oven over medium heat, stirring constantly, 1 minute. Add 1 1/3 cups cream; bring to a boil. Remove from heat; add spinach and shallots.
- Pour 1/2 cup sauce mixture in a 13- x 9-inch baking dish coated with cooking spray; top with 3 lasagna noodles. Layer half of spinach

mixture, half of roasted peppers, 3 lasagna noodles, and half of ricotta mixture over pasta. Repeat layers; top with 3 lasagna noodles. Pour remaining sauce mixture over top. Place baking dish on a foil-lined baking sheet.

- Bake at 350° for 1 hour. Top with 1 cup Parmesan, and bake 15 minutes. Let stand 30 minutes.

252. Spinach Lasagna Rollups

Serving: Makes 6 servings | Prep: 60mins | Cook: 68mins | Ready in:

Ingredients

- 14 uncooked lasagna noodles
- 1 large onion, finely chopped
- 2 teaspoons olive oil
- 2 garlic cloves, minced
- 3 1/2 tablespoons all-purpose flour
- 3 1/2 cups 1% low-fat milk
- 1 3/4 teaspoons salt, divided
- 1/2 teaspoon freshly ground pepper, divided
- 1/8 teaspoon ground nutmeg
- 1 (16-oz.) bag frozen cut-leaf spinach, thawed
- 1 (24-oz.) container small-curd cottage cheese
- 1 cup grated part-skim mozzarella cheese
- 1 large egg
- 1/4 cup freshly grated Parmesan cheese

Direction

- Cook 7 lasagna noodles according to package directions; remove with tongs or a slotted spoon to a large bowl of cold water. Repeat with remaining noodles. Drain noodles, and arrange in a single layer on clean kitchen towels. Cover with plastic wrap.
- Cook onion in hot oil in a saucepan over medium heat, stirring occasionally, 8 minutes or until onion is caramel colored. Add garlic, and sauté 1 minute. Reserve 1/4 cup onion mixture. Whisk flour into remaining onion mixture in saucepan, and cook, whisking constantly, 1 minute. Gradually whisk in milk. Cook over medium heat, whisking constantly, 8 to 10 minutes or until sauce is thickened and bubbly. Remove from heat; stir in 3/4 tsp. salt, 1/4 tsp. pepper, and 1/8 tsp. nutmeg. Spoon 1/2 cup sauce into a lightly greased 13- x 9-inch baking dish.
- Drain spinach well, pressing between paper towels.
- Preheat oven to 425°. Stir together spinach, cottage cheese, mozzarella cheese, egg, reserved 1/4 cup onion mixture, and remaining 1 tsp. salt and 1/4 tsp. pepper.
- Spread about 3 Tbsp. spinach mixture over 1 noodle; roll up firmly, and place, seam side down, in prepared baking dish. Repeat with remaining noodles and spinach mixture. Spoon remaining sauce over rollups, and sprinkle with Parmesan cheese.
- Bake at 425° for 20 to 25 minutes or until golden and bubbly. Let stand 5 minutes before serving.

253. Spinach Manicotti

Serving: 8 servings (serving size: 1 shell and about 1/2 cup sauce) | Prep: 7mins | Cook: 30mins | Ready in:

Ingredients

- 8 manicotti shells, uncooked
- 1 1/2 cups part-skim ricotta cheese
- 1 cup (4 ounces) pre-shredded part-skim mozzarella cheese
- 1/3 cup (1.3 ounces) grated fresh Parmesan cheese
- 1/4 teaspoon salt
- 1/4 teaspoon pepper
- 1 teaspoon dried Italian seasoning
- 1 (10-ounce) package frozen chopped spinach, thawed, drained, and squeezed dry
- 1 large egg, lightly beaten
- 1 large egg white
- Olive oil-flavored cooking spray
- 2 1/2 cups low-fat roasted garlic pasta sauce

Direction

- Preheat oven to 350°.
- Cook pasta according to package directions, omitting salt and fat. Drain and rinse.
- Combine ricotta cheese and next 8 ingredients in a medium bowl, stirring well. Spoon mixture evenly into pasta shells. Place shells in an 11 x 7-inch baking dish coated with cooking spray. Spoon pasta sauce evenly over shells. Cover and bake at 350° for 20 minutes or until thoroughly heated. Serve warm.

Nutrition Information

- Calories: 221
- Sodium: 654 mg
- Fiber: 5.7 g
- Protein: 15.4 g
- Total Carbohydrate: 17.7 g
- Saturated Fat: 5.1 g
- Cholesterol: 54 mg
- Total Fat: 9.8 g

254. Spinach Stuffed Shells

Serving: Serves: 8 | Prep: 35mins | Cook: | Ready in:

Ingredients

- Salt and pepper
- 1 12-oz. box jumbo shell pasta
- 15 ounces ricotta
- 1 10-oz. box frozen chopped spinach, thawed and squeezed dry
- 1/2 cup grated Parmesan
- 1/4 cup grated pecorino
- 1 large clove garlic, minced
- 1 tablespoon chopped parsley
- 4 cups shredded mozzarella
- 1 large egg, beaten
- 5 cups jarred tomato sauce (about 2 24-oz. jars)

Direction

- Preheat oven to 400°F. In a large pot of boiling, salted water, cook shells 2 minutes less than time specified on package, about 9 minutes. Drain and rinse with cool water.
- In a large bowl, mix ricotta, spinach, Parmesan, pecorino, garlic, parsley and 2 cups mozzarella. Season with salt and pepper. Stir in egg.
- Spread half of tomato sauce in a 9-by-13-inch dish. Fill each shell with 1 heaping Tbsp. ricotta mixture and place open side up in dish. Spoon remaining sauce over shells; sprinkle with remaining mozzarella. Cover with foil and bake 30 minutes. Remove foil and bake 20 to 30 minutes, until bubbling. Let stand 5 minutes; serve.

Nutrition Information

- Calories: 532
- Saturated Fat: 13 g
- Total Fat: 22 g
- Fiber: 4 g
- Total Carbohydrate: 50 g
- Sodium: 1622 mg
- Cholesterol: 86 mg
- Protein: 34 g

255. Spinach And Mushroom Lasagna

Serving: 9 servings (serving size: 1 piece) | Prep: | Cook: | Ready in:

Ingredients

- 9 uncooked gluten-free lasagna noodles
- 1 teaspoon olive oil
- 7 cups sliced mushrooms
- 3 cups sliced shiitake mushroom caps
- 1/2 teaspoon ground nutmeg
- 3 garlic cloves, minced
- 2 (15-ounce) containers part-skim ricotta cheese

- 2 (10-ounce) packages frozen chopped spinach, thawed, drained, and squeezed dry
- 6 tablespoons grated fresh Parmesan cheese, divided
- 1 teaspoon dried Italian seasoning
- 1 teaspoon freshly ground black pepper
- 3 large egg whites
- 1 (25.5-ounce) jar gluten-free marinara sauce
- Cooking spray
- 3 cups (12 ounces) shredded part-skim mozzarella cheese, divided
- Fresh oregano leaves (optional)

Direction

- Cook lasagna noodles according to package directions, omitting salt and fat. Drain; set aside.
- Heat oil in a nonstick skillet over medium heat. Add mushrooms; sauté 3 minutes. Add nutmeg and garlic; sauté 5 minutes. Set aside.
- Combine ricotta, spinach, 1/4 cup Parmesan cheese, Italian seasoning, pepper, and egg whites; set aside.
- Preheat oven to 375°.
- Spread 1/2 cup marinara sauce in bottom of a 13 x 9-inch baking dish coated with cooking spray. Arrange 3 lasagna noodles over sauce; top with half of ricotta cheese mixture, half of mushroom mixture, 1 1/2 cups sauce, and 1 cup mozzarella cheese. Repeat layers, ending with noodles. Spread 1/2 cup sauce over noodles.
- Cover and bake at 375° for 40 minutes. Uncover; sprinkle with remaining 1 cup mozzarella cheese and remaining 2 tablespoons Parmesan cheese; bake 10 minutes. Let stand 10 minutes before serving. Garnish with oregano leaves, if desired.

Nutrition Information

- Calories: 430
- Total Carbohydrate: 39.1 g
- Saturated Fat: 10.1 g
- Sodium: 741 mg
- Cholesterol: 52 mg
- Protein: 30.4 g
- Total Fat: 17.1 g
- Fiber: 4.3 g

256. Spinach And Ricotta Stuffed Shells

Serving: 6 servings (serving size: 4 stuffed shells and about 1/3 cup sauce) | Prep: | Cook: | Ready in:

Ingredients

- 2 cups Basic Marinara, divided
- Cooking spray
- 2 1/2 cups part-skim ricotta cheese
- 1/2 cup (2 ounces) grated fresh Parmesan cheese
- 1/2 teaspoon onion powder
- 1/2 teaspoon dried oregano
- 1/4 teaspoon salt
- 1/4 teaspoon freshly ground black pepper
- 1 (10-ounce) package frozen chopped spinach, thawed, drained, and squeezed dry
- 1 large egg yolk
- 1 garlic clove, minced
- 24 cooked jumbo pasta shells

Direction

- Preheat oven to 350°.
- Spread 1/2 cup Basic Marinara over bottom of a 13 x 9-inch baking dish coated with cooking spray.
- Combine ricotta and next 8 ingredients (through garlic) in a large bowl, stirring well. Spoon about 1 1/2 tablespoons filling into each pasta shell. Arrange stuffed shells in prepared dish; spread with remaining 1 1/2 cups Basic Marinara. Cover and bake at 350° for 30 minutes. Let stand 5 minutes before serving.

Nutrition Information

- Calories: 329
- Total Fat: 9.8 g
- Saturated Fat: 4.8 g
- Cholesterol: 67 mg
- Protein: 19.6 g
- Total Carbohydrate: 39.4 g
- Fiber: 4.2 g
- Sodium: 552 mg

257. Spinach Ravioli Lasagna

Serving: Makes 6 to 8 servings | Prep: 10mins | Cook: 35mins | Ready in:

Ingredients

- 1 (6-oz.) package fresh baby spinach, thoroughly washed
- 1/3 cup refrigerated pesto sauce
- 1 (15-oz.) jar Alfredo sauce
- 1/4 cup vegetable broth*
- 1 (25-oz.) package frozen cheese-filled ravioli (do not thaw)
- 1 cup (4 oz.) shredded Italian six-cheese blend
- Garnishes: chopped fresh basil, paprika

Direction

- Preheat oven to 375°. Chop spinach, and toss with pesto in a medium bowl.
- Combine Alfredo sauce and vegetable broth. Spoon one-third of alfredo sauce mixture (about 1/2 cup) into a lightly greased 2-qt. or 11- x 7-inch baking dish. Top with half of spinach mixture. Arrange half of ravioli in a single layer over spinach mixture. Repeat layers once. Top with remaining Alfredo sauce.
- Bake at 375° for 30 minutes. Remove from oven, and sprinkle with shredded cheese. Bake 5 minutes or until hot and bubbly. Garnish, if desired.
- *Chicken broth may be substituted.
- Note: For testing purposes only, we used Santa Barbara Original Basil Pesto and Bertolli Alfredo Sauce.

258. Spinach And Ricotta Stuffed Shells

Serving: Serves 6 | Prep: 20mins | Cook: 60mins | Ready in:

Ingredients

- 24 jumbo pasta shells
- 1 15-oz. container ricotta
- 2 cups shredded mozzarella
- 1/2 cup shredded Parmesan
- 1 10-oz. package frozen chopped spinach, thawed and squeezed dry
- 1 large egg, lightly beaten
- Salt and pepper
- 1 teaspoon Italian seasoning
- Pinch of ground nutmeg
- 1 26-oz. jar spaghetti sauce

Direction

- Preheat oven to 375°F. Mist a 9-by-13-inch baking dish with cooking spray. Cook pasta shells according to package label directions; drain and set aside to cool. While pasta cooks, in a large bowl, stir together ricotta, 1 cup mozzarella, Parmesan, spinach, egg, salt, pepper, Italian seasoning and nutmeg.
- Spread 3/4 cup spaghetti sauce over bottom of baking dish. Stuff shells with cheese-and-spinach mixture and place in dish. Spoon remaining sauce over shells and sprinkle with remaining 1 cup mozzarella.
- Cover baking dish with foil and bake for 35 minutes. Remove foil and bake about 10 minutes longer, until bubbly and cheese begins to brown.

Nutrition Information

- Calories: 498
- Sodium: 1253 mg
- Total Carbohydrate: 41 g
- Protein: 28 g
- Fiber: 7 g
- Cholesterol: 88 mg
- Total Fat: 26 g
- Saturated Fat: 13 g

259. Sticky Noodle Bowl

Serving: Makes 4 servings | Prep: 15mins | Cook: 15mins | Ready in:

Ingredients

- 1 (11-oz.) box Asian-style noodles with soy-ginger sauce
- 1 (6-oz.) package fresh snow peas
- 1 small red bell pepper, thinly sliced
- 1/2 medium onion, thinly sliced
- 2 tablespoons freshly grated ginger
- 1 tablespoon olive oil
- 1 (8-oz.) package MORNINGSTAR FARMS Meal Starters Steak Strips
- 1 teaspoon minced garlic
- 1/3 cup vegetable broth
- 1 tablespoon creamy peanut butter
- Toppings: chopped peanuts, chopped fresh cilantro, bean sprouts, lime wedges

Direction

- Remove and reserve sauce and sesame seed topping packets from box of noodles. Cook noodles according to package directions, stirring in snow peas during last minute of cooking; drain and rinse.
- Sauté bell pepper, onion, and ginger in hot oil in a large skillet over medium-high heat 3 minutes or until crisp-tender. Stir in strips and garlic; sauté 3 minutes or until thoroughly heated. Stir in cooked noodles, reserved sauce packet, vegetable broth, and peanut butter, tossing to coat. Cook, stirring constantly, 2 minutes or until peanut butter is melted and mixture is thoroughly heated.
- Transfer noodle mixture to a large serving platter, and serve with desired toppings. Top with reserved sesame seed topping, if desired.

260. Stuffed Shells

Serving: Serves 9 (serving size: 4 stuffed shells and 1/3 cup sauce) | Prep: | Cook: | Ready in: 73mins

Ingredients

- 1 (12-ounce) package jumbo pasta shells
- 2 teaspoons olive oil
- 2 medium zucchini, halved lengthwise and cut into 1/4-inch-thick slices (3 cups)
- 1 (8-ounce) package mushrooms, cut into 1/4-inch-thick slices
- 2 garlic cloves, minced
- 1 (5-ounce) package fresh baby spinach
- 1/2 teaspoon kosher salt
- 1/4 cup chopped fresh basil
- 2 tablespoons dried parsley
- 1 1/2 teaspoons dried oregano
- 1/2 teaspoon crushed red pepper
- 1 (15-ounce) container part-skim ricotta cheese
- 6 ounces part-skim mozzarella cheese, shredded (about 1 1/2 cups), divided
- 1 (24.5-ounce) jar lower-sodium marinara sauce, divided
- Cooking spray
- 1/2 cup (2 ounces) grated fresh Parmesan cheese

Direction

- Preheat oven to 350°.
- Cook pasta according to package directions, omitting salt and fat; drain.
- While pasta cooks, heat a large nonstick skillet over medium-high heat. Add oil to pan; swirl to coat. Add zucchini and mushrooms; sauté 6 minutes or until vegetables are tender and

beginning to brown. Add garlic; sauté 1 minute. Add spinach and salt; cover, and cook 1 minute or until spinach wilts. Remove pan from heat; cool 10 minutes.

- Combine basil, next 4 ingredients (through ricotta cheese), and 1/2 cup mozzarella cheese in a large bowl; stir in vegetable mixture.
- Spread 1 cup marinara sauce over bottom of a 13 x 9-inch glass or ceramic baking dish coated with cooking spray. Stuff cheese mixture evenly into shells. Place shells on top of sauce in dish. Pour remaining sauce over shells. Top with 1 cup mozzarella cheese and Parmesan cheese. Cover with a sheet of foil coated with cooking spray, coated side down.
- Bake at 350° for 40 minutes or until sauce is bubbly and cheese melts. Let stand 15 minutes before serving.

Nutrition Information

- Calories: 384
- Total Carbohydrate: 40.1 g
- Total Fat: 14 g
- Sodium: 603 mg
- Cholesterol: 43 mg
- Protein: 24.1 g
- Fiber: 3.3 g
- Saturated Fat: 7.2 g

261. Summer Tortellini Salad

Serving: Makes 4 servings | Prep: 10mins | Cook: 10mins | Ready in:

Ingredients

- 1 (19-oz.) package frozen cheese tortellini
- 2 cups chopped cooked chicken
- 1/4 cup sliced green olives
- 1/4 cup sliced black olives
- 1/4 cup diced red bell pepper
- 2 tablespoons chopped sweet onion
- 2 tablespoons chopped fresh parsley
- 2 tablespoons mayonnaise
- 1 tablespoon red wine vinegar
- 1 teaspoon herbes de Provence*
- 1/4 cup canola oil
- Salt to taste
- Garnish: fresh parsley sprigs

Direction

- Cook tortellini according to package directions; drain. Plunge into ice water to stop the cooking process; drain and place in large bowl. Stir in chicken and next 5 ingredients.
- Whisk together mayonnaise, red wine vinegar, and herbes de Provence. Add oil in a slow, steady stream, whisking constantly until smooth. Pour over tortellini mixture, tossing to coat. Stir in salt to taste. Cover and chill at least 25 minutes. Garnish, if desired.
- *1 tsp. dried Italian seasoning may be substituted.
- Note: For testing purposes only, we used Rosetto Cheese Tortellini.
- Tuna Tortellini Salad: Substitute 1 (12-oz.) can albacore tuna, rinsed and drained well, for chicken. Prepare recipe as directed.

262. Summer Vegetable Rigatoni With Chicken

Serving: Serves 6 (serving size: about 1 1/2 cups) | Prep: | Cook: | Ready in: 40mins

Ingredients

- 12 ounces uncooked rigatoni
- 1 1/2 cups diagonally sliced sugar snap peas
- Cooking spray
- 3 (6-ounce) skinless, boneless chicken breast halves
- 1 teaspoon freshly ground black pepper, divided
- 3/4 teaspoon kosher salt, divided
- 1/4 cup olive oil
- 2 tablespoons sliced garlic

- 2 oregano sprigs
- 2 thyme sprigs
- 1/2 cup unsalted chicken stock
- 3 ounces Parmigiano-Reggiano cheese, grated and divided (about 3/4 cup)
- 2 cups multicolored cherry tomatoes, halved
- 1/4 cup small fresh basil leaves
- 1 teaspoon fresh oregano leaves
- 1 teaspoon fresh thyme leaves

Direction

- Cook pasta according to package directions for 10 minutes, omitting salt and fat. Add peas; cook 2 minutes. Drain mixture over a bowl, reserving 1 1/2 cups cooking liquid; rinse with cold water. Drain.
- Heat a grill pan over medium-high heat; coat with cooking spray. Sprinkle chicken with 1/2 teaspoon pepper and 1/4 teaspoon salt. Add chicken to pan; cook 5 minutes on each side or until done. Let stand 10 minutes; cut chicken into 1-inch pieces.
- Combine oil, garlic, oregano sprigs, and thyme sprigs in a large skillet over medium heat; cook 4 minutes or just until garlic begins to brown. Add reserved 1 1/2 cups cooking liquid, 1/4 teaspoon pepper, remaining 1/2 teaspoon salt, and stock to pan; bring to a boil. Cook until reduced to 3/4 cup (about 10 minutes); discard herb sprigs. Stir in 2 ounces cheese; stir until cheese melts. Stir in pasta mixture. Stir in chicken, remaining 1 ounce cheese, and tomatoes. Sprinkle with remaining 1/4 teaspoon pepper, basil, oregano, and thyme leaves.

Nutrition Information

- Calories: 428
- Total Carbohydrate: 47 g
- Total Fat: 13.7 g
- Protein: 28 g
- Saturated Fat: 2.5 g
- Sodium: 370 mg
- Cholesterol: 56 mg
- Fiber: 3 g

263. Swedish Meatballs With Red Currant Pan Sauce

Serving: Serves 4 (serving size: 5 meatballs, 3/4 cup noodles, and about 1/3 cup sauce) | Prep: | Cook: | Ready in: 23mins

Ingredients

- 6 ounces egg noodles
- 1 teaspoon unsalted butter
- 1/4 cup grated red onion
- 1/4 cup whole-wheat panko breadcrumbs
- 1/4 cup 2% reduced-fat milk
- 3 tablespoons chopped fresh dill
- 1 teaspoon freshly ground black pepper, divided
- 3/4 teaspoon salt, divided
- 1/2 teaspoon ground allspice
- 1/4 teaspoon grated whole nutmeg
- 1 pound 90% lean ground sirloin
- Cooking spray
- 4 teaspoons all-purpose flour
- 1 cup unsalted beef stock
- 2 tablespoons red currant or lingonberry jelly
- 2 tablespoons sour cream

Direction

- Cook noodles according to package directions, omitting salt and fat. Drain; toss with butter, cover, and set aside.
- Combine grated onion, panko, milk, dill, 1/2 teaspoon pepper, 1/4 teaspoon salt, allspice, and nutmeg in a large bowl; stir to moisten panko. Add beef; stir with your hands until combined. Gently form beef mixture into 20 balls (about 1 tablespoon each).
- Heat a large skillet over medium-high heat. Coat pan with cooking spray. Add meatballs to pan; cook 6 minutes, turning occasionally, or just until cooked through (thermometer inserted into center of a meatball should

register 160°). Transfer meatballs to a paper towel-lined plate; leave browned bits in pan.

- Place flour in a medium bowl; gradually whisk in stock. Return pan to medium heat; add stock mixture and jelly to pan. Cook 2 minutes or until thickened and bubbly, stirring constantly with a whisk. Remove pan from heat; whisk in sour cream, remaining 1/2 teaspoon pepper, and remaining 1/2 teaspoon salt. Serve meatballs and sauce with noodles.

Nutrition Information

- Calories: 459
- Total Carbohydrate: 45 g
- Cholesterol: 130 mg
- Protein: 31 g
- Saturated Fat: 6.9 g
- Total Fat: 16.4 g
- Fiber: 2 g
- Sodium: 576 mg

264. Sweet Potato Gnocchi With Mushrooms

Serving: Makes 8 servings | Prep: | Cook: | Ready in: 25mins

Ingredients

- 1 (16-oz.) package sweet potato gnocchi
- 6 tablespoons butter, divided
- 1 (8-oz.) package sliced baby portobello mushrooms
- 4 garlic cloves, thinly sliced
- 3 tablespoons sliced fresh shallots
- 2 tablespoons chopped fresh flat-leaf parsley
- 1 tablespoon thinly sliced fresh sage
- 1 teaspoon kosher salt
- 1/4 teaspoon freshly ground pepper
- Toppings: freshly shaved Parmesan cheese, freshly ground pepper, chopped fresh parsley

Direction

- Prepare gnocchi according to package directions. Keep warm.
- Melt 2 Tbsp. butter in a large skillet over medium-high heat. Add mushrooms; sauté 3 to 5 minutes or until lightly browned. Add garlic and shallots; sauté 2 minutes or until tender. Remove from skillet. Wipe skillet clean.
- Melt remaining 4 Tbsp. butter in skillet over medium-high heat; cook 2 to 3 minutes or until lightly browned. Stir in parsley, sage, and mushroom mixture. Add hot cooked gnocchi, and toss gently. Stir in salt and pepper. Serve immediately with desired toppings.

265. Sweet Potato Noodle Kugel

Serving: Makes 6 servings (serving size: 1 cup) | Prep: | Cook: | Ready in:

Ingredients

- 8 ounces egg noodles made for Passover
- 1/4 cup butter
- 2 medium sweet potatoes (1 1/4 pounds), peeled and grated (about 4 cups)
- 2 large eggs
- 2 large egg whites
- 1/2 cup reduced-fat sour cream
- 1/2 cup apricot jam
- 1 teaspoon salt
- 1/4 cup chopped pecans, toasted

Direction

- Preheat oven to 350°.
- Cook noodles according to package directions; drain and rinse with cold water. Drain again, and set aside.
- Meanwhile, melt butter in a large nonstick skillet over medium heat. Add the sweet potatoes; sauté until tender, 8 minutes. Let cool 5 minutes.

- Beat together eggs and egg whites in a large bowl. Add sour cream, jam, and salt; mix well. Add the sweet-potato mixture; mix well. Stir in noodles. Transfer mixture to an 8-inch square glass baking dish that has been coated with nonstick cooking spray; cover dish with foil.
- Bake 30 minutes or until heated through. Top with pecans; let stand for 5 minutes before serving.

Nutrition Information

- Calories: 427
- Saturated Fat: 7 g
- Total Fat: 17 g
- Fiber: 4 g
- Protein: 10 g
- Sodium: 453 mg
- Total Carbohydrate: 61 g
- Cholesterol: 129 mg

266. Sweet Hot Asian Noodle Bowl

Serving: Makes 8 servings | Prep: 35mins | Cook: 15mins | Ready in:

Ingredients

- 3/4 cup rice wine vinegar
- 1/3 cup lite soy sauce
- 1/3 cup honey
- 2 tablespoons minced fresh ginger
- 2 tablespoons dark sesame oil
- 1 tablespoon Asian chili-garlic sauce
- 16 ounces uncooked spaghetti
- 1 (15-ounce) can cut baby corn, rinsed and drained
- 1 (8-ounce) can sliced water chestnuts, rinsed and drained
- 1 large red bell pepper, thinly sliced
- 1 cup (about 4 ounces) thinly sliced snow peas
- 1/3 cup finely chopped green onions
- 1/4 cup chopped fresh cilantro
- 1 tablespoon toasted sesame seeds (optional)

Direction

- Whisk together first 6 ingredients in a medium bowl; set aside.
- Cook spaghetti according to package directions in a large Dutch oven; drain and return pasta to Dutch oven.
- Pour vinegar mixture over hot cooked pasta. Add baby corn and next 5 ingredients, and toss to combine. Sprinkle with sesame seeds, if desired. Serve hot or cold.
- Note: For testing purposes only, we used Lee Kum Kee Chili Garlic Sauce, found in the Asian section of large supermarkets.

267. Take Two Turkey Noodle Soup With Ginger And Chile

Serving: Serves 4 to 6 | Prep: | Cook: | Ready in: 25mins

Ingredients

- 12 cups reduced-sodium or homemade chicken broth
- About 2 oz. fresh ginger, peeled and thinly sliced (1/3 cup)
- 8 ounces cooked turkey
- 9 ounces fresh Chinese-style egg noodles or 5 oz. dried*
- 6 ounces fresh shiitake mushrooms, stemmed and sliced (2 1/2 cups)
- 6 ounces broccolini, large stems halved lengthwise, then all of it cut into 1-in. lengths
- 2 tablespoons hoisin sauce
- 1 to 1 1/2 tbsp. Asian chili garlic sauce
- 2 cups coarsely chopped cilantro leaves and tender stems
- 8 green onions, thinly sliced

Direction

- Bring broth and ginger to a boil, covered, over high heat. Meanwhile, tear turkey into large shreds; set aside.
- Add noodles, mushrooms, and broccolini to broth (if using dried noodles, cook noodles first for 2 minutes, then add vegetables). Cook noodles until almost tender, about 2 minutes for fresh and 4 to 5 minutes for dried.
- Keep soup at a simmer and add turkey. Stir in hoisin and chili garlic sauces, then most of cilantro and green onions. Ladle into large, deep bowls and top with remaining cilantro and green onions.
- *Find fresh noodles in the refrigerated section of most grocery stores and Asian markets, and dried noodles in your grocery store's Asian-foods aisle.

Nutrition Information

- Calories: 288
- Fiber: 3.1 g
- Cholesterol: 93 mg
- Sodium: 626 mg
- Total Carbohydrate: 33 g
- Total Fat: 4.7 g
- Protein: 28 g
- Saturated Fat: 1.4 g

268. Tex Mex Lasagna

Serving: 4 servings | Prep: | Cook: | Ready in:

Ingredients

- 3/4 cup bottled salsa
- 1 1/2 teaspoons ground cumin
- 1 (14.5-ounce) can no salt-added diced tomatoes
- 1 (8-ounce) can no salt-added tomato sauce
- Cooking spray
- 6 precooked lasagna noodles (such as Barilla or Vigo)
- 1 cup frozen whole-kernel corn, thawed
- 1 (15-ounce) can black beans, rinsed and drained
- 2 cups (8 ounces) preshredded reduced-fat 4-cheese Mexican blend cheese
- 1/4 cup chopped green onions

Direction

- Preheat oven to 450°.
- Combine first 4 ingredients; spread 2/3 cup sauce in bottom of an 8-inch square baking dish coated with cooking spray. Arrange 2 noodles over sauce; top with 1/2 cup corn and half of beans. Sprinkle with 1/2 cup cheese; top with 2/3 cup sauce. Repeat layers once; top with remaining 2 noodles. Spread remaining sauce over noodles. Sprinkle with remaining 1 cup cheese. Cover and bake at 450° for 30 minutes or until noodles are tender and sauce is bubbly. Let stand 15 minutes. Sprinkle with onions.

Nutrition Information

- Calories: 415
- Saturated Fat: 6.1 g
- Protein: 27.2 g
- Total Carbohydrate: 55.2 g
- Sodium: 970 mg
- Cholesterol: 41 mg
- Total Fat: 13.3 g
- Fiber: 10.4 g

269. Tex Mex Ravioli Casserole

Serving: Makes 6 servings | Prep: 20mins | Cook: | Ready in:

Ingredients

- 1 (16-ounce) jar mild salsa
- 1 (10 3/4-ounce) can tomato puree
- 1/2 teaspoon ground cumin

- 1 (28-ounce) bag frozen cheese ravioli, unthawed
- 2 (19-ounce) cans black beans, rinsed and drained
- 1/2 cup chopped fresh cilantro
- 1 bunch green onions, thinly sliced
- 2 cups (8 ounces) shredded sharp Cheddar cheese
- 1 cup (4 ounces) shredded Monterey Jack cheese

Direction

- Combine first 3 ingredients. Pour 1/2 cup sauce mixture on the bottom of a lightly greased 2-quart oval or 11- x 7-inch baking dish. Top evenly with frozen cheese ravioli. Layer with black beans, chopped cilantro, green onions, and remaining sauce mixture; top evenly with shredded Cheddar and Monterey Jack cheeses.
- Bake, covered with aluminum foil, at 350° for 45 minutes or until bubbly. Remove foil, and bake 5 more minutes. Let stand 5 minutes.

270. Thai Chicken Noodle Bowls

Serving: Serves 6 | Prep: | Cook: | Ready in: 532mins

Ingredients

- Marinade:
- 1/2 cup chopped fresh cilantro
- 2 tablespoons brown sugar
- 2 tablespoons minced peeled fresh ginger
- 2 tablespoons lower-sodium soy sauce
- 2 tablespoons rice vinegar
- 1 tablespoon fresh lime juice
- 1 1/2 teaspoons roasted red chile paste
- 1/3 cup finely chopped green onions (4 onions)
- 3 garlic cloves, minced
- 6 (6-ounce) skinless, boneless chicken breast halves
- 6 ounces uncooked rice sticks (rice-flour noodles)
- Sauce:
- 1/4 cup rice vinegar
- 2 tablespoons brown sugar
- 2 tablespoons chopped fresh cilantro
- 2 tablespoons fresh lime juice
- 1 tablespoon fish sauce
- 1 tablespoon minced peeled fresh ginger
- 1 teaspoon roasted red chile paste
- Cooking spray
- Toppings:
- 2 carrots, peeled and cut into ribbons (about 2 cups)
- 1/2 English cucumber, halved lengthwise and thinly sliced (about 1 1/4 cups)
- 1/4 cup chopped fresh basil
- 2 tablespoons finely chopped unsalted dry-roasted peanuts
- Additional ingredients:
- 6 lime wedges

Direction

- To prepare marinade, combine first 9 ingredients in a large heavy-duty zip-top plastic bag; add chicken. Seal bag; marinate in refrigerator overnight.
- Remove chicken from bag; discard marinade. Let stand at room temperature 30 minutes.
- While chicken stands, cook noodles according to package directions, omitting salt and fat. Drain.
- To prepare sauce, combine 1/4 cup rice vinegar and next 6 ingredients (through chile paste) in a small bowl.
- Preheat grill to medium-high heat.
- Place chicken on grill rack coated with cooking spray. Cook 6 minutes on each side or until done. Let stand 5 minutes. Cut chicken crosswise into slices.
- Place 3/4 cup noodles and slices from 1 chicken breast half in each of 6 bowls. Top each serving with 1/3 cup carrot, about 3 tablespoons cucumber, 2 teaspoons basil, and 1 teaspoon peanuts. Drizzle each serving with

1 1/2 teaspoons sauce, and serve with 1 lime wedge.

- Tips: To make carrot ribbons, use a vegetable peeler.

Nutrition Information

- Calories: 356
- Total Fat: 3.9 g
- Sodium: 469 mg
- Saturated Fat: 0.8 g
- Cholesterol: 99 mg
- Protein: 41.1 g
- Total Carbohydrate: 37.3 g
- Fiber: 1.7 g

271. Thai Crunch Bowl With Salmon

Serving: Serves 1 | Prep: | Cook: | Ready in:

Ingredients

- 2/3 cup cooked quinoa
- 2 tablespoons matchstick-cut carrot
- 2 tablespoons chopped red bell pepper
- 2 tablespoons steamed edamame
- 1/4 cup shredded red cabbage
- 3 ounces broiled salmon
- 1 teaspoon chopped dry-roasted peanuts
- Sesame-Peanut Sauce:
- 1 teaspoon creamy peanut butter
- 1 teaspoon lower-sodium soy sauce
- 1/2 teaspoon rice vinegar
- 1/2 teaspoon dark sesame oil
- 1/2 teaspoon fresh lime juice

Direction

- Top cooked quinoa with carrot, red bell pepper, edamame, cabbage, and salmon. Sprinkle with peanuts.
- In a small bowl, combine peanut butter, soy sauce, vinegar, sesame oil, and lime juice, stirring well with a whisk. Drizzle over bowl.

Nutrition Information

- Calories: 397
- Total Fat: 15.3 g
- Sugar: 4 g
- Cholesterol: 54 mg
- Fiber: 6 g
- Saturated Fat: 1.9 g
- Protein: 31 g
- Sodium: 302 mg
- Total Carbohydrate: 34 g

272. Three Cheese Lasagna

Serving: Serves 6 | Prep: | Cook: | Ready in: 85mins

Ingredients

- 1 cup part-skim ricotta cheese
- 1/4 cup fresh flat-leaf parsley, divided
- 1 tablespoon chopped fresh oregano
- 1 teaspoon chopped fresh thyme
- 1/2 teaspoon kosher salt
- 1/2 teaspoon freshly ground black pepper
- 6 ounces shredded part-skim mozzarella cheese, divided (about 1 1/2 cups)
- 1 ounce fresh Parmesan cheese, grated and divided (about 1/4 cup)
- 1 egg, lightly beaten
- 1/4 cup torn fresh basil
- 1/8 teaspoon ground red pepper
- 4 garlic cloves, minced
- 1 (24-ounce) jar lower-sodium pasta sauce
- 9 cooked lasagna noodles
- Cooking spray

Direction

- Preheat oven to 375°.

- Combine ricotta, 2 tablespoons parsley, oregano, thyme, salt, black pepper, 1 cup mozzarella, 1 tablespoon Parmesan cheese, and egg in a small bowl. Combine basil, red pepper, garlic, and pasta sauce in a medium bowl.
- Cut the noodles into 9 (7 x 2-inch) pieces; discard remaining pieces. Spread 1/2 cup pasta sauce mixture in bottom of an 8-inch square glass or ceramic baking dish coated with cooking spray. Arrange 3 noodles over pasta sauce mixture; top with about 2/3 cup ricotta mixture and 3/4 cup pasta sauce mixture. Repeat layers twice, ending with 1/2 cup pasta sauce mixture. Top evenly with the remaining 1/2 cup mozzarella and remaining 3 tablespoons Parmesan cheese. Bake at 375° for 40 minutes.
- Preheat broiler to high. (Keep lasagna in oven.)
- Broil lasagna for 2 minutes or until cheese is golden brown and sauce is bubbly. Let stand 10 minutes. Sprinkle with remaining 2 tablespoons parsley.

Nutrition Information

- Calories: 339
- Saturated Fat: 6 g
- Cholesterol: 66 mg
- Sodium: 564 mg
- Total Fat: 11.8 g
- Total Carbohydrate: 39.2 g
- Fiber: 2.6 g
- Protein: 20.2 g

273. Three Cheese Spaghetti Gratin

Serving: Serves: 6 | Prep: 10mins | Cook: 25mins | Ready in:

Ingredients

- 1 1/2 cups cooked spaghetti
- 1 cup shredded mozzarella
- 1/2 cup grated Swiss cheese, preferably Gruyère
- 3 scallions, white parts only, thinly sliced
- 4 large eggs
- 1/2 cup milk
- 1/2 teaspoon salt
- 1/4 teaspoon pepper
- 1 cup panko
- 1/2 cup grated Parmesan
- 3 tablespoons unsalted butter, melted and cooled

Direction

- Preheat oven to 375°F and generously mist a 9-inch glass or ceramic pie dish with cooking spray.
- Combine spaghetti, mozzarella and Swiss cheese in a large bowl. Add scallions and toss to blend. In a small bowl, beat eggs with milk until blended. Pour over spaghetti, season with 1/2 tsp. salt and 1/4 tsp. pepper, mix well and pour into baking dish.
- Combine panko and Parmesan in a small bowl. Add melted butter; toss with a fork to coat crumbs. Spread evenly over top of spaghetti mixture and bake until golden brown on top, about 25 minutes. Let stand for 5 minutes. Cut into wedges and serve.

Nutrition Information

- Calories: 371
- Total Fat: 22 g
- Total Carbohydrate: 22 g
- Cholesterol: 183 mg
- Protein: 21 g
- Saturated Fat: 12 g
- Sodium: 578 mg
- Fiber: 1 g

274. Tofu And Edamame Noodle Bowl With Caramelized Coconut Broth

Serving: Serves 4 (serving size: about 1 1/2 cups) | Prep: | Cook: | Ready in:

Ingredients

- 2 teaspoons grated fresh jalapeño pepper
- 1 teaspoon grated peeled fresh ginger
- 1 (13.5-ounce) can light coconut milk
- 1 garlic clove, grated
- 1 (14-ounce) package extra-firm water-packed tofu, drained and cut into 1/2-inch cubes
- 6 ounces dried brown rice noodles (such as Annie Chun's)
- 1 1/2 cups frozen edamame
- 1/2 cup unsalted vegetable stock
- 1 1/2 tablespoons fresh lime juice
- 3/4 teaspoon kosher salt
- 6 ounces baby spinach
- 1/4 cup chopped unsalted, dry-roasted peanuts

Direction

- Combine first 4 ingredients in a large skillet; bring to a boil. Add tofu to pan. Cook 12 minutes or until liquid is reduced to about 1/3 cup and starts to turn light golden, stirring frequently.
- Prepare rice noodles according to package directions, omitting salt and fat. Add edamame to noodles during last minute of cooking time. Reserve 1/2 cup cooking liquid. Drain noodle mixture; rinse with cold water. Drain.
- Add noodle mixture, stock, and 1/2 cup reserved cooking liquid to pan; toss to coat. Remove from heat; stir in juice, salt, and spinach. Sprinkle with peanuts.

Nutrition Information

- Calories: 393
- Total Fat: 13.6 g
- Total Carbohydrate: 52 g
- Cholesterol: 0.0 mg
- Fiber: 5 g
- Protein: 18 g
- Saturated Fat: 2.8 g
- Sodium: 469 mg

275. Tomato Ravioli

Serving: Serves 4 (serving size: about 6 ravioli and 1/2 cup tomato mixture) | Prep: | Cook: | Ready in: 55mins

Ingredients

- 1 pound cherry tomatoes
- 2 shallots, cut into wedges
- Cooking spray
- 3 tablespoons extra-virgin olive oil, divided
- 2 tablespoons balsamic vinegar
- 1/4 teaspoon kosher salt
- 1/4 teaspoon black pepper
- 12 ounces cheese ravioli
- 2 tablespoons chopped fresh basil

Direction

- Preheat oven to 425°.
- Halve half of tomatoes. Arrange cut tomatoes, whole tomatoes, and shallots on a jelly-roll pan coated with cooking spray. Drizzle with 1 tablespoon oil; toss. Bake at 425° for 35 minutes.
- Add 2 tablespoons oil, vinegar, salt, and pepper to pan. Bake 10 minutes.
- Cook ravioli according to package directions, omitting salt and fat. Drain ravioli, reserving 1/4 cup cooking liquid. Add ravioli to tomatoes; toss. Add cooking liquid, if needed. Garnish with chopped basil.

Nutrition Information

- Calories: 406
- Fiber: 3.9 g

- Saturated Fat: 6.3 g
- Protein: 13.4 g
- Sodium: 572 mg
- Cholesterol: 49 mg
- Total Fat: 18.7 g
- Total Carbohydrate: 47.8 g

276. Tomato Basil Lasagna Rolls

Serving: Makes 10 servings | Prep: | Cook: | Ready in: 95mins

Ingredients

- 10 uncooked lasagna noodles
- 1 cup finely chopped sweet onion
- 2 teaspoons olive oil
- 3 garlic cloves, minced and divided
- 1 (24-oz.) jar tomato-and-basil pasta sauce
- 1 1/2 teaspoons sugar
- 1/4 teaspoon dried crushed red pepper
- 1 cup low-fat ricotta cheese
- 2 ounces 1/3-less-fat cream cheese, softened
- 1 (14-oz.) can baby artichoke hearts, drained and quartered
- 1 large egg white, lightly beaten
- 1/4 cup torn fresh basil
- 1/4 cup (1 oz.) freshly shredded Parmesan cheese
- Toppings: fresh basil, Parmesan cheese

Direction

- Preheat oven to 350°. Cook pasta according to package directions for al dente. Drain pasta (do not rinse); arrange in a single layer on a piece of lightly greased aluminum foil or wax paper.
- Sauté onion in hot oil in a 3-qt. saucepan over medium heat 7 to 8 minutes or until caramelized. Add two-thirds of minced garlic, and cook, stirring constantly, 1 minute. Stir in tomato sauce and next 2 ingredients. Bring mixture to a boil, stirring often. Reduce heat to low; simmer, stirring often, 5 minutes. Remove from heat.
- Stir together ricotta and cream cheese until smooth. Stir in artichoke hearts, next 3 ingredients, and remaining minced garlic. Spread 1/4 cup cheese mixture on 1 noodle. Roll up firmly, and place, seam side down, into a lightly greased 11- x 7-inch baking dish. Repeat with remaining noodles and cheese. Spoon tomato sauce over lasagna rolls.
- Bake, covered, at 350° for 45 to 50 minutes or until thoroughly heated and bubbly. Let stand 5 minutes. Sprinkle with desired toppings.
- Note: We tested with Classico Tomato & Basil pasta sauce.
- Note: Nutritional analysis is per serving (not including toppings).

Nutrition Information

- Calories: 190
- Saturated Fat: 1.5 g
- Fiber: 0.0 g
- Sodium: 590 mg
- Total Fat: 5 g
- Cholesterol: 11 mg
- Total Carbohydrate: 28 g
- Protein: 9 g

277. Tomato Tortellini Soup

Serving: Serves 8 to 10 | Prep: | Cook: | Ready in:

Ingredients

- 1 tablespoon margarine
- 3 cloves garlic, minced
- 3 10 1/2 oz. cans chicken broth
- 1 8-oz. pkg. cheese tortellini
- 1/4 cup grated Parmesan cheese
- salt and pepper to taste
- 2/3 cup frozen chopped spinach, thawed and drained
- 1 14 1/2 oz. can Italian stewed tomatoes

- 1/2 cup tomato sauce

Direction

- Melt margarine in a saucepan over medium heat; add garlic. Saute for 2 minutes; stir in broth and tortellini. Bring to a boil; reduce heat.
- Mix in Parmesan cheese, salt and pepper; simmer until tortellini is tender.
- Stir in spinach, tomatoes and tomato sauce; simmer for 5 minutes.

278. Tortellini Caprese Bites

Serving: Makes 12 servings | Prep: | Cook: | Ready in: 167mins

Ingredients

- 1 (9-oz.) package refrigerated cheese-filled tortellini
- 3 cups halved grape tomatoes
- 3 (8-oz.) containers fresh small mozzarella cheese balls
- 60 (6-inch) wooden skewers
- Basil Vinaigrette

Direction

- Prepare tortellini according to package directions. Rinse under cold running water.
- Thread 1 tomato half, 1 cheese ball, another tomato half, and 1 tortellini onto each skewer. Place skewers in a 13- x 9-inch baking dish. Pour Basil Vinaigrette over skewers, turning to coat. Cover and chill 2 hours. Transfer skewers to a serving platter, and sprinkle with salt and pepper to taste. Discard any remaining vinaigrette.

279. Tortellini Tapenade Salad

Serving: Makes 1 serving (serving size: 2 1/2 cups) | Prep: 12mins | Cook: | Ready in:

Ingredients

- 2/3 cup cooked chicken tortellini
- 2 teaspoons green or black olive tapenade
- 2/3 cup canned low-sodium white cannellini beans, rinsed and drained
- 1/2 cup thinly sliced red, orange, or yellow bell pepper
- 3/4 cup raw sugar-snap peas, halved if large, trimmed
- 1/2 ounce (1 1/2 TBSP) goat cheese, crumbled
- Freshly ground black pepper, to taste

Direction

- In a portable container, combine all ingredients and toss well.
- Refrigerate up to 24 hours. Serve at room temperature.

Nutrition Information

- Calories: 401
- Total Fat: 9.3 g
- Total Carbohydrate: 59 g
- Fiber: 11 g
- Protein: 21 g
- Saturated Fat: 3 g
- Cholesterol: 30 mg
- Sodium: 499 mg

280. Tortellini And White Bean Soup

Serving: Serves 4 | Prep: 10mins | Cook: 15mins | Ready in: 25mins

Ingredients

- 1 tablespoon olive oil

- 2 ribs celery, sliced
- 1 15-oz. can diced tomatoes, drained
- 1/2 teaspoon dried oregano
- 2 cloves garlic, minced
- 6 cups low-sodium chicken broth
- 1 8-oz. package fresh cheese or meat tortellini
- 1 15-oz. can white beans, drained and rinsed
- Salt, optional
- 1/4 cup grated Parmesan

Direction

- Warm oil in a large saucepan over medium-high heat. Add celery, tomatoes and oregano and cook, stirring occasionally, until celery begins to soften, about 3 minutes. Add garlic and sauté until fragrant, 2 minutes longer.
- Stir in broth and bring soup to a boil. Carefully add tortellini and beans and cook, stirring occasionally, until soup is heated through and tortellini are tender, about 7 minutes. Season with salt, if desired. Divide soup among 4 bowls, sprinkle each with 1 Tbsp. Parmesan and serve immediately.

Nutrition Information

- Calories: 383
- Protein: 24 g
- Cholesterol: 20 mg
- Fiber: 7 g
- Sodium: 760 mg
- Total Carbohydrate: 53 g
- Total Fat: 10 g
- Saturated Fat: 4 g

281. Tortellini With Snap Peas And Pesto

Serving: Serves 4 (serving size: about 1 1/4 cups) | Prep: | Cook: | Ready in:

Ingredients

- 1 (9-ounce) package refrigerated three-cheese tortellini (such as Buitoni)
- 8 ounces sugar snap peas, trimmed and halved diagonally (about 1 1/2 cups)
- 1 cup fresh mint leaves
- 1 cup fresh basil leaves
- 3 tablespoons sliced almonds, toasted
- 2 tablespoons grated Parmesan cheese
- 1 teaspoon grated lemon rind
- 1/4 teaspoon freshly ground black pepper
- 1/8 teaspoon kosher salt
- 1 garlic clove, minced
- 3 tablespoons olive oil
- 1 tablespoon fresh lemon juice

Direction

- Cook tortellini according to package directions, omitting salt and fat. Add snap peas to pan during last 3 minutes of cooking; cook 3 minutes. Drain.
- Place mint and next 7 ingredients (through garlic) in a mini food processor; process until finely chopped, scraping sides of bowl once. Combine oil and juice in a small bowl, stirring with a whisk. With processor on, slowly pour oil mixture through food chute; process until well blended. Combine tortellini mixture and mint mixture; toss gently to coat.

Nutrition Information

- Calories: 351
- Cholesterol: 26 mg
- Total Carbohydrate: 37 g
- Saturated Fat: 4.1 g
- Total Fat: 17.4 g
- Fiber: 5 g
- Protein: 13 g
- Sodium: 392 mg

282. Tuna Noodle Bowl

Serving: Serves 4 | Prep: 20mins | Cook: | Ready in:

Ingredients

- 1/2 pound bow-tie pasta
- 2 medium carrots, thinly sliced
- 1 cup sugar snap or snow peas, trimmed
- 1 red bell pepper, thinly sliced
- 1/3 cup extra-virgin olive oil
- 2 tablespoons red wine vinegar
- 1 shallot, finely chopped
- 1 teaspoon dried thyme
- 3 tablespoons capers, drained
- 2 6-ounce cans light tuna, preferably in olive oil, drained
- Parmesan cheese for grating

Direction

- Cook pasta in boiling salted water until almost done, about 8 minutes. Add the carrots and peas to the pot and continue cooking until pasta and carrots are firm-tender, about 2 minutes. Transfer pasta with carrots and peas along with the bell pepper to a large bowl. Whisk together the oil, vinegar, shallot, thyme, and salt and freshly ground pepper to taste. Drizzle over pasta and toss with capers and tuna. Taste and adjust seasonings. Divide among four bowls and shave or grate Parmesan over top.

Nutrition Information

- Calories: 552
- Fiber: 4 g
- Protein: 32 mg
- Sodium: 501 mg
- Total Fat: 25 g
- Cholesterol: 14 mg
- Saturated Fat: 4 g
- Total Carbohydrate: 49 g

283. Turkey Chili Mac

Serving: 6 servings (serving size: 1 1/3 cups) | Prep: 10mins | Cook: 20mins | Ready in:

Ingredients

- 1 cup uncooked enriched multigrain elbow macaroni (such as Barilla Plus)
- Cooking spray
- 1 pound ground turkey breast
- 1 medium onion, chopped
- 3 garlic cloves, minced
- 1 teaspoon chili powder
- 1/2 teaspoon black pepper
- 1/2 teaspoon ground cumin
- 1/4 teaspoon salt
- 1 (16-ounce) can kidney beans, rinsed and drained
- 1 (14.5-ounce) can stewed tomatoes, chopped and undrained
- 1 (8-ounce) can tomato sauce
- 3/4 cup (3 ounces) shredded 2% reduced-fat sharp Cheddar cheese

Direction

- Cook pasta according to package directions, omitting salt and fat; drain.
- While pasta cooks, heat a Dutch oven over medium-high heat. Coat pan with cooking spray; add turkey, onion, and next 5 ingredients. Cook 7 minutes or until turkey is browned, stirring to crumble.
- Add cooked pasta, beans, tomatoes, and tomato sauce. Cook 5 minutes or until thoroughly heated. Sprinkle evenly with cheese.

Nutrition Information

- Calories: 306
- Protein: 23 g
- Cholesterol: 70 mg
- Saturated Fat: 3.8 g
- Total Carbohydrate: 28.3 g
- Total Fat: 9.9 g

- Sodium: 718 mg
- Fiber: 4.8 g

284. Turkey Sausage Gnocchi Soup

Serving: 7 servings (serving size: 1 cup soup and about 1 tablespoon cheese) | Prep: 1mins | Cook: 14mins | Ready in:

Ingredients

- 1 (4.5-ounce) link hot turkey Italian sausage
- 2 cups water
- 1 (16-ounce) package vacuum-packed gnocchi (such as Bellino or Vigo)
- 1 (14-ounce) can fat-free, less-sodium beef broth
- 1 (14 1/2-ounce) can Italian-style stewed tomatoes, undrained and chopped
- 1/2 cup (2 ounces) grated fresh Parmesan cheese

Direction

- Remove casings from sausage. Cook sausage in a large Dutch oven over medium-high heat until sausage is browned, stirring to crumble.
- Add 2 cups water and next 3 ingredients to pan; bring to a boil. Reduce heat, and simmer 4 to 5 minutes or until gnocchi float to the top of pan. Ladle soup into bowls; sprinkle each serving evenly with cheese.

Nutrition Information

- Calories: 182
- Saturated Fat: 1.7 g
- Cholesterol: 22 mg
- Total Carbohydrate: 25.1 g
- Sodium: 809 mg
- Total Fat: 4 g
- Fiber: 0.5 g
- Protein: 10.5 g

285. Turkey Tetrazzini

Serving: Makes 8 servings | Prep: | Cook: | Ready in: 60mins

Ingredients

- 5 tablespoons butter
- 3 leeks, trimmed, sliced lengthwise, rinsed under cold running water and sliced crosswise into thin half-moons
- 2 portabella mushroom caps, cut into cubes
- 1 1/2 cups (4 oz.) sliced button mushrooms
- 5 teaspoons salt, plus more to taste
- 1/4 teaspoon nutmeg
- 1 pound medium egg noodles
- 3 tablespoons flour
- 2 cups chicken broth
- 1/2 cup dry sherry
- 1 cup half-and-half
- 1/2 cup parmesan cheese
- 2 cups cubed or shredded cooked turkey, in 1/2-in. pieces
- 1/3 cup chopped fresh flat-leaf parsley, plus extra for garnish
- 3/4 cup chopped radicchio leaves

Direction

- Melt 2 tbsp. of butter in a 14-in. frying pan or 5-qt. saucepan over medium heat. Add leeks, mushrooms, 1 tsp. salt, and nutmeg; cook, stirring often, until vegetables are soft and beginning to brown, about 12 minutes. Using a slotted spoon, transfer vegetables to a bowl and set aside.
- Bring a large pot of water to a boil. Add 3 tsp. salt and egg noodles. Cook until barely tender to the bite. Drain noodles and set aside, covered.
- While noodles are cooking, melt remaining 3 tbsp. butter in the same pan. Sprinkle in flour and stir until mixture looks glossy and golden brown, about 3 minutes. Whisk in chicken

broth and sherry and simmer until thickened, about 3 minutes. Remove from heat and whisk in half-and-half, parmesan, and remaining 1 tsp. salt. Reduce heat to low, return pan to heat, and stir in vegetable mixture, turkey, and parsley. Just before serving, stir in radicchio. Serve over cooked noodles and garnish with parsley.

- Note: Nutritional analysis is per serving.

Nutrition Information

- Calories: 455
- Cholesterol: 115 mg
- Fiber: 2.8 g
- Sodium: 1148 mg
- Total Carbohydrate: 53 g
- Total Fat: 16 g
- Protein: 24 g
- Saturated Fat: 8.6 g

286. Ultimate Spaghetti And Meatballs

Serving: 4 Servings | Prep: 10mins | Cook: 30mins | Ready in:

Ingredients

- 1/2 pound ground beef, preferably chuck
- 1/2 pound ground veal or turkey
- 1/2 pound ground pork
- 2 tablespoons grated onion
- 1 large egg
- 1/2 cup dry bread crumbs
- Salt and pepper
- 2 tablespoons olive oil
- 1 (28 oz.) jar pasta sauce
- 3/4 pound spaghetti
- Grated Parmesan, optional

Direction

- Combine meats, onion, egg, bread crumbs, salt and pepper in a large bowl. Mix gently with your hands until well-blended (do not overmix). Shape mixture into 8 meatballs, each about 2 1/2 inches in diameter.
- Warm olive oil in a large skillet over medium-high heat. Cook meatballs until brown all over, 6 to 8 minutes, turning carefully with tongs. Remove skillet from heat and carefully pour pasta sauce over meatballs. Place skillet over medium heat and bring to a simmer. Cook gently until there is no trace of pink in center of meatballs, about 20 minutes.
- Cook spaghetti according to package directions. Drain well and divide among 4 shallow pasta bowls or plates. Top each portion with 2 meatballs and ladle on sauce. If desired, top with grated Parmesan.

Nutrition Information

- Calories: 986
- Sodium: 733 mg
- Total Carbohydrate: 85 g
- Total Fat: 46 g
- Protein: 55 g
- Saturated Fat: 13 g
- Cholesterol: 189 mg
- Fiber: 7 g

287. Uncle Jack's Mac And Cheese

Serving: Makes 8 to 10 servings | Prep: | Cook: | Ready in: 265mins

Ingredients

- 1 (16-oz.) package elbow macaroni
- 1 1/2 cups heavy cream
- 1 (12-oz.) can evaporated milk
- 4 large eggs, lightly beaten
- 1/2 cup butter, melted
- 1 1/2 teaspoons table salt

- 1/2 teaspoon freshly ground black pepper
- 4 cups (16 oz.) shredded extra-sharp Cheddar cheese, divided
- Vegetable cooking spray

Direction

- Cook macaroni according to package directions. Stir together cream, next 5 ingredients, cooked macaroni, and 2 1/2 cups cheese in a large bowl.
- Pour macaroni mixture into a lightly greased (with cooking spray) 6-qt. slow cooker; sprinkle remaining 1 1/2 cups cheese over macaroni mixture.
- Cover and cook on HIGH 3 hours; reduce slow cooker to LOW, and cook 1 hour.

288. Vegetable Lasagna With Butternut Béchamel

Serving: Serves 6 (serving size: 1 piece) | Prep: | Cook: | Ready in: 94mins

Ingredients

- 3 cups cubed peeled butternut squash
- 1 cup plus 1 tablespoon organic vegetable broth, divided
- 1 cup fat-free milk
- 4 garlic cloves
- 1/2 teaspoon kosher salt
- 1/4 teaspoon freshly ground black pepper
- Dash of ground nutmeg
- 2 ounces cave-aged Gruyère cheese, shredded (about 1/2 cup)
- 3 ounces part-skim mozzarella cheese, shredded (about 3/4 cup), divided
- 1 tablespoon olive oil
- 1 small onion, chopped (about 3/4 cup)
- 1 pound sliced cremini mushrooms
- 1 bunch Swiss chard, trimmed and very thinly sliced (about 5 cups)
- 3 tablespoons pine nuts, toasted and chopped
- Cooking spray
- 6 whole-wheat lasagna noodles (such as Bionaturae), cooked
- 3/4 cup part-skim ricotta cheese
- 1 ounce finely grated fresh Parmigiano-Reggiano cheese (about 1/4 cup)

Direction

- Preheat oven to 375°.
- Combine squash, 1 cup broth, milk, and garlic in a medium saucepan; bring to a boil. Reduce heat to medium; simmer until squash is tender (about 20 minutes). Remove from heat.
- Place squash mixture in a blender. Add salt, pepper, and nutmeg. Remove center piece of blender lid (to allow steam to escape); secure blender lid on blender. Place a clean towel over opening in blender lid (to avoid splatters). Blend until smooth. Place blended squash mixture in a bowl; add Gruyère cheese and 5 ounces mozzarella cheese, stirring until cheese melts and mixture is smooth.
- Heat a large skillet over medium heat. Add oil to pan; swirl to coat. Add onion and mushrooms; cook 7 minutes or until browned and liquid evaporates. Add chard and remaining 1 tablespoon broth. Cover and cook 2 minutes or until chard wilts. Place chard mixture in a fine sieve; drain 5 minutes. Place chard mixture in a bowl. Add pine nuts; toss to combine.
- Spread 1/2 cup squash sauce in bottom of a broiler-safe 11 x 7-inch glass or ceramic baking dish coated with cooking spray. Arrange 3 noodles over sauce; top with half of chard mixture. Dollop ricotta cheese on top of chard. Spread half of remaining sauce over top. Arrange 3 noodles over sauce. Top with remaining chard mixture; top with remaining sauce. Sprinkle evenly with remaining 5 ounces mozzarella cheese and Parmigiano-Reggiano cheese. Cover with foil coated with cooking spray. Bake at 375° for 35 minutes. Uncover and bake an additional 10 minutes or until bubbly.
- Preheat broiler to high. (Keep lasagna in oven.

- Broil lasagna 3 minutes or until cheese is golden brown. Remove from oven; let stand 10 minutes.

Nutrition Information

- Calories: 363
- Protein: 22 g
- Total Fat: 16.2 g
- Total Carbohydrate: 36 g
- Sugar: 7 g
- Saturated Fat: 6.3 g
- Sodium: 584 mg
- Cholesterol: 33 mg
- Fiber: 7 g

289. Vegetarian Bolognese With Whole Wheat Penne

Serving: 6 servings | Prep: | Cook: | Ready in: 70mins

Ingredients

- 1/4 cup dried porcini mushrooms (about 1/4 ounce)
- 1 tablespoon olive oil
- 1 1/2 cups finely chopped onion
- 1/2 cup finely chopped carrot
- 1/2 cup finely chopped celery
- 1 (8-ounce) package cremini mushrooms, finely chopped
- 1/2 cup dry red wine
- 1/4 cup warm water
- 1/2 teaspoon salt
- 1/2 teaspoon freshly ground black pepper
- 1 (28-ounce) can organic crushed tomatoes with basil, undrained
- 1 (2-inch) piece Parmigiano-Reggiano cheese rind
- 12 ounces uncooked whole-wheat penne (tube-shaped pasta)
- 1/2 cup (2 ounces) shaved Parmigiano-Reggiano cheese

Direction

- Place dried mushrooms in a spice or coffee grinder; process until finely ground.
- Heat oil in a large saucepan over medium-high heat. Add onion, carrot, celery, and mushrooms; sauté 10 minutes. Add wine; simmer 2 minutes or until liquid almost evaporates. Add 1/4 cup warm water and next 4 ingredients (through cheese rind) to onion mixture. Stir in ground porcini. Cover, reduce heat, and simmer 40 minutes. Keep warm. Remove rind; discard.
- Cook pasta according to package directions, omitting salt and fat. Place 1 cup of pasta in each of 6 bowls. Top each portion with 3/4 cup sauce and about 1 tablespoon cheese.

Nutrition Information

- Calories: 334
- Cholesterol: 9 mg
- Total Carbohydrate: 57.7 g
- Fiber: 9.7 g
- Sodium: 542 mg
- Total Fat: 7.2 g
- Protein: 14.8 g
- Saturated Fat: 2.1 g

290. Vietnamese Beef Noodle Bowl

Serving: 6 servings (serving size: 1/2 cup noodles and 2 cups broth mixture) | Prep: | Cook: | Ready in:

Ingredients

- 8 cups water
- 2 (14 1/4-ounce) cans fat-free beef broth
- 3 whole star anise (optional)
- 2 (3-inch) cinnamon sticks
- 1 (1 1/2-inch) piece peeled fresh ginger, sliced
- 4 ounces uncooked rice stick noodles or vermicelli

- 1 1/2 pounds boned sirloin steak, thinly sliced
- 2 1/2 tablespoons minced shallots
- 2 tablespoons sake (rice wine) or rice vinegar
- 1 tablespoon minced peeled fresh ginger
- 2 cups fresh bean sprouts
- 1 cup sliced fresh basil leaves
- 1/3 cup minced fresh cilantro
- 1/4 cup minced green onions
- 3 tablespoons fish sauce
- 1/2 teaspoon salt
- 1/4 teaspoon black pepper
- 1 teaspoon thinly sliced red chile (optional)
- 6 lime wedges (optional)

Direction

- Combine first 5 ingredients in a large Dutch oven; bring to a boil. Reduce heat; simmer 30 minutes. Strain broth; discard solids. Return broth to pan.
- Place rice noodles in a large bowl; cover with hot water. Let stand 15 minutes; drain. Cook noodles in boiling water 1 minute or until tender; drain.
- Combine the beef, shallots, sake, and minced ginger in a large zip-top plastic bag; seal and marinate in refrigerator 10 minutes. Add beef mixture to broth in pan; bring to a boil. Reduce heat to medium; cook 3 minutes. Stir in bean sprouts and next 6 ingredients (bean sprouts through black pepper); cook 1 minute.
- Place the noodles into each of 6 large bowls; top with broth mixture. Garnish with sliced chile and lime wedges, if desired.

Nutrition Information

- Calories: 264
- Saturated Fat: 2.1 g
- Sodium: 967 mg
- Total Carbohydrate: 20.8 g
- Cholesterol: 70 mg
- Fiber: 1.2 g
- Protein: 31.1 g
- Total Fat: 6 g

291. Vietnamese Salt And Pepper Shrimp Rice Noodle Bowl (Bun Tom Xao)

Serving: Serves 4 | Prep: | Cook: | Ready in: 45mins

Ingredients

- 5 ounces uncooked rice vermicelli noodles
- 1/2 cup lukewarm water
- 3 tablespoons granulated sugar
- 1/4 cup fresh lime juice
- 1 tablespoon rice vinegar
- 5 teaspoons fish sauce (such as Three Crabs)
- 2 serrano chiles, thinly sliced
- 4 cups (1/4-inch) slices green leaf lettuce
- 3 cups diagonally cut slices seeded Kirby (pickling) cucumber (about 2)
- 1/4 cup cilantro leaves
- 1/4 cup torn Thai basil leaves
- 1/4 cup torn mint leaves
- 2 teaspoons cornstarch
- 1 teaspoon dark brown sugar
- 1/4 teaspoon salt
- 3/4 teaspoon white pepper
- 1 pound large shrimp, peeled and deveined
- 2 tablespoons canola oil, divided
- 1/3 cup (1/4-inch) slices green onions
- 3 garlic cloves, finely chopped
- 1/2 cup unsalted, dry-roasted peanuts, coarsely chopped

Direction

- Cook rice vermicelli noodles according to package directions. Drain and rinse with cold water; drain.
- Combine 1/2 cup lukewarm water and granulated sugar in a medium bowl, stirring until sugar dissolves. Add lime juice, vinegar, fish sauce, and chiles; set aside.
- Combine lettuce, cucumber, and herbs; set aside.
- Combine cornstarch, brown sugar, salt, and pepper in a large bowl; stir until well

combined. Add shrimp; toss to coat. Heat a wok or large skillet over high heat. Add 1 1/2 teaspoons oil, and swirl to coat. Add half of shrimp; cook for 1 1/2 minutes on each side or until shrimp are seared. Remove from pan. Add 1 1/2 teaspoons oil to wok; repeat procedure with remaining shrimp. Reduce heat to medium-high. Add remaining 1 tablespoon oil to wok; swirl to coat. Add onions and garlic; stir-fry 30 seconds. Return shrimp to pan; stir-fry 1 minute.

- Arrange about 1 cup lettuce mixture in each of 4 large bowls, and top each serving with about 1 cup noodles and 2 tablespoons chopped peanuts. Divide the shrimp evenly among servings, and serve each with 1/4 cup sauce.

Nutrition Information

- Calories: 462
- Fiber: 4.4 g
- Sodium: 802 mg
- Cholesterol: 143 mg
- Total Fat: 17.6 g
- Saturated Fat: 1.9 g
- Total Carbohydrate: 52.9 g
- Protein: 24.6 g

292. Vietnamese Style Pork Noodle Salad

Serving: Serves 6 (serving size: about 1 1/2 cups spinach mixture and 3 ounces pork) | Prep: | Cook: | Ready in: 22mins

Ingredients

- 4 ounces thin brown rice noodles (such as Annie Chun's)
- 1 cup sliced red onion
- 5 tablespoons fresh lime juice, divided
- 2 tablespoons fish sauce
- 2 teaspoons minced fresh garlic
- 3 tablespoons sugar, divided
- 1/2 teaspoon black pepper
- 1 (1-pound) pork tenderloin, trimmed and cut into 1-inch pieces
- 1/4 cup hot water
- 1/4 teaspoon crushed red pepper
- 5 ounces baby spinach (about 7 cups)
- 1 1/4 cups matchstick-cut carrots (4 ounces)
- 1/2 cup fresh cilantro leaves
- 2 tablespoons canola oil

Direction

- Bring a medium saucepan of water to a boil. Add noodles; cook 3 minutes. Drain; rinse under cold water. Drain.
- Place onion in a bowl of ice water; let stand 10 minutes. Drain. Combine 2 tablespoons juice, 1 tablespoon fish sauce, garlic, 1 1/2 tablespoons sugar, and black pepper. Add pork; toss.
- Combine remaining 1 1/2 tablespoons sugar and 1/4 cup hot water, stirring until sugar dissolves. Add remaining 3 tablespoons juice, remaining 1 tablespoon fish sauce, and crushed red pepper. Add noodles, onion, spinach, carrot, and cilantro; toss.
- Heat a wok or large skillet over high heat. Add oil; swirl. Add pork mixture; stir-fry 4 minutes. Divide spinach mixture among 6 plates; top evenly with pork.

Nutrition Information

- Calories: 250
- Protein: 17 g
- Total Carbohydrate: 31 g
- Sodium: 569 mg
- Total Fat: 6.4 g
- Fiber: 2 g
- Cholesterol: 49 mg
- Saturated Fat: 0.9 g

293. Vietnamese Style Spicy Crab With Garlic Noodles

Serving: Makes 4 to 6 servings | Prep: | Cook: | Ready in: 90mins

Ingredients

- 1 cup flour
- 1 1/2 teaspoons plus 1 tbsp. salt
- 1 1/2 teaspoons freshly ground black pepper
- 1/2 teaspoon cayenne
- 2 Dungeness crabs, cooked, cleaned, quartered, and cracked
- Vegetable oil for frying, plus 3 tbsp.
- 10 cloves garlic, chopped
- 1/2 pound spaghettini (thin spaghetti)
- 3 tablespoons butter, at room temperature
- 6 small dried red chiles
- 2 tablespoons grated fresh ginger
- 4 green onions, chopped
- 4 serrano chiles, stemmed, seeded, and chopped
- 1/3 cup sake or other rice wine
- 1 cup basil leaves, chopped
- 1/2 cup mint leaves, chopped
- 1/2 cup cilantro leaves

Direction

- Combine flour, 1 tsp. salt, 1 tsp. pepper, and the cayenne in a large bowl. Pat crab pieces dry with paper towels and toss (in batches) with flour mixture. Remove crab and shake off excess flour. Set aside.
- In a wok or large pot, heat 3 in. oil to 375°. Lay out paper towels for draining crab and garlic. Fry crab in batches (do not crowd wok) until golden, about 5 minutes per batch. Drain on paper towels.
- Using the same hot oil, fry garlic until golden brown, 2 to 3 minutes. Remove with a slotted spoon and drain on paper towels. Set garlic aside; cool and discard oil.
- Bring a large pot of water to a boil. Add 1 tbsp. of the salt and the spaghettini. Cook until tender to the bite, 5 to 10 minutes. Drain, transfer to a serving bowl, and toss with butter and half of the fried garlic. Cover and put in a warm place.
- Heat a wok or pot large enough to hold all the crab over high heat. Add remaining 3 tbsp. oil, dried chiles, and ginger. Cook, stirring constantly, until fragrant, about 30 seconds. Add green onions, serrano chiles, and remaining 1/2 tsp. salt. Cook, stirring, until onions wilt, about 1 minute. Add sake and cook, stirring, until sake is reduced by about half. Stir in crab and cover. Cook until crab is heated through, about 3 minutes.
- Remove lid and cook, stirring, until any liquid evaporates. Stir in basil, mint, cilantro, and remaining 1/2 tsp. pepper. Cook, stirring, until herbs have wilted. Stir in remaining fried garlic. Transfer crab to a warm platter and serve hot, with garlic noodles.
- Note: Nutritional analysis is per serving.

Nutrition Information

- Calories: 610
- Total Fat: 29 g
- Cholesterol: 105 mg
- Fiber: 4.2 g
- Saturated Fat: 7.1 g
- Sodium: 1292 mg
- Protein: 27 g
- Total Carbohydrate: 56 g

294. Warm Soba Noodle Bowl

Serving: Serves 4 | Prep: | Cook: | Ready in: 40mins

Ingredients

- 2 eggs
- 6 cups liquid dashi (or use concentrate)*
- 4 shiitake mushrooms, stemmed and thinly sliced
- 1 tablespoon mirin
- 1 tablespoon soy sauce

- 16 ounces dried soba noodles
- 20 thin slices daikon, peeled
- 1 sheet nori seaweed, cut into 1/4- by 1-in. strips
- 2 green onions, finely sliced diagonally

Direction

- Put eggs in a small pot of cold water. Bring to a boil, remove from heat, cover, and let sit 15 minutes. Drain; rinse with cold water.
- Bring dashi to a boil. Reduce heat to low and add mushrooms, mirin, and soy sauce.
- Bring a 3-qt. saucepan of water to a boil. Add soba and cook, stirring to separate noodles, until softened, about 5 minutes. Drain but don't rinse. Divide noodles among 4 serving bowls.
- Pour 1 1/2 cups of dashi over noodles in each bowl. Arrange mushrooms and daikon over noodles, dividing evenly so each bowl has a neat row of both. Peel eggs and cut each in half lengthwise, placing 1 half in each bowl. Divide nori and green onions among bowls.
- *Find liquid dashi in containers in Japanese groceries and some gourmet stores. It's more widely available as a dry concentrate called dashi-no-moto; reconstitute according to package directions.
- Note: Nutritional analysis is per serving.

Nutrition Information

- Calories: 436
- Cholesterol: 106 mg
- Sodium: 1534 mg
- Total Fat: 3.3 g
- Saturated Fat: 0.9 g
- Total Carbohydrate: 88 g
- Fiber: 0.4 g
- Protein: 20 g

295. Watercress, Prosciutto, And Goat Cheese Linguine

Serving: Serves 4 | Prep: | Cook: | Ready in: 17mins

Ingredients

- 1 (9-ounce) package refrigerated fresh linguine
- 1 tablespoon olive oil
- 1 3/4 ounces chopped prosciutto
- 1/4 teaspoon crushed red pepper
- 4 ounces soft goat cheese, divided (about 1/2 cup)
- 1/4 teaspoon kosher salt
- 1 tablespoon grated lemon rind
- 5 cups trimmed watercress (about 3 bunches)
- 1/2 teaspoon freshly ground black pepper

Direction

- Cook pasta according to package directions. Drain in a colander over a bowl; reserve 1 1/4 cups cooking liquid.
- Heat a large skillet over medium-high heat. Add olive oil to pan; swirl to coat. Add prosciutto; sauté for 3 minutes or until browned and crisp. Remove prosciutto from pan with a slotted spoon; drain on a paper towel. Add red pepper to drippings in pan; cook 30 seconds, stirring constantly. Add reserved cooking liquid to pan; bring to a boil. Add 3 ounces goat cheese and salt, and cook for 2 minutes, stirring until smooth. Stir in grated lemon rind. Add pasta; toss gently to coat. Add watercress, and toss gently to combine.
- Place about 1 1/2 cups pasta mixture on each of 4 plates. Top each serving evenly with remaining 1 ounce cheese, prosciutto, and black pepper.

Nutrition Information

- Calories: 323
- Saturated Fat: 5.3 g
- Total Fat: 12.2 g

- Sodium: 591 mg
- Total Carbohydrate: 37 g
- Protein: 17 g
- Cholesterol: 69 mg
- Fiber: 3 g

296. Whole Grain Spaghetti With Veggi Fied Meat Sauce

Serving: Serves 4 (serving size: about 3/4 cup pasta, 1 cup sauce, and 1 1/2 teaspoons cheese) | Prep: | Cook: | Ready in: 34mins

Ingredients

- 6 ounces whole-grain spaghetti (such as Barilla)
- Cooking spray
- 1 cup finely chopped onion
- 8 ounces 93% lean ground beef
- 6 garlic cloves, minced
- 1 cup finely chopped zucchini
- 8 ounces cremini mushrooms, finely chopped
- 1 (14.5-ounce) can unsalted diced tomatoes
- 1 tablespoon unsalted tomato paste
- 1/2 teaspoon dried oregano
- 1/4 teaspoon crushed red pepper
- 3/4 teaspoon kosher salt
- 1/4 teaspoon freshly ground black pepper
- 2 tablespoons finely grated Parmigiano-Reggiano cheese

Direction

- Cook pasta according to package directions, omitting salt and fat. Drain pasta, and keep warm.
- While pasta cooks, heat a large skillet over medium-high heat. Coat pan with cooking spray. Add onion, beef, and garlic; cook 4 minutes, stirring to crumble beef. Add zucchini and mushrooms; cook 10 minutes or until most of liquid evaporates, stirring occasionally. Place tomatoes in a mini food processor; pulse 4 times or until almost smooth. Add tomato paste, oregano, and red pepper to pan; cook 1 minute, stirring frequently. Stir in tomatoes; reduce heat, and simmer 5 minutes or until slightly thickened. Stir in salt and black pepper. Serve sauce over pasta; top with cheese.

Nutrition Information

- Calories: 324
- Cholesterol: 38 mg
- Total Fat: 6.8 g
- Fiber: 6 g
- Protein: 25 g
- Sodium: 524 mg
- Saturated Fat: 2.3 g
- Total Carbohydrate: 43 g

297. Whole Wheat Fettuccine With Arugula Pesto

Serving: 4 first-course servings | Prep: | Cook: | Ready in: 60mins

Ingredients

- 3/4 cup whole-wheat flour
- 3/4 cup all-purpose flour
- Salt
- 3 large egg yolks
- 1/3 cup water
- 1/3 cup plus 1 tablespoon extra-virgin olive oil
- 2 tablespoons pine nuts
- 2 cups (2 ounces) packed baby arugula
- 1/4 cup Parmigiano-Reggiano cheese, freshly grated
- 1 garlic clove, chopped
- 1 cup cherry tomatoes, halved

Direction

- In a food processor, pulse the whole-wheat and all-purpose flours with 1/2 teaspoon of salt. In a bowl, whisk the egg yolks, water and the 1 teaspoon of oil. With the processor on, add the egg yolk mixture and process until a ball forms. Transfer the dough to a work surface and knead until smooth. Cover with plastic wrap and let stand at room temperature for 20 minutes. Wipe out the processor.

- In a small skillet, toss the pine nuts over moderate heat until toasted, 1 minute; let cool. In the food processor, pulse the arugula, pine nuts, cheese, garlic and the remaining 1/3 cup of oil to a paste. Season the pesto with salt and add to a large skillet.
- Cut the dough into 3 pieces; work with 1 piece at a time and keep the rest covered. Flatten the dough slightly and run it through progressively narrower settings in a pasta machine until you reach the thinnest setting. Cut the pasta into 10-inch lengths. Using the pasta machine, cut each length into fettuccine. Transfer to a baking sheet, leaving space between the pasta so it doesn't stick.
- In a pot of boiling, salted water, cook the pasta, stirring, until al dente, about 30 seconds. Drain the pasta, reserving 1/3 cup of the cooking water. Stir the reserved water into the pesto. Add the pasta and tomatoes to the pesto, toss over moderate heat and serve.

298. Whole Wheat Pasta With Mushrooms

Serving: Makes 6 servings | Prep: | Cook: | Ready in:

Ingredients

- Pinch garlic salt
- 12 ounces whole-wheat pasta
- 1 1/2 tablespoons olive oil, divided
- 1 sliced shallot
- 1 (3.5-ounce) package presliced shiitake mushrooms
- 1 (4-ounce) package presliced mixed mushroom blend
- 1 (16-ounce) package presliced baby portobello mushrooms
- 1 teaspoon salt, divided
- 1 teaspoon pepper, divided
- 1 1/2 tablespoons truffle oil
- 1/3 cup grated Parmesan
- 2 tablespoons freshly chopped parsley

Direction

- Bring large pot of water to boil. Add garlic salt to water, and cook pasta according to directions.
- Heat 1/2 tablespoon olive oil in large nonstick pan; sauté shallot. Add all mushrooms, and cook over medium-high heat for 5-6 minutes or until brown; turn to brown on opposite side for another 5-6 minutes. Season with 1/2 teaspoon salt and 1/4 teaspoon pepper.
- Drain pasta. Toss in a large bowl with mushroom mixture. Add the truffle oil, remaining 1 tablespoon olive oil, and remaining salt and pepper. Toss to combine.
- Top with Parmesan and parsley; serve hot.

Nutrition Information

- Calories: 310
- Total Fat: 9 g
- Cholesterol: 4 mg
- Protein: 13 g
- Sodium: 280 mg
- Total Carbohydrate: 49 g
- Fiber: 6 g
- Saturated Fat: 2 g

299. Whole Wheat Penne With Eggplant Tomato Sauce

Serving: Serves 6 | Prep: 20mins | Cook: 360mins | Ready in:

Ingredients

- 2 tablespoons unsalted butter, cut into small pieces
- 1 small onion, finely chopped
- 1 rib celery, finely chopped
- 1 carrot, finely chopped
- 1 clove garlic, minced
- 1 medium eggplant, peeled, cut into 1/2-inch dice
- 10 ounce mushrooms, chopped
- Salt
- 1 28-oz. can crushed tomatoes
- 1 pound whole-wheat penne
- 1/4 cup finely chopped fresh basil leaves

Direction

- Mist a slow-cooker insert with cooking spray. Combine butter, onion, celery, carrot and garlic in slow cooker. Add eggplant, mushrooms and 1 tsp. salt. Stir in tomatoes, cover and cook on high for 4 hours or on low for 6 hours. Stir once or twice during cooking.
- Bring a large pot of salted water to a boil and cook penne until just tender, about 10 minutes. Drain pasta, toss with sauce, sprinkle with basil (and grated Parmesan, if desired) and serve.

Nutrition Information

- Calories: 359
- Protein: 14 g
- Total Carbohydrate: 74 g
- Cholesterol: 10 mg
- Total Fat: 7 g
- Fiber: 14 g
- Saturated Fat: 3 g
- Sodium: 579 mg

300. Whole Wheat Spaghetti With Garlic, Parsley, And Lemon

Serving: Makes: 4 servings (serving size: 1 1/4 cups) | Prep: 12mins | Cook: 15mins | Ready in:

Ingredients

- 8 ounces whole-wheat spaghetti
- 3 tablespoons extra-virgin olive oil, divided
- 1/2 cup chopped garlic
- 1 3/4 cups chopped flat-leaf parsley
- 3/4 teaspoon black pepper
- 1 tablespoon freshly grated lemon zest
- 1/4 teaspoon kosher salt
- 1/2 ounce Asiago, Pecorino, or Parmesan cheese, shaved with a vegetable peeler

Direction

- Cook the pasta according to the label until al dente. Reserve 3 TBSP cooking liquid; drain.
- Meanwhile, heat 2 TBSP oil in a large skillet over medium heat. Reduce the heat to low, add the garlic, and cook, stirring frequently, until golden brown and fragrant (3-4 minutes). Stir in the parsley, pepper, and lemon zest. Cook, stirring often, until the parsley is tender (3-4 minutes).
- Add the pasta and cooking liquid to the skillet with the salt and remaining TBSP oil. Toss until well mixed. Top with the cheese and serve.

Nutrition Information

- Calories: 331
- Total Carbohydrate: 49 g
- Total Fat: 12.3 g
- Protein: 11 g
- Sodium: 152 mg
- Saturated Fat: 2.2 g
- Cholesterol: 4 mg
- Fiber: 8 g

301. Ziti With Spinach, Cherry Tomatoes, And Gorgonzola Sauce

Serving: 2 servings (serving size: 1 1/4 cups) | Prep: 40mins | Cook: | Ready in:

Ingredients

- 4 ounces uncooked ziti
- 1/2 teaspoon extra-virgin olive oil
- 1 cup cherry tomatoes, halved
- 1/4 teaspoon salt
- 1/8 teaspoon crushed red pepper
- 1 garlic clove, minced
- 6 tablespoons half-and-half
- 3 tablespoons Gorgonzola cheese, crumbled
- 1 cup fresh spinach

Direction

- Cook pasta according to package directions, omitting salt and fat; drain.
- Heat extra-virgin olive oil in a large nonstick skillet over medium heat. Add cherry tomatoes, salt, crushed red pepper, and minced garlic to pan; cook 1 minute, stirring occasionally. Stir in half-and-half and Gorgonzola cheese; cook 2 minutes or until slightly thick, stirring constantly. Stir in spinach and pasta; cook 1 minute or until spinach wilts, tossing occasionally.

Nutrition Information

- Calories: 335
- Sodium: 485 mg
- Total Carbohydrate: 49.9 g
- Saturated Fat: 5.9 g
- Fiber: 3.6 g
- Cholesterol: 26 mg
- Total Fat: 10.4 g
- Protein: 12.3 g

302. Zucchini Eggplant Lasagna

Serving: 12 servings | Prep: | Cook: | Ready in:

Ingredients

- 1 large eggplant, cut crosswise into 1/4-inch-thick slices
- 3/4 teaspoon salt, divided
- 2 teaspoons olive oil
- 3/4 cup chopped onion (about 1 medium onion)
- 3 garlic cloves, chopped
- 3/4 teaspoon freshly ground black pepper, divided
- 1/2 teaspoon chopped fresh oregano
- 1/8 teaspoon ground red pepper
- 1 (28-ounce) can crushed tomatoes
- 1 cup fresh basil leaves, chopped
- 1 cup (8 ounces) part-skim ricotta cheese
- Cooking spray
- 1 (8-ounce) package precooked lasagna noodles
- 2 medium zucchini, cut into 1/4-inch-thick slices
- 2 1/2 cups (10 ounces) shredded part-skim mozzarella cheese

Direction

- Preheat oven to 350°.
- Arrange eggplant slices in a single layer on several layers of paper towels. Sprinkle evenly with 1/2 teaspoon salt; let stand 15 minutes.
- Heat oil in a large skillet over medium-high heat. Add onion and garlic to pan; sauté 2 minutes, stirring frequently. Add remaining 1/4 teaspoon salt, 1/4 teaspoon black pepper, oregano, red pepper, and tomatoes; bring to a boil. Reduce heat, and simmer for 10 minutes, stirring occasionally.
- Combine basil, ricotta, and remaining 1/2 teaspoon black pepper in a small bowl. Spread 1/2 cup tomato mixture into the bottom of a

13 x 9-inch baking dish coated with cooking spray. Arrange 4 noodles over tomato mixture; top with half of eggplant and half of zucchini. Spread ricotta mixture over vegetables; cover with 4 noodles. Spread 1 cup tomato mixture over noodles; layer with remaining eggplant and zucchini slices. Arrange remaining 4 noodles over vegetables, and spread remaining tomato mixture over noodles. Top evenly with mozzarella. Cover with foil coated with cooking spray. Bake at 350° for 35 minutes. Uncover and bake an additional 25 minutes or until browned. Cool for 5 minutes.

Nutrition Information

- Calories: 216
- Cholesterol: 21 mg
- Total Fat: 7.7 g
- Fiber: 4.2 g
- Total Carbohydrate: 25.7 g
- Saturated Fat: 4.2 g
- Protein: 12.7 g
- Sodium: 393 mg

303. Zucchini And Corn Lasagna

Serving: Serves 8 | Prep: | Cook: | Ready in: 120mins

Ingredients

- 3 1/2 pounds green or yellow zucchini (10 medium), ends trimmed, thinly sliced lengthwise
- 1 3/4 teaspoons kosher salt, divided
- 3 tablespoons olive oil, divided
- 1/2 cup chopped shallot
- 2 garlic cloves, chopped
- 2 cups raw corn kernels (from 2 or 3 ears corn)
- 1 teaspoon fresh thyme leaves
- 15 ounces ricotta cheese
- 1 1/4 cups shredded parmesan cheese, divided
- 1 large egg, beaten to blend
- 1/4 cup chopped basil leaves
- 2 tablespoons chopped chives
- 1/4 teaspoon pepper
- 1 1/2 tablespoons butter, divided

Direction

- Line 3 rimmed baking sheets with paper towels and arrange zucchini in a single layer on top. Sprinkle with 1 1/2 tsp. salt and set aside 30 minutes.
- Meanwhile, heat a grill to medium (350° to 450°). Heat 1 tbsp. oil in a medium frying pan over medium heat. Add shallot and garlic and cook, stirring constantly, until beginning to brown, about 2 minutes. Add corn and thyme and cook until corn is just hot, 2 to 3 minutes. Transfer to a medium bowl. Stir in ricotta, half of parmesan, the egg, basil, chives, pepper, and remaining 1/4 tsp. salt.
- Preheat oven to 375°. Press water out of zucchini with more paper towels and remove all paper towels from baking sheets. Brush zucchini all over with remaining 2 tbsp. oil. Grill half of zucchini, turning once, until grill marks appear, 2 to 4 minutes; transfer to rimmed baking sheets as cooked. Repeat with remaining zucchini.
- Butter bottom of a 9- by 13-in. baking dish with 1/2 tbsp. butter. Arrange a quarter of zucchini ribbons crosswise in -bottom of dish, overlapping slightly. Evenly spread a third of corn-ricotta mixture over zucchini. Repeat process 2 more times, ending with zucchini. Sprinkle remaining parmesan on top and dot with remaining 1 tbsp. butter.
- Bake until lasagna turns golden brown, about 45 minutes, rotating dish halfway through for even browning. Let rest 20 minutes before serving.
- Make ahead: Through step 4, up to 1 day, chilled; bake about 55 minutes.

Nutrition Information

- Calories: 283

- Sodium: 492 mg
- Protein: 15 g
- Saturated Fat: 9.1 g
- Cholesterol: 68 mg
- Total Fat: 19 g
- Total Carbohydrate: 15 g
- Fiber: 2.5 g

Index

P

Q

R

S

Conclusion

Thank you again for downloading this book!

I hope you enjoyed reading about my book!

If you enjoyed this book, please take the time to share your thoughts and post a review on Amazon. It'd be greatly appreciated!

Write me an honest review about the book – I truly value your opinion and thoughts and I will incorporate them into my next book, which is already underway.

Thank you!

If you have any questions, **feel free to contact at:** *author@rosemaryrecipes.com*

Rosalie Walston

rosemaryrecipes.com

Printed in Great Britain
by Amazon

67825742R00115